Second Edition

THE INSTANT EXAM REVIEW
for the USMLE STEP 3

Handwritten annotations:

B thallasemia major (Cooley anemia)
homozygous

Hollenhorst Plaque ... EMBOLI
FUNDOSCOPIC EXAM

Mesenteric ischemia
- pain out prop to exam
- thumbprinting

Review RBC

CoMA
- T trauma, temperature
- I infection (CNS, systemic)
- P psychiatric,
- S space occupying lesion, stroke
     subarachnoid hms, shock

- A alcohol; other drugs
- E endocrine, exocrine electrolyts
- I insulin (diabetic)
- O oxygen (hypoxia) opiates
- U uremia

Vasovagal

Ectopic pregnancy (Hypovolemic)
S site

① testicular vein → ② renal vein
② testicular vein → IVC

oral hairy leukoplakia
assoc HIV
EBV

Syncopy
- H Hypoxic Hypoglycemic
- E epilepsy
- A Anxiety
- D Dys brain stem

- H Heart Attack
- E Emb of pulm artery
- A Aortic obstruction
- R Rhythm disturbance
- T tachycardic (ventricular)

- V Vasovagal
- E Ectopic (Hypovolemic)
- S Situational
- S Carotid sinus sensitiv
- L low systemic vasc. resistance
- S Subclavian steal

Menieres
VERTIGO
TINNITUS
DEAFness

SIADH
  must R/o renal, adrenal, thyroid D3 prior to this dx
  must Be euvolemic

RBC CAST ≡ Glomerulonephritis

ATN vs prerenal Azotemia

$$FE_{N2} = \left(U_{Na}/U_{Cr}\right) / \left(P_{Na}/P_{Cr}\right) \times 100$$

    <1 prerenal
    >2 ATN

AR is associated c Rheumatoid Arthritis
AR assoc AS, Reiters, Psoriatic Arthrits Enteropathic Arthrits

Caplan Syndrome
      nodular infiltrates in rheumatoid lungs
      c pneumoconiosy.

  Felty: Chronic RA
            Splenomegaly
            Neutropenic

Anaphylaxis— IgE mediated

PERIORBITAL   ORBITAL CELLULITIS

Preseptal   Behind septum
  soft tissue infection   post eye structures may form
of ant. eye structures   ABscess.
usually localized to
eyelids; conjunctivae   direct spread from ethmoid sinus

  Hematogenous spread
of Bact

CENTRAL RETINAL ARTERY
      Dilated nonreactive pupil
      milky to pale retina c
            cherry red spot @ macula
      sudden painless loss vision

Second Edition

THE INSTANT EXAM REVIEW

for the USMLE STEP 3

Joel S. Goldberg, DO
Assistant Professor of Medicine
Department of Medicine
Allegheny University of the Health Sciences
MCP ◆ Hahnemann School of Medicine
Philadelphia, Pennsylvania

Appleton & Lange
Stamford, Connecticut

Handwritten annotations:

CAVERNOUS SINUS
TOXIC APPEARANCE
HIGH FEVER
3RD/6th nerve palsy
retinal engorgement
Bil chemosis & ptosis

LP: cell ct/diff
(#2) GS, c&s
③ Glucose/Protein
④ cell ct/diff

CSF/serum glu <0.5
bac meningitis

B₂ agonist-
albuterol
Fenoterol
Antimuscarinics
ipratropium

Kawasaki
    mucocutaneous lymph node syndrome
    Risk coronary artery aneurysm 10-20%
    5/6 systemic vasculitis - affects skin, mucous membrane
                    and heart

① Fever ≥5days
② Δ peripheral extremities (erythema palms/soles)
        desquamation fingertips
③ polymorphous exanthema
④ Bil. conjunctival congestion
⑤ chg lips and oral cavity
        erythema
        strawberry tongue
    diffuse injection
    of mucosa
⑥ acute nonpurulent cervical lymphadenopathy

97 98 99 00 01 / 10 9 8 7 6 5 4 3 2 1

Prentice Hall International (UK) Limited, *London*
Prentice Hall of Australia Pty. Limited, *Sydney*
Prentice Hall Canada, Inc., *Toronto*
Prentice Hall Hispanoamericana, S.A., *Mexico*
Prentice Hall of India Private Limited, *New Delhi*
Prentice Hall of Japan, Inc., *Tokyo*
Simon and Schuster Asia Pte. Ltd., *Singapore*
Editora Prentice Hall do Brasil Ltda., *Rio de Janeiro*
Prentice Hall, *Upper Saddle River, New Jersey*

Library of Congress Cataloging-in-Publication Data

The instant exam review for the USMLE, step 3 / [edited by] Joel S.
    Goldberg. — 2nd ed.
        p. cm.
    Includes bibliographical references.
    ISBN 0–8385–4337–5 (pbk. : alk. paper)
    1. Medicine—Examinations, questions, etc. 2. Medicine—Outlines,
syllabi, etc. I. Goldberg, Joel S. II. Title: USMLE, step 3.
III. Title: USMLE, step three.
    [DNLM: 1. Medicine—examination questions. W 18.2 I59 1997]
R834.5.I55 1997
610'.76—DC21
DNLM/DLC
for Library of Congress   96–46590
                                                           CIP

Acquisitions Editor: Marinita Timban
Production Editor: Eileen L. Pendagast
Designer: Libby Schmitz

ISBN 0-8385-4337-5

90000

9 780838 543375

PRINTED IN THE UNITED STATES OF AMERICA

PERIPHERAL NEUROPATHIES

D DiAbetes
A Alcohol
N Utritional
G uillen Barre

T ·rauma (Cerpal tunnel)
H Hereditary
E nvironmental

R Remote effect Cencer
A Amyloid
P orphyric
I nflammation
S. yphillis
T umors

Poly neuropathy –
Predominently Symmetric
Usually distal –
longest nerve
are most
metabolic Active

HCO_3/Na pump together in prox tubule.
Kidney maintains Na^+ homeostasis at expense of other ions.

| RTA |

Type I (Fanconi) ≡ Proximal Tubule ACIDOSIS
  Defect CARDONIC AnHyDRASE
  HCO_3 not regenerate, POT in blood –passes thru DT
  Problem ē AA, Glu, PO reabsorption
      S/S
        metabolic hyper choleremic ACIDOSIS
      ACIDURIA
        HCO_3 requirement
Type II = Distal CLASSIC RTA
        H^+ not secreted in exchy Na^+, so K^+ excreted.
      S/S
      1) metabolic hyper choremic acidoss
      2) Hypo kalemie
      3) alkaline urine ($pH > 5.5$)
      4) HCO_3 requirement
      5) Nephrocalcinous/stony

RTA 4 - Hypoaldosterone
  Na+ not reabsorb
  K+ not excreted → ↑K+
  H+ not secreted ⇒ ACIDOSIS
  HCO3 not generated

Hyperchloremic nonAnion GAP metabolic ACIDOSIS
  ACIDURIA
  ↓GFR

Contents

Contributors

Doris G. Bartuska, MD, FACP
Professor of Medicine
Director, Division of Endocrinology, Diabetes
  and Metabolism
Department of Medicine
Allegheny University of the Health Sciences
MCP ◆ Hahnemann School of Medicine
Philadelphia, Pennsylvania

Amy Brodkey, MD
Assistant Professor of Psychiatry
Department of Psychiatry
Eastern Pennsylvania Psychiatric Institute
Philadelphia, Pennsylvania

Guy H. Chan, MD, FACS
Professor
Department of Ophthalmology
Temple University School of Medicine
Philadelphia, Pennsylvania

Christopher A. Clyne, MD
Assistant Professor of Medicine
Cardiovascular Division
Department of Medicine
University of Pennsylvania School of Medicine
Director, Clinical Electrophysiology
Cardiovascular Division
Department of Medicine
Hospital of the University of Pennsylvania
Philadelphia, Pennsylvania

David P. Coll, MD
Clinical Instructor in Surgery
Allegheny University of the Health Sciences
MCP ◆ Hahnemann School of Medicine
Philadelphia, Pennsylvania

Jeffrey M. Finkelstein, MD, DMD, FACS
Assistant Professor of Otolaryngology and
  Bronchoesophagology
Department of Otolaryngology and
  Bronchoesophagology
Temple University School of Medicine
Philadelphia, Pennsylvania

Joel S. Goldberg, DO
Assistant Professor of Medicine
Department of Medicine
Allegheny University of the Health Sciences
MCP ◆ Hahnemann School of Medicine
Philadelphia, Pennsylvania

Jeffrey Greenstein, MD
Professor and Chair
Department of Neurology
Temple University Hospital
Philadelphia, Pennsylvania

Samuel L. Jacobs, MD
Assistant Professor
Division of Reproductive Endocrinology
Department of Obstetrics and Gynecology
Allegheny University of the Health Sciences
MCP ◆ Hahnemann School of Medicine
Philadelphia, Pennsylvania

Gary R. Kantor, MD
Associate Professor of Medicine
Division of Dermatology
Department of Medicine
Allegheny University of the Health Sciences
MCP ◆ Hahnemann School of Medicine
Philadelphia, Pennsylvania

Morris D. Kerstein, MD
Professor of Surgery
Clinical Instructor in Surgery
Department of Surgery
Allegheny University of the Health Sciences
MCP ◆ Hahnemann School of Medicine
Philadelphia, Pennsylvania

Margaret R. Khouri, MD, FACP
Associate Professor of Clinical Medicine
Allegheny University of the Health Sciences
MCP ◆ Hahnemann School of Medicine
Center City, Pennsylvania

Carey Kimmelstiel, MD
Assistant Professor of Medicine
Division of Cardiology
Tufts University School of Medicine
Boston, Massachusetts

Kurt S. Kodroff, MD
Clinical Instructor in Medicine
Department of Medicine
Medical College of Pennsylvania
Philadelphia, Pennsylvania

Mary Ann Kuzma, MD
Assistant Professor of Medicine
Director of Student Clerkship
Division of General Medicine
Allegheny University of the Health Sciences
MCP ◆ Hahnemann School of Medicine
Philadelphia, Pennsylvania

Joan A. Lit, MD
Assistant Professor of Medicine
Division of Endocrinology, Diabetes and
    Metabolism
Department of Medicine
Allegheny University of the Health Sciences
MCP ◆ Hahnemann School of Medicine
Philadelphia, Pennsylvania

S. Bruce Malkowicz, MD
Associate Professor of Urology
University of Pennsylvania
Philadelphia, Pennsylvania

Joseph R. McClellan, MD
Assistant Professor of Medicine
Division of Cardiology
Department of Medicine
University of Pennsylvania
Director, Cardiac Care Unit and Nuclear
    Cardiology
Division of Cardiology
Department of Medicine
Hospital of the University of Pennsylvania
Philadelphia, Pennsylvania

Pekka A. Mooar, MD
Chief, Sports Medicine
Traumatology
Allegheny University of the Health Sciences
MCP ◆ Hahnemann School of Medicine
Philadelphia, Pennsylvania

Stephen D. Nimer, MD
Acting Head, Division of Hematologic Oncology
Associate Professor of Medicine, Cornell
    University
New York, New York

Anna Parlick, MD
Hematologic Oncology Fellow
Division of Hematologic Oncology
Department of Medicine
Memorial Sloan-Kettering Cancer Center
New York, New York

Charles A. Pohl, MD
Clinical Assistant Professor
Co-Director In Patient Services
Pediatric Sleep Disorders and Infant Apnea
    Program
Department of Pediatrics
Thomas Jefferson University
Philadelphia, Pennsylvania

R. Douglas Ross, MD
Associate Professor and Vice Chairman
Department of Obstetrics and Gynecology
Allegheny University of the Health Sciences
MCP ◆ Hahnemann School of Medicine
Philadelphia, Pennsylvania

Richard Rubin, MD
Director of Medical Students Education
Department of Ophthalmology
Temple University School of Medicine
Philadelphia, Pennsylvania

Andrea M. Saxon, MD
Assistant Professor of Ophthalmology
Division of Ophthalmology
Allegheny University of the Health Sciences
MCP ◆ Hahnemann School of Medicine
Philadelphia, Pennsylvania

Edward S. Schulman, MD
Professor of Medicine
Division Chief, Pulmonary and Critical Care
  Medicine
Allegheny University of the Health Sciences
MCP ◆ Hahnemann School of Medicine
Philadelphia, Pennsylvania

Michael Sherman, MD
Assistant Professor of Medicine
Medical Director of Pulmonary Services
Allegheny University of the Health Sciences
MCP ◆ Hahnemann School of Medicine
Philadelphia, Pennsylvania

Regina Simonetti, MD
Associate Residency Director
Inpatient Coordinator

Department of Pediatrics
AI duPont Childrens Hospital
Wilmington, Delaware

Richard Spielvogel, MD
Professor and Chair
Department of Medicine
Director, Division of Dermatology
Allegheny University of the Health Sciences
MCP ◆ Hahnemann School of Medicine
Philadelphia, Pennsylvania

Gerado R. Torres, MD
Assistant Professor of Medicine
Director, Neurology Residency Program
Temple University Hospital
Philadelphia, Pennsylvania

Craig A. Wood, MD
Assistant Professor of Medicine
Division of Infectious Diseases
Department of Medicine
Allegheny University of the Health Sciences
MCP ◆ Hahnemann School of Medicine
Philadelphia, Pennsylvania

Preface

The typical review book is written in a question-and-answer type format. It has long existed as the sole product for student examinations, until now. In 1992 I formulated my concept of a rapid-reading review manual, conceived out of the tremendous need for a succinct, yet complete review text. The key component was the extensive coverage of the USMLE "high-impact" disease list, with the inclusion and incorporation of all pertinent test material. In addition, it was necessary to present this material in a concise, easily assimilated format, to allow for a swift and highly effective review.

This text, *The Instant Exam Review for USMLE Step 3,* 2nd edition exists as a result of the tremendous popularity and widespread use of the Step 2 text, called *The Instant Exam Review for USMLE Step 2.* After the Step 2 text received extraordinary acceptance and acclaim by students and educators across the United States and abroad, I was asked by Appleton & Lange to create a new study book for the Step 3 exam. Thus, *The Instant Exam Review for USMLE Step 3!*

In this review manual, my original concept and ideals remain unchanged. Once again, the material in this book encompasses the key test facts, diseases, and disorders listed by the National Board of Medical Examiners for the new Step 3 examination. Our categories in this revised edition have changed to reflect the new examination content, with each chapter encompassing the Board's new list of diseases and disorders.

Finally, I have enlisted as contributors an exceptional group of physicians, widely renowned for their clinical and educational proficiency.

Please note that this text was not designed to teach general medicine, nor was it to be a substitute for accepted methods of medical education. Like its predecessor, it was designed as a unique study tool, to assist you, the student, in passing the Step 3 examination.

neuroblastoma nmyc

α_1 Antitrypsin d3
    Serum protease inhibitor syn in liver
    abn Pi 3 3

Obstructive
    Asthma
    CF
    emphysema
    FB
    Pneumoni
    Drowng
    Tuma

Acknowledgments

I would like to extend my sincere appreciation to Ms. Marinita Timban for her editorial assistance and to Ms. Amy Schermerhorn for her additional guidance. They were always available for counsel and support during the task of manuscript preparation, copyediting, review of page proofs, and production of bound books.

I wish to thank my coauthors for their willingness to participate in this complex endeavor and investing extensive time and effort in the construction of their chapters, despite their busy professional and personal schedules. They are a group of physicians dedicated to medicine, and their commitment to education is clear.

Finally, I would like to express my gratitude to the staff and faculty of Allegheny University of the Health Sciences, MCP ◆ Hahnemann School of Medicine for their assistance and unselfish dedication to both the clinical practice of medicine and the education of young physicians in training.

1° ↑ PTH   Parathyroid

2° ↑   R/O MEN I

THYROID

① PAPILLARY –
  Gardner (AD)
  x ray
  Psammoa   (lymph spread)
  slow spread
  TK thyroidectomy

② Follicular
  Hematogenous
  DO NOT FNA
  Thyroidectomy

③ Medullary –
  assoc MEN II
  Secrets Calcitonin
  from parafollicular
  thyr; lymph nodedis

④ Anaplastic
  poor

MEN (AD)

I : Wermers

        Parathyroid hyperplasia = $\uparrow Ca^+$

P   Pancreatic Islet cell

P   Gastrome : 3E

P   Insulinome

        Pituitary tumor

            optic

II   Sepples

M   Medullary

P   Calcitonin secretn

H   (Penagastrin)

    Pheochromocytoma

    Parathyroid hyperplasic

    Hyperparathyroid = $\uparrow Cg$

IIB   Mucosal neuroma

    Medullary thyroid

m   Marfomaid body habit

m   Pheoch.. bul

m

P

How to Use This Book

This book is an innovative and practical study guide designed to be utilized in both the initial phase of USMLE Step 3 examination preparation as a comprehensive study outline, and in the final few days and hours before the exam as a quick review manual.

USING THE BOOK AS A STUDY OUTLINE

When you begin to study, turn to the Contents to obtain an overview of this test. Review the material supplied by your school and the National Board of Medical Examiners, including the "Step 3 General Instructions, Content Description and Sample Items." It is important to have a full understanding of the design of the exam and the type of questions that will be asked.

Once you begin to study, *do not* omit any chapters in this text, but instead start at the beginning and read the book in its entirety. Notice that the outline format is streamlined to allow the rapid assimilation of facts in a minimal amount of reading time. Because extraneous and time-consuming information and phrasing have been omitted, working with *The Instant Exam Review for the USMLE Step 3*, 2nd edition for 1 hour will provide a database equivalent to that procured from several hours study of any other review text. Since the text is concise, it is vital that you be well rested and in a proper frame of mind for study and concentration. A quiet, comfortable, bright study area without glare is vital (with plenty of snacks nearby, of course!).

USING THE BOOK AS A QUICK REVIEW

In the final several weeks and days prior to your examination, *The Instant Exam Review for USMLE Step 3*, 2nd edition will serve as a rapid review tool. As in the *Step 2* text, this revolutionary new format, which completely covers the "high-impact" fact list, will allow the handbook to be read quickly, with successful, easy assimilation of the core facts necessary for exam success.

Joel S. Goldberg

1

Cardiovascular Medicine

Christopher A. Clyne, MD, Joseph R. McClellan, MD,
and Carey Kimmelstiel, MD

I. ISCHEMIC HEART DISEASE

A. ACUTE

S_4 ($\downarrow$ LV compliance)

1. Unstable Angina

• **H&P Keys**
Chest pain with accelerating pattern including new onset or rest symptoms. Often a midsternal squeezing or heaviness that may radiate to the left shoulder or arm, jaw, neck, etc. Symptoms may be similar to those present previously; however, usual alleviating factors (eg, nitroglycerin [NTG], rest) may no longer be effective. Associated symptoms, eg, diaphoresis, nausea, dyspnea, are

common. Reduction in left ventricular (LV) compliance may allow auscultation of an S_4 gallop. With coexisting LV dysfunction an S_3 may be heard. In the presence of global ischemia or LV dysfunction, a dyskinetic cardiac impulse may be palpated. Ischemia-induced papillary muscle dysfunction may cause the murmur of mitral regurgitation (MR). Ischemia-induced elevations in cardiac filling pressures often cause pulmonary congestion, allowing auscultation of rales.

• **Diagnosis**
Electrocardiogram (ECG): ST depression or elevation or T wave inversion. Exercise stress testing (ETT; not performed in patients with unstable angina). ETT or phar-

macologic stress testing is combined with an imaging agent, such as thallium, that permits the visualization of myocardial perfusion, coronary angiography.

- **Disease Severity**
Response to therapy and duration of symptoms dictate evaluation. Patients easily stabilized on medical therapy can often be closely followed clinically. Patients not medically stabilized or whose symptoms reemerge on therapy and those with prominent ischemic ECG findings usually undergo coronary angiography. Location and severity of stenoses (eg, left main, three-vessel) dictate management.

- **Concept and Application**
Vast majority of patients with unstable angina have underlying coronary atherosclerosis (CAD). Conversion from stable to unstable symptoms is usually caused by plaque rupture with superimposed thrombosis. Platelet aggregation at site of plaque rupture with release of vasoconstricting mediators plays an important role.

- **Management**
Continuous ECG monitoring. Bed rest, mild sedation, and treatment of extra cardiac precipitants of increased oxygen demand (eg, hypoxia, sepsis, anemia, uncontrolled hypo- or hypertension, etc). Nitrates, heparin, and aspirin (acetylsalicylic acid [ASA]) are of proven efficacy. Intravenous NTG often is successful when other routes fail. β- and calcium channel blockers are useful added to nitrates when necessary. Intra-aortic balloon counterpulsation (IABP) is often used as a bridge to percutaneous transluminal coronary angioplasty (PTCA) or coronary artery bypass graft (CABG) and is effective in stabilizing medically refractory patients.

2. Myocardial Infarction

- **H&P Keys**
Chest pain, often midsternal squeezing or crushing. The pain may radiate to the neck, jaw, shoulders, arms, etc. Diaphoresis is frequent. Approximately 20% of episodes occur in the absence of pain (silent). Displaced and even dyskinetic cardiac impulse can be palpated. Ischemia-induced papillary muscle dysfunction may allow auscultation of MR murmur. In the presence of associated right ventricular (RV) infarction, jugular venous distention (JVD) can be seen. Elevations in cardiac filling pressures often cause pulmonary congestion, allowing auscultation of pulmonary rales.

- **Diagnosis**
ECG: transmural or Q wave myocardial infarction (MI): ST segment elevation and T wave inversions with subsequent evolution of Q waves. Nontransmural or non-Q MI: ST depression and T wave inversions are seen. Elevations in cardiac enzymes: creatine kinase (CK), specifically CK-MB, peaks at 24 hours; aspartate aminotransferase (AST, or SGOT) peaks at 48 to 72 hours; L-lactate dehydrogenase (LDH) peaks at 3 to 5 days after MI. A ratio of $LDH_1 : LDH_2$ greater than $1 : 0$ suggests that MI has occurred. If a question of diagnosis of MI exists, technetium (infarct-avid) scanning can localize MIs.

- **Disease Severity**
Cardiac imaging with echocardiography (echo) or radionuclide ventriculography (RVG) can help assess extent and prognosis of infarction by measuring LV systolic function. Echo aids in diagnosis of MI complications, eg, LV thrombus or aneurysm, pericardial effusion, free wall and septal rupture, and MR.

- **Concept and Application**
MI results from myocardial O_2 supply–demand imbalance. The vast majority of cases of MI are due to CAD. Plaque rupture leads to thrombosis and coronary occlusion. Platelet aggregation and release of mediators further hinder flow and contribute to spasm. Elevation of myocardial oxygen demand (eg, tachycardia) can lead to MI. Irreversible cell death occurs, usually within 6 hours, if therapy is not given or if spontaneous improvement does not occur. Nonatherosclerotic causes of MI, such as embolism, trauma, vasculitis, or hypercoagulable states, are less common.

- **Management**
Continuous monitoring in the cardiac care unit (CCU) is important. Thrombolysis

(streptokinase, tissue plasminogen activator [TPA], acylated streptokinase-plasminogen complex [APSAC]), especially early administration, reduces mortality. PTCA is effective, especially if thrombolysis is contraindicated. Heparin and ASA are useful (in conjunction) with thrombolysis. In the absence of thrombolysis, ASA and beta-blockade are efficacious. Nitrates are helpful in decreasing oxygen demand and increasing supply. Analgesia should be administered as necessary. Coronary angiography is recommended, especially if the patient is unresponsive to medical therapy or needs IABP, PTCA, or CABG. Catheterization may be required for the diagnosis and treatment of complications.

3. Spasm (Prinzmetal's or Variant Angina)

NITRATES
Ca Channel Blockers

- **H&P Keys**
Anginal-type chest pain, typically occurring at rest. High percentage of patients with isolated coronary spasm are cigarette smokers or cocaine abusers. Patients tend to be younger than those with exertional angina. If patient is asymptomatic, the cardiac exam is usually normal.

- **Diagnosis**
ECG: typically shows ST elevation during symptomatic periods. Coronary spasm in response to the vasoconstrictor ergonovine, usually during coronary angiography, is the gold standard diagnostic test.

- **Disease Severity**
Severity judged by symptom frequency and response to ergonovine.

- **Concept and Application**
Most patients have CAD, and spasm occurs in close proximity to a diseased segment, although approximately one third have angiographically normal coronaries. Diseased coronary vasculature loses the ability to manifest endothelial-dependent vasodilation and may react paradoxically to what are normally vasorelaxant stimuli.

- **Management**
Nitrates and calcium channel blockers are usually effective; the effect of β-blockers is unpredictable; in some they can precipitate spasm. β-Blockers (eg, prazosin) can be helpful. Cigarette smoking and cocaine use are to be avoided.

B. Chronic

1. Stable Angina Pectoris

- **H&P Keys**
Episodic chest discomfort, often described as heaviness or squeezing. Pain may radiate to the jaw, neck, shoulder, or the left arm. Symptoms typically are precipitated by exertion, cold weather, or emotional upset, often relieved by rest. Family history of premature CAD, diabetes, hyperlipidemia, hypertension, cigarette smoking. Exam may be normal, but if the patient is examined during an ischemic episode, reduction in LV compliance may allow auscultation of an S_4. An S_3 may be heard if coexisting LV dysfunction is present. In the presence of global ischemia or LV dysfunction, a dyskinetic cardiac impulse may be palpated. Ischemia-induced papillary muscle dysfunction may give rise to MR murmur. Ischemia-induced elevations in filling pressures often lead to pulmonary congestion with auscultation of rales.

- **Diagnosis**
ECG may be normal if patient is asymptomatic, but evidence of prior MI may be seen. If patient is symptomatic, ischemic ST and T wave changes may be noted. ETT, pharmacologic stress testing, or exercise echo are useful.

- **Disease Severity**
Global ECG changes suggest multivessel CAD. Quantitation of ischemic burden can be accomplished with perfusion imaging. Coronary arteriography documents presence, extent, and severity of CAD.

- **Concept and Application**
Angina results from myocardial oxygen supply–demand imbalance. Obstructive cor-

onary lesions cause blood flood limitation to myocardial segments. Dilatation of myocardial arteriolar resistance vessels mitigates ischemia, but this mechanism eventually is inadequate as stenosis severity increases. Angina can be precipitated in the absence of CAD in patients with augmented myocardial oxygen demand, eg, hypertrophy or aortic stenosis.

- **Management**

  NITRATE
  B Blockers
  Ca Chennel Bl.
  ASA

  Reduction of ischemic precipitants. Therapy with nitrates, β- and calcium channel blockers, as well as ASA. Secondary risk reduction with control of lipids, discontinuation of smoking. Treatment of coexisting illnesses (eg, hyperthyroidism) that increase oxygen demand. PTCA and CABG in appropriate patients.

2. Silent Ischemia

- **H&P Keys**
  Patients are most frequently asymptomatic, and the physical exam in the absence of ischemia is usually normal.

- **Diagnosis**
  Holter monitoring can uncover ambulatory ST changes indicative of ischemia, as can ETT.

- **Disease Severity**
  Degree of ST segment depression and number of leads involved can suggest disease extent; nocturnal ST segment often means multivessel CAD.

- **Concept and Application**
  Two populations exist, those with entirely asymptomatic ischemia and those with both symptomatic and asymptomatic episodes. In patients with symptomatic CAD, most episodes are asymptomatic. Whether an abnormal pain mechanism or a heightened pain threshold is responsible for silent ischemia is unknown; however, it appears to occur with higher frequency in diabetics.

- **Management**
  Medical therapy is often used; however, specific therapy depends on extent of disease, patient's age, occupation, etc.

II. HEART FAILURE

A. Left-Sided

1. Low Output

- **H&P Keys**
  History may elicit cause, eg, CAD, history MI, hypertension, or valvular disease. Symptoms: fatigue, weakness, reduced exercise tolerance, exertional or rest dyspnea, paroxysmal nocturnal dyspnea (PND), orthopnea. Physical findings: displaced cardiac impulse; S_3 or S_4; murmurs, especially MR; rales; rarely Cheyne-Stokes respiration.

- **Diagnosis**
  Most often made by history and exam. Confirmation can be made by chest roentgenogram, echo, or RVG. In patients with prior MI, Q waves may be seen on ECG. Pulmonary artery catheterization documents hemodynamic derangement.

- **Disease Severity**
  Determined by degree of symptomatic incapacity and of LV impairment (systolic dysfunction), degree of hemodynamic impairment, indicated by elevated filling pressures (systolic and diastolic dysfunction).

- **Concept and Application**
  In systolic dysfunction, the heart delivers inadequate oxygen to meet metabolic needs; in diastolic dysfunction ventricular filling is compromised. Systolic and diastolic dysfunction commonly coexist. In predominantly systolic dysfunction, activation of sympathetic nervous system, renin-angiotensin-aldosterone axis, and hormonal (antidiuretic hormone [ADH]) elaboration occurs.

- **Management**
  Search and therapy for precipitating causes of decompensation (infection, MI, uncontrolled hypertension, dietary indiscretion, etc). Correction underlying diseases, eg, valvular disease, ischemia, arrhythmia. Salt restriction. Medical therapy with diuretics, reduction of afterload with vasodilators, eg, angiotensin-converting enzyme (ACE) in-

hibitors; augmentation of contractility with digoxin. With severe decompensation, sympathomimetic amines may be necessary.

2. High Output *Left Sided.*

- **H&P Keys**
Signs of hyperdynamic circulation, eg, brisk pulses. Dyspnea, orthopnea often present. Angina in patients with CAD.

- **Disease Severity**
Assessed primarily on degree of disability.

- **Concept and Application**
Patients often have an underlying syndrome causing elevation in metabolic demands, eg, arteriovenous fistulas, Paget's disease, hyperthyroidism, anemia.

- **Management**
Treatment of underlying cause, medical therapy: often diuresis.

B. Right-Sided

- **H&P Keys**
Seen with history LV failure, RV infarction, lung disease, pulmonic stenosis, pulmonary emboli, myocarditis, etc. Clinical findings: fatigue, RV heave and gallops, JVD, hepatomegaly, edema, atrial arrhythmias.

- **Diagnosis**
Signs and symptoms of RV failure in setting of predisposing condition. ECG may show RV or right atrial (RA) hypertrophy. Echo may show RV dilatation and hypokinesis.

- **Disease Severity**
Often suggested by degree of edema and JVD on exam. Ascites suggests more severe decompensation. Echo and RVG can quantitate the degree of functional impairment and dilatation. Right heart catheterization quantitates the degree of hemodynamic impairment and response to therapy. Arterial blood gases (ABG) and pulmonary function tests (PFTs) document the degree of pulmonary disability, if any.

- **Concept and Application**
RV outflow obstruction (eg, pulmonic stenosis), pulmonary hypertension resulting from chronic LV failure, obstructive lung disease, chronic pulmonary emboli (cor pulmonale), etc, lead to chronic overload of the RV. Elevated pressures in systemic vasculature lead to accumulation of fluid in the extravascular space.

- **Management**
Treatment of underlying condition. Diuretics lead to symptomatic improvement. Oxygen supplementation, antiarrhythmics, anti-ischemics, anticoagulation as needed.

III. HYPOTENSION AND ACUTE CIRCULATORY COLLAPSE (SHOCK)

Occurs in a wide array of conditions that ultimately lead to inadequate oxygen delivery to the organs, tissues, and cells. Impairment in oxygen transport results from increases in demand or inability to maintain normal oxygen supply. Shock is classified according to the primary hemodynamic derangement as cardiogenic, hypovolemic, obstructive, and distributive. In all forms, physical examination reveals hypotension defined as mean pressure less than 60 mm Hg with evidence of peripheral hypoperfusion, including vasoconstriction, with cool and mottled extremities and other evidence of poor organ perfusion, including abnormal mentation and decreased urine output.

A. Cardiogenic Shock

Inadequate cardiac output as a result of an abnormality in intrinsic cardiac function or an anatomic derangement in cardiac structure, for example, acute valvular heart disease.

- **H&P Keys**
During an MI, patients will have acute chest pain, dyspnea, diaphoresis, evidence of peripheral hypoperfusion, S_3 gallop, elevated venous pressure, or a murmur of MR or ventricular septal defect.

- **Diagnosis**
ECG to confirm MI, echo to evaluate global LV function, regional abnormalities, and

[handwritten margin notes top-left: SHOCK / CARDIOGENIC / HYPOVOLEMIC / OBSTRUCTIVE / DISTRIBUTING]

structural abnormalities, eg, ventricular septal defect or acute MR. Hemodynamic monitoring with Swan-Ganz catheter often required for characterization.

- **Disease Severity**

  [handwritten margin note: LACTATE]

  Level of blood pressure, organ perfusion including urine output, metabolic acidosis, or elevated serum lactate.

- **Concept and Application**

  With fatal cardiogenic shock, 40% of the functioning myocardium is lost. Reduction in coronary perfusion pressure leads to a downward spiral, with progressive loss of contractility. Mechanical derangements, including rupture of the ventricular septum or mitral valve apparatus at any level, eg, papillary muscle or chordae, result in elevation of venous pressure, pulmonary congestion, reduced cardiac output, and organ hypoperfusion.

- **Management**

  [handwritten margin notes: Thrombolysis / Angioplasty]

  Most effective therapy is acute restoration of blood flow with thrombolysis or coronary angioplasty. Hemodynamic management is guided by placement of a balloon flotation catheter with determinations of pulmonary capillary wedge pressure and cardiac output. If pulmonary capillary wedge pressure is low, volume is administered; if pulmonary capillary wedge pressure is high and cardiac output is low, treatment is needed to augment cardiac output and improve organ perfusion at reduced filling pressures. Intra-aortic balloon pump augments coronary perfusion and produces systolic unloading of the ventricle. Dopamine or dobutamine may be helpful to produce augmentation of cardiac output and maintenance of peripheral perfusion. Oxygenation must be maintained. Mortality remains high, in spite of modern management techniques, unless effective myocardial blood flow can be restored.

B. Hypovolemic Shock

Inadequate circulatory volume caused by hemorrhage or dehydration. Common with trauma, surgery, vomiting, diarrhea, and some skin disorders.

- **H&P Keys**

  Weakness, postural light-headedness in setting of blood loss or fluid loss, eg, history of hemorrhage, melena. Postural hypotension and tachycardia, low jugular venous pressure.

- **Diagnosis**

  Measurement of postural blood pressure and heart rate changes, nasogastric aspiration, hemoglobin, blood urea and nitrogen (BUN) : creatinine ratio.

- **Disease Severity**

  Level of blood pressure, severity of impaired organ perfusion, hourly urine output.

- **Concept and Application**

  Cardiac output is dependent on preload or venous return. An initial reduction in volume is compensated by an increase in heart rate and arterial and venous vasoconstriction. As volume reduction progresses, compensatory mechanisms are unable to compensate, and blood pressure falls.

- **Management**

  Acute, rapid volume restoration with blood, crystalloid, or colloid solutions and maintenance of peripheral perfusion pressure with vasoconstrictors. Next, identification of cause or source of blood loss or fluid loss and control of site of bleeding, eg, with endoscopy, arterial cauterization, surgery.

C. Obstructive Shock

[handwritten margin notes: PG / Pericardial effusion / TAMPONADE]

Impairment of venous return to the right ventricle or left ventricle occurs secondary to obstruction in the venous system, pulmonary artery, or pericardium. Observed with acute pulmonary embolus, pericardial effusion, or tamponade. Effusion is caused by trauma, infections, malignancy, connective tissue disease, and renal failure.

- **H&P Keys**

  Dyspnea, orthopnea, elevated venous pressure, chest pain, hemoptysis, pulsus paradoxus, faint and distant heart sounds, or pulmonary hypertension.

- **Diagnosis**
Echo for effusion or tamponade, ECG with electrical alternans, analysis of pericardial fluid for etiology. Analysis for source of embolus, venous Doppler probe, ventilation-perfusion lung scan.

- **Concept and Application**
During pericardial tamponade, elevation of the intrapericardial pressure raises pressure in the cardiac chambers, leading to a reduction in venous return to the right and left heart and reduced cardiac output. Venous obstruction or pulmonary artery embolus also prevents adequate flow and venous return to the left heart with reduction in cardiac output.

- **Disease Severity**
Level of blood pressure, mentation, peripheral perfusion.

- **Management**
Acute volume administration, administration of beta-agonist to increase heart rate and stroke volume. Definitive therapy requires drainage by pericardiocentesis, guided by hemodynamic monitoring or two-dimensional echo, or subxiphoid or anterior pericardiectomy. Pulmonary embolus with shock has a high mortality. Thrombolytic therapy with streptokinase infusion over 24 hours is favored over acute embolectomy.

D. Distributive Shock

Characteristic of sepsis, also anaphylaxis and neurogenic, toxic, or endocrinologic shock.

- **H&P Keys**
Fever, chills, rigor, respiratory alkalosis, bee sting or other toxic ingestion, hypotension, peripheral vasodilation with warm extremities.

- **Disease Severity**
Level of blood pressure, evidence of poor organ perfusion.

- **Diagnosis**
Blood cultures, white blood count, ABG, pH, lactate, toxin screen, hemodynamic monitoring to determine venous pressure and cardiac output.

- **Concept and Application**
Diffuse arterial and venous dilatation in response to endotoxins, exotoxins, and cytokines. Other mediators include kinins, histamine, and prostaglandins. Cardiac output is increased and peripheral oxygen demand also markedly increased. Inadequate tissue oxygen delivery and failure of microcirculation, with inappropriate vasodilatation and vasoconstriction. Later, sepsis leads to depression in myocardial function.

- **Management**
Initial characterization of site of infection; antibiotic coverage, including two bacteriocidal agents for likely organisms. Initial rapid volume infusion with crystalloid and colloid solutions and blood to maintain hemoglobin- and oxygen-carrying capacity. Vasoactive drugs including dopamine to maintain perfusion pressure of 60 mm Hg.

IV. MYOCARDIAL DISEASES

A. Dilated Cardiomyopathy

- **H&P Keys**
Symptoms suggest low cardiac output and congestion of systemic and pulmonary vasculature: dyspnea, fatigue, orthopnea, PND, edema. Exam often reveals hypotension, tachycardia, cool extremities, pulmonary rales, displaced cardiac impulse often of diminished intensity, S_3, mitral, or tricuspid murmur. Signs of RV failure (edema, ascites, elevated JVD) often present.

- **Diagnosis**
Chest roentgenogram often shows cardiomegaly, often with signs of congestion, possibly with pleural effusions. ECG often shows signs of ventricular or atrial enlargement, atrial fibrillation; premature ventricular complexes (PVCs) are often seen. Echo and RVG often show ventricular or four chamber enlargement with diffuse hypocontractility.

- **Disease Severity**
Symptoms may correlate poorly with degree of ventricular impairment. Echo and

RVG document degree of ventricular dilatation and dysfunction. Echo documents associated valvular abnormalities. Cardiac catheterization documents degree of hemodynamic abnormality and presence of CAD. In absence of CAD, catheterization rarely alters therapy.

- **Concept and Application**
ischemic
viral
peripartum
Toxic
Various etiologies, most common being idiopathic. Other etiologies include ischemic (postinfarction), viral (eg, Coxsackie), peripartum, toxic (eg, alcohol, doxorubicin). Myocyte injury occurs, causing reduction in contractility, leading to ventricular dilation, with compensation by activation of sympathetic nervous system and renin-angiotensin-aldosterone axis. ·
PATTOPH

- **Management**
Removal of inciting cause (eg, discontinue alcohol) if one can be found. Diuresis improves symptoms and relieves pulmonary and systemic congestion. Salt restriction. Enhancement of myocardial contractility with digoxin. ACE inhibition has been shown to improve survival and quality of life. Anticoagulation in patients with atrial fibrillation or cardiac embolism. Implantable cardioverter-defibrillator in select patients with severe ventricular arrhythmias.
DIG
ACE

B. Hypertrophic Cardiomyopathy

- **H&P Keys**
Often patients are younger; history of sudden death of a relative during exertion may be obtained. Symptoms: exertional dyspnea, chest pain, syncope, light-headedness, sudden death, especially during exertion. Exam may reveal S_4, double or triple apical impulse, crescendo–decrescendo systolic murmur, increased by Valsalva maneuver and by rising from recumbency, decreased by squatting.
↑VALSA
↓SQUATTINL

- **Diagnosis**
ECG may show left ventricular hypertrophy (LVH) and possibly large Q waves in inferior and lateral leads; giant negative T waves are occasionally seen in the mid-precordium. Echo or Doppler may document signs of LV outflow obstruction

(including an intraventricular pressure gradient and systolic anterior motion of the mitral valve) as well as MR. Holter monitoring may document atrial fibrillation, which is poorly tolerated, or ventricular arrhythmias, which may precede sudden death.

- **Disease Severity**
Echocardiography can quantitate degree of hypertrophy, especially in asymmetric septal hypertrophy (ASH), the most common variant. Intraventricular gradient can be calculated by Doppler; if one does not exist at rest, the presence and magnitude of gradient can be documented in catheterization lab with use of IV isoproterenol.

- **Concept and Application**
A massively hypertrophied LV wall results in a noncompliant, stiffened chamber with impaired filling. Increased myocardial mass leads to increased myocardial oxygen demand and frequently angina. Patients with ASH often have dynamic LV obstruction and frequently MR. Hypertrophic cardiomyopathy (HCM) can be both spontaneous, inherited, or the result of long-standing hypertension.

- **Management**
Competitive sports are generally prohibited because of the risk of sudden death. β- and calcium channel blockers are effective in decreasing the intraventricular gradient, myocardial oxygen demand, and ventricular stiffness. Surgery (septal myectomy) is effective in patients with obstructive HCM; more recently, dual-chamber pacing has been shown to be effective in these patients.
B B
auc B₂

C. Restrictive Cardiomyopathy

- **H&P Keys**
Patient may have an underlying disease (eg, hemachromatosis, sarcoid, amyloid, or cancer). Symptoms: fatigue, weakness, dyspnea. Physical findings: elevated jugular venous pressure; Kussmaul's sign; edema; ascites; enlarged, tender liver; distant heart sounds; S_3 and S_4 are common.

- **Diagnosis**
  ECG often shows low voltage, with echo showing thickened LV walls, often with a "speckled" appearance.

- **Disease Severity**
  Echo shows degree of LV thickening and degree of systolic impairment (if any). Doppler and cardiac catheterization can show augmented early diastolic filling. Catheterization demonstrates lowered cardiac output and typical "dip and plateau" morphology in ventricular diastole. RV biopsy can identify a specific cause.

- **Concept and Application**
  Restrictive cardiomyopathy is the least common of the cardiomyopathies. Systemic disorders (eg, hemachromatosis, sarcoid, amyloid, metastatic cancer), patients with thoracic radiation or with other disorders (eg, endomyocardial fibrosis) caused by myocardial infiltration, fibrosis, etc, have elevated filling pressures, which lead to signs and symptoms of right and left heart congestion. Reduced cavity size causes decreased cardiac output.

- **Management**
  Unless—and sometimes even with—a known underlying cause, prognosis is poor. Treatment of underlying cause (eg, steroids in sarcoid, chelation therapy in hemachromatosis). Symptomatic treatment includes diuretics, salt restriction. Digoxin is often not helpful and may be harmful in these disorders.

V. CARDIAC ARRHYTHMIAS

A. Supraventricular Arrhythmias

Rhythm disturbances involving sinus node, atria, and atrioventricular (AV) node.

1. Bradyarrhythmias

a. Sinus Node Dysfunction (Sick Sinus Syndrome). Heart rates less than 60 beats per minute (bpm) or inappropriate rise in rate for level of activity (chronotropic incompetence). Includes sinus arrest, sinus exit block, bradycardia-tachycardia syndrome (rapid atrial fibrillation or flutter with long pauses).

- **H&P Keys**
  Fatigue, dizziness, weakness, syncope, slow rhythm and pulse.

- **Diagnosis**
  ECG, carotid sinus massage > 3-second pauses and symptoms, electrophysiologic studies.

- **Disease Severity**
  Depressed mental status, fatigue, limitation of activity, shortness of breath.

- **Concept and Application**
  Disruption of normal structures and conduction pathways resulting from collagen deposition, hypertension, ischemia, atrial stretch, idiopathic causes, autonomic nervous system.

- **Management**
  Acute symptomatic: temporary pacemaker; Chronic symptomatic: permanent pacemaker, withdrawal of offending drugs.

b. AV Node

First-Degree AV Block. PR interval > 0.20 seconds. May or may not be associated with bradyarrhythmia.

Second-Degree AV Block. Intermittent failure of atrial activity to reach ventricles:

Mobitz Type I (Wenckebach). Usually at level of AV node, progressive PR prolongation prior to blocked QRS. Does not include blocked premature atrial contraction.

Mobitz Type II Block. Usually distal to AV node (bundle of His). High risk for complete AV block. Often associated with wide QRS.

Complete (Third-Degree) AV Block. May be at level of AV node, bundle of His, or bundle branches. Atrial and ventricular activity are independent and atrial rate faster than ventricular escape rate. QRS usually wide. Often associated with symptoms.

- **H&P Keys**
Fatigue, shortness of breath, congestive heart failure, dizziness, syncope. Slow or irregular pulse.

- **Diagnosis**
ECG, intermittent cannon A waves and complete heart block, carotid sinus massage with > 3-second pauses and symptoms, electrophysiologic studies.

- **Disease Severity**
Heart rate, blood pressure, mentation, level of activity.

- **Concept and Application**
Influence of autonomic nervous system, medications, hypertension, associated valve diseases (calcific), ischemic heart disease, Lev's and Lenegre's diseases, electrolyte disturbances (potassium).

- **Management**
Withdrawal of offending medications, temporary pacemaker in unstable patients, permanent pacemakers for patients with symptomatic bradycardia or asymptomatic Mobitz II or third-degree heart block.

2. Tachyarrhythmias

a. **Premature Atrial Complex (PAC).** Found in over 60% of normal adults. Usually benign and asymptomatic. May be associated with the initiation of atrial fibrillation, flutter, or atrial tachycardias.

b. **Premature Junctional Complex (PJC).** Early beat originating in AV node. Narrow QRS.

c. **Sinus Tachycardia.** Rate > 100 bpm. Normal or abnormal response to metabolic demand.

d. **Atrial Fibrillation.** Relatively common disorder characterized by irregularly irregular rhythm and absence of identifiable P waves. Sometimes seen in normal patients, often associated with various cardiac abnormalities and thyroid disease.

e. **Atrial Flutter.** Usually associated with atrial fibrillation. Organized atrial activity with rates 250 to 300 bpm. Sawtooth atrial activity on ECG. Variable conduction to ventricles (2 : 1, 3 : 1, 4 : 1).

f. **Atrial Tachycardia.** Rates > 100 bpm inappropriate for activity level. Originate from within left or right atrium.

g. **AV Reentry (AVRT; Wolff-Parkinson-White Syndrome) and AV Nodal Reentrant Tachycardias (AVNRT).** Reentrant arrhythmias dependent on the AV node. Classic models for reentry.

- **H&P Keys**
Palpitations: rapid heart rate is irregularly irregular for atrial fibrillation and often regular for other forms of sustained supraventricular tachycardia. Fatigue, shortness of breath, dizziness, syncope.

- **Diagnosis**
Long-term ECG recording, electrophysiologic studies.

- **Disease Severity**
Frequency of symptoms, including fatigue, lethargy, dizziness, chest pain, shortness of breath, syncope. Stroke is associated with atrial fibrillation.

- **Concept and Application**
Automatic mechanism for PACs, PJCs, and some atrial tachycardia. Reentry is predominant mechanism for most supraventricular tachycardia. May be congenital (Wolff-Parkinson-White) or associated with other forms of structural heart disease, eg, hypertension, ischemic heart disease, congenital heart disease (atrial septal defect). May be seen in normal patients.

- **Management**
Maintenance of sinus rhythm. Digoxin, calcium channel blockers, and β-blockers, antiarrhythmic drugs, direct-current cardioversion if unstable, radiofrequency ablation.

B. Ventricular Arrhythmias

Disorders of rhythm isolated to ventricles.

1. Bradyarrhythmias

Conduction disturbances within the His-Purkinje system and bundle branches. Often symptomatic. Usually caused by second- and third-degree heart block.

- **H&P Keys**
  Light-headedness, fatigue, syncope, intermittent cannon A waves in jugular venous pulse exam (third-degree heart block), slow pulse (intermittent or chronic).

- **Diagnosis**
  ECG, auscultation (dissociation of atrial [S_4] and ventricular [S_1 and S_2] activity), electrophysiologic studies.

- **Disease Severity**
  Frequency of symptoms including dizziness, light-headedness, fatigue, shortness of breath, chest pain, syncope. Trifascicular block may be asymptomatic but predictive of complete heart block.

- **Concept and Application**
  Lenegre's disease (sclerodegenerative disease of the conduction system), myocardial infarction, cardiomyopathies, drugs, infections (myocardial abscess).

- **Management**
  Temporary pacemaker for stabilization of symptomatic patients. Permanent pacemaker for patients at high risk of developing third-degree heart block, patients with trifascicular block or symptomatic bradycardia. Withdrawal of offending medications.

2. Tachyarrhythmias

PVCs may be seen in normal patients. Often associated with ischemic heart disease, congestive heart failure, electrolyte abnormalities, and cardioactive drugs.

- **a. Ventricular Tachycardia (VT).** May be nonsustained, eg, 3 beats ≤ 30 seconds, or sustained, eg, > 30 seconds. May be uniform (regular); or polymorphic (irregular). Rate > 100 bpm and usually < 250 bpm.

- **b. Ventricular Fibrillation.** Chaotic ventricular tachycardia with rate > 250 bpm. Most common cause of cardiac arrest.

- **H&P Keys**
  Palpitations, sudden-onset weakness, dizziness, syncope, and cardiac arrest. Often associated with ischemia, congestive heart failure, cardiomyopathy. Cardiac arrest victim is pulseless and without respirations.

- **Diagnosis**
  ECG, signal-averaged ECG, invasive electrophysiologic studies.

- **Disease Severity**
  Cardiac arrest has high recurrence rate if untreated. Prognosis related to LV function, CAD. Two-dimensional echo, cardiac catheterization.

- **Concept and Application**
  Most ventricular arrhythmias are due to reentry and are associated with acute or chronic ischemic heart disease or congestive heart failure (CHF). Rarely seen in structurally normal heart. Other forms (automatic, triggered activity) are associated with medications or electrolyte abnormalities (torsade de pointes) or are idiopathic.

- **Management**

  Sustained Ventricular Tachycardia. Low-energy cardioversion (50 to 200 J) or antiarrhythmic drugs, including lidocaine and procainamide.

  Ventricular Fibrillation. Rapid defibrillation with 200 to 360 J.

  Chronic Management. Stabilization of underlying disease, correction of electrolyte imbalances, antiarrhythmic drugs, implantable cardioverter defibrillator in some patients.

VI. PERICARDIAL DISEASES

A. Acute Pericarditis

Most common pericardial disorder, consisting of acute inflammation of the pericardium with a variety of causes.

- **H&P Keys**

  Retrosternal and left precordial sharp chest pain, often radiating to the back and left trapezius, with strong pleuritic component. Dyspnea is common. Symptoms often are worse in supine position, alleviated by sitting forward. Friction rub (three-component) best heard in left precordium while patient sitting forward during held exhalation.

- **Diagnosis**

  ECG can show evolutionary changes consisting of widespread ST elevations with upward concavity and depressed PR interval, reduction of T wave amplitude or T wave inversion; with large associated pericardial effusions, reduction in R wave amplitude. Tests for etiology, eg, antinuclear antibodies (ANA), purified protein derivative (PPD).

- **Disease Severity**

  Predominantly involves testing for etiology. Echo used to assess for presence and degree of associated pericardial effusion.

- **Concept and Application**

  Pericardial inflammation caused by a variety of factors. Most common cause is idiopathic, although serologic studies have suggested these cases may be due to viral infection. Tuberculous pericarditis now reemerging, especially in AIDS patients. Purulent (bacterial) pericarditis is a fulminant disease with a poor prognosis. Other causes are post-MI injury (eg, Dressler's syndrome), malignant neoplasia, radiation, uremia, collagen vascular diseases, etc.

- **Management**

  In idiopathic or viral cases, anti-inflammatory agents are used; rarely, steroids are used in recalcitrant cases. Purulent pericarditis requires drainage and antibiotics. Other treatment depends on specific etiology.

B. Pericardial Effusion   Water bottle

Fluid accumulation in the pericardial space. The rapidity with which this occurs in large measure determines the symptomatic impairment.

- **H&P Keys**

  Symptoms of pericarditis, or patient may be asymptomatic. Previously present friction rub may diminish in intensity. In large effusion, heart sounds may be muffled; Ewart's sign may be seen.

- **Diagnosis**

  Chest roentgenogram shows cardiomegaly with "water bottle" shape. ECG, especially in large effusions, shows reduced QRS amplitude; electrical alternans may be seen. Echo for direct visualization of size and presence of effusion.

- **Disease Severity**

  Determined by rapidity of accumulation and size of effusion. Echo documents size of effusion and can suggest hemodynamic impairment; hemodynamic effects can be documented by cardiac catheterization.

- **Concept and Application**

  Any cause of pericarditis can cause the formation of a pericardial effusion. Aside from causes previously noted, pericardial effusion can occur with systemic disorders such as hypothyroidism.

- **Management**

  Treatment of underlying cause. Pericardiocentesis for diagnosis and treatment.

C. Cardiac Tamponade

An accumulation of pericardial fluid under high pressure, which limits the ability of the heart to fill.

- **H&P Keys**

  May have antecedent history of pericarditis or chest trauma. Symptoms: dyspnea, fatigue. Physical findings: JVD, hypotension, distant heart sounds, tachycardia, pulsus paradoxus.

- **Diagnosis**

  Echo documents effusion, often with diastolic collapse of RA and RV. Cardiac catheterization documents elevated pericardial pressure and equivalence of this pressure to diastolic pressures in all four chambers. RA tracing typically shows amputation of the Y descent (compromised early ventricular filling).

- **Disease Severity**
  Can be assessed by degree of symptomatic or hemodynamic impairment.

- **Concept and Application**
  Pericardial fluid under high pressure compresses the heart, impairing its ability to fill. This leads to signs and symptoms of pulmonary and systemic venous congestion and ultimately shock.

- **Management**
  Removal of fluid, usually during hemodynamic monitoring. In recurrent cases, surgical or balloon pericardiectomy may be necessary.

D. Constrictive Pericarditis   *SQUARE ROOT SIGN*

TB

Obliteration of pericardial space or scarring of pericardial tissue, causing cardiac enclosure, resulting in compromised cardiac filling.

- **H&P Keys**
  Symptoms: fatigue, hypotension, weakness. Physical signs: ascites, edema, JVD, often with Kussmaul's sign, pericardial knock in diastole, reduced amplitude of apical impulse.

- **Diagnosis**
  ECG may show low voltage, QRS with diffuse T wave changes. Chest roentgenogram may show pericardial calcification, present in approximately 50% of patients. Echo and Doppler demonstrate normal cavity size with enhanced early diastolic filling. Pericardial thickening can be suggested by echo; however, computed tomography (CT) and magnetic resonance imaging (MRI) are more diagnostic of this change.

- **Disease Severity**
  Degree of thickening can be judged noninvasively, but confirmation is by catheterization. Hemodynamic features seen during catheterization include elevation and equalization of all diastolic pressures; LV

and RV tracings track closely in diastole and have a dip and plateau configuration (square root sign); RA tracing shows an M configuration with prominence of the Y descent.

- **Concept and Application**
  Formerly, tuberculosis was the most common cause; current common causes are idiopathic pericarditis, radiation, etc. The scarred encasing pericardium restricts cardiac filling, leading to signs of reduced cardiac output and systemic venous congestion.

- **Management**
  Pericardial resection is the definitive therapy. Diuretics can afford symptomatic improvement. Risks of the operation and prognosis postoperatively depend on degree of involvement of the epicardium in the scarring calcific process.

VII. VALVULAR DISEASES

A. Acute

1. Rheumatic Fever   *GROUP A STREP*

Delayed sequel to pharyngeal infections with group A streptococci. Involves the heart, joints, central nervous system (CNS), skin, and subcutaneous tissues.

2. Endocarditis

Native valve endocarditis; endocarditis in IV drug abusers; and prosthetic valve endocarditis. May be acute or subacute. *Acute endocarditis* is often caused by *Staphylococcus aureus* and is rapidly destructive. Often fatal (if untreated) in less than 6 weeks. *Subacute endocarditis* is frequently caused by *viridans* streptococci and takes longer than 6 weeks to months when untreated to be fatal.

3. Myopathic

Acute valvular decompensation resulting from ischemic heart disease, eg, acute ischemia or

Acute - staph aureus
Subacute - viridans strep
MR

myocardial infarction: may lead to cardiac decompensation and death. Usually acute MR caused by posterior papillary muscle ischemia or infarct.

Aschoff bodies - myocardium

- **H&P Keys**

Acute Rheumatic Fever. Arthritis, heart murmurs, congestive heart failure, fever, arrhythmias, CNS disorders, subcutaneous nodules, and skin rash.

Endocarditis. Fever, malaise, weakness, congestive heart failure, cardiac murmurs, splinter hemorrhages under fingernails, skin manifestations (Ossler's nodes, Janeway lesions), embolic episodes, and petechiae.

Myopathy-Related Acute Valvular Decompensation. Acute-onset CHF and hypotension (shock); new cardiac murmur may not be heard.

- **Diagnosis**
  Blood cultures, elevated white blood cell count, erythrocyte sedimentation rate (ESR), liver and muscle enzyme levels. Streptococcal antibody titer for rheumatic fever. Echocardiography, cardiac catheterization.

- **Disease Severity**
  Involves infecting organism, chronicity of infection with acute rheumatic fever and infective endocarditis. Degree of involvement of subvalvular apparatus (papillary muscle) determines severity in CHF patients with ischemia-related MR.

- **Concept and Application**
  Destruction of valvular and subvalvular apparatus, and the production of inflammatory myocarditis. Systemic embolization, as well as involvement of other organ systems, with both the infecting agent and inflammatory response responsible for other disease manifestations. Acute volume overload results in acute mitral or aortic valve rupture.

- **Management**
  Hemodynamic stabilization in the acutely ill patient. Long-term antibiotic therapy and (possibly) surgical valvular replacement.

Erythema Marginatum = pink, evanescent rash over trunk

B. Chronic

Degeneration of cardiac valvular structures over a prolonged time. Progressive dilation of the LV or RV. Chronic degenerative disorders including mitral valve prolapse (myxomatous degeneration) and calcific valvular disease in the elderly. Mitral and aortic valves most commonly involved for endocarditis and degenerative valvular disorders (MR, mitral stenosis [MS], aortic regurgitation [AR], aortic stenosis [AS]). Pulmonary and tricuspid valves less often involved. Bicuspid aortic valve (congenital) associated with AS later in life.

- **H&P Keys**
  CHF, shortness of breath, fatigue, pedal edema, murmurs.

- **Diagnosis**
  Chest roentgenogram, echo, cardiac catheterization.

- **Disease Severity**
  Heart rate, respiratory rate, peripheral edema, pulmonary rales, blood pressure, oxygen saturation, level of consciousness.

- **Concept and Application**
  AS and MS (congenital, rheumatic, calcific): limitation of blood exiting and entering the heart, respectively. AR and MR (most often associated with ischemic heart disease, cardiomyopathy).

AR. Dilated aorta, hypertension; large volume of blood in reverse direction from aorta to left ventricle.

MR. Mitral valve prolapse; large volume of blood in reverse direction from left ventricle to left atrium and pulmonary veins.

- **Management**
  Acute MR and AR: diuretics, afterload reduction, IABP, surgery (valve replacement).

Chronic MR and AR. In less severe cases, diuretics, afterload reduction.

Symptomatic AS and MS. Treated surgically with valve replacement.

VIII. CARDIAC TRANSPLANTATION

Reserved for patients who are severely compromised by CHF despite maximal medical therapy. Approximately 2500 heart transplants are performed worldwide yearly; limitation to wider application of transplantation is primarily due to an undersupply of donor hearts. Major contraindications to cardiac transplantation include factors that increase short- and intermediate-term morbidity or mortality, eg, associated diseases such as diabetes with end-organ complications or lung disease with pulmonary hypertension. A compliant patient able to adhere to the rigorous post-transplant rejection surveillance program and a strong social support system are important factors in selecting potential candidates for this therapy.

Immunosuppression is critical in preventing rejection in the post-transplant period, and cyclosporin has been a major advancement since its introduction in 1980. Sequential endomyocardial biopsies are performed to assess transplant rejection; based on biopsy results, doses of cyclosporin, prednisone, and azathioprine are adjusted. Severe rejection is often treated with short courses of T-cell suppression. One- and 5-year survival rates are approximately 90% and 70%, respectively.

Complications associated with cardiac transplantation include rejection, infection, accelerated atherosclerosis, and hypertension.

[margin handwritten: cyclosporin]

IX. CONGENITAL HEART DISEASE

Result of aberrant embryonic development of a normal structure or failure of such structure to develop beyond early stage of embryonic or fetal development. Malformations are complex and multifactorial and include genetic (chromosomal), environmental (maternal rubella infection), and toxic (anticoagulants) factors.

A. Ventricular Septal Defect

[handwritten: most common / Endocarditis Prophylexis]

Opening in membranous septum (VSD). Most common congenital heart disease in adult.

- **H&P Keys**
  Harsh systolic murmur at left sternal border radiating to right percordium, palpable thrill over percordium. Large shunt associated with CHF, and reversal of flow (right to left), resulting in Eisenmenger's syndrome (cyanosis, pedal edema, syncope, CHF).

- **Diagnosis**
  Chest roentgenogram, oxygen saturation, two-dimensional echo, cardiac catheterization, and oxymetry.

- **Disease Severity**
  Mentation, heart rate, cyanosis, growth retardation. In children, 30% to 50% spontaneous closure. May be asymptomatic if shunt is small.

- **Concept and Application**

  Left-to-Right Shunt. Large volume of blood from LV to RV, causing volume overload of pulmonary circulation and decreased LV output.

  Right-to-Left Shunt. Large volume of unsaturated blood from RV to LV and systemic circulation, causing cyanosis, fatigue, right heart failure, embolic phenomenon.

- **Management**
  Small shunts do not require treatment. Large shunts undergo surgical repair. Because bacterial endocarditis may be associated with VSD, endocarditis prophylaxis is warranted.

B. Atrial Septal Defect

Persistent opening in septum (ASD).

1. Secundum ASD

In region of fossa ovalis.

2. Primum ASD

Involves lower atrial septum.

[handwritten: MV/TV D/O]

VSD - LSB → Ⓡ percordium

3. Sinus Venosus ASD   *upper Ⓛ SB SPLIT S_2*

In region of sinus node. Shunting at the level of atria.

- **H&P Keys**

  TRISOMY 21

  Often asymptomatic. Murmur heard at upper left sternal border. Associated with fixed and widely split S_2. May be associated with trisomy 21. Dyspnea, fatigue, atrial arrhythmias, right heart failure. May be associated with severe pulmonary hypertension and Eisenmenger's syndrome. Primum ASD may be associated with mitral and tricuspid valve disorders.

- **Diagnosis**

  Chest roentgenogram, ECG, two-dimensional echo, cardiac catheterization, and oxymetry.

- **Disease Severity**

  CHF, pedal edema, elevated jugular venous pulse, fatigue, palpitations, dizziness, paradoxic emboli.

- **Concept and Application**

  Shunting of blood at level of atria. Usually left-to-right shunt, but reversal of flow may develop, limiting right heart output. Disease severity correlates with size of shunt and symptoms.

- **Management**

  Observation of small shunts in asymptomatic patients. Surgical repair for larger and symptomatic shunts.

C. Tetralogy of Fallot   *BACT ENDOCARD PROPHYLAXIS*

Most common congenital heart lesion over the age of 1 year characterized by the following four signs:

1. VSD
2. RV outflow narrowing
3. Overriding aorta
4. RV hypertrophy

- **H&P Keys**

  Growth retardation, cardiac murmurs, cardiac arrhythmias, polycythemia and cyanosis, exercise limitation with squat maneuver to restore normal breathing, clubbing, thrill at left sternal border.

- **Diagnosis**

  Physical exam, chest roentgenogram, ECG (RV hypertrophy), two-dimensional echo, cardiac catheterization.

- **Disease Severity**

  Activity level, growth, ABG, mentation, heart rate, cyanosis and pedal edema, heart size, CHF, syncope.

- **Concept and Application**

  Caused by the combination and severity of characteristic abnormalities; degree of obstruction at right ventricular outflow tract (RVOT), shunting at level of VSD, amount of blood from RV and LV to aorta.

- **Management**

  Bacterial endocarditis prophylaxis, total surgical correction.

D. Coarctation of the Aorta

Narrowing of aortic lumen, usually at level just below left subclavian artery (ligamentum arteriosum).

- **H&P Keys**

  More common in males. Differential development of upper and lower body, differential pulses in upper and lower extremities, a cause of secondary hypertension.

- **Diagnosis**

  Brachial and femoral artery pulses, blood pressure in upper versus lower extremities, chest roentgenogram (rib notching), two-dimensional echo in children, aortography, CT scan.

- **Disease Severity**

  Depends on extent of luminal narrowing. Severe hypertension may result, producing headache, CHF, CNS hemorrhage. Lower extremity claudication, aortic rupture possible. May be associated with bicuspid aortic valve (AS or AR).

- **Concept and Application**

  Congenital. Narrowing of aorta at the level of the ligamentum arteriosum.

- **Management**

  Surgical correction optimally at age 4 to 8. Bacterial endocarditis prophylaxis.

X. CARDIAC LIFE SUPPORT

Cardiopulmonary arrest is the cessation of effective cardiac function resulting in hemodynamic collapse. In children, pulmonary etiology is most common, whereas in adults cardiac etiology (ventricular tachycardia or ventricular fibrillation) is the most common.

- **H&P Keys**

  Dizziness, dyspnea, palpitations, chest pain may precede cardiac arrest and loss of consciousness that is not spontaneously terminated. Examination: cyanotic, pulseless, unconscious, or unarousable patient. Children often are cyanotic.

- **Diagnosis**

  Most cardiopulmonary arrests occur outside the hospital and are fatal. Only 25% of cardiopulmonary arrest victims survive to hospital admission. Cardiopulmonary arrest victims are identified as unresponsive and pulseless patients. ECG, electrolytes, myocardial enzymes, and cyanosis.

- **Disease Severity**

  Duration of cardiopulmonary arrest time, ie, time to resuscitation.

- **Concept and Application**

  Children. Sudden infant death syndrome (SIDS) may be multifactorial; pulmonary failure may be secondary to obstruction of airways.

  Adult. VT or ventricular fibrillation (VF) secondary to acute and chronic CAD. Often associated with depressed LV function resulting from acute or past MI.

- **Management**

  Basic Life Support (BLS). ABC: (1) *Air*way: Check for patency and obstruction. (2) *Breathing*: Ventilate. (3) *Circulation*: Reestablish with external compression. Repetitive cycles of ventilation and external compression, punctuated by assessing for spontaneous ventilation and pulse, continued until Advanced Cardiac Life Support team available.

  Advanced Cardiac Life Support (ACLS). Continued BLS. Use of adjunctive equipment including endotracheal tube and intravenous lines. Arrhythmia recognition ("quick look" with defibrillator paddles or ECG) and appropriate treatment with electrical cardioversion (VT : 50 to 200 J), or defibrillation (VF: 200 to 360 J). Initiation of pharmacologic therapy, including IV fluids (normal saline) epinephrine (1 : 10 000), lidocaine, procainamide, bretylium, dopamine, norepinephrine. Rapid intubation.

XI. HYPERTENSION

Hypertension is defined as a diastolic pressure greater than 90 and a systolic pressure greater than 140. Severe hypertension includes a diastolic blood pressure greater than 115. Hypertension is an important public health problem. It is a major cause of CHF, and uncontrolled hypertension is associated with marked reduction in life expectancy (20 to 25 years).

A. Essential Hypertension

The etiology is unknown in 95% of patients with essential hypertension. There is a strong family occurrence.

- **H&P Keys**

  The vast majority of patients are asymptomatic. Symptoms of occipital headache are seen with severe hypertension. Other associated symptoms reflect end-organ damage, eg, hematuria, blurring of vision, CHF. Exam is tailored to detect evidence of end-organ damage, eg, retinal hemorrhages, S_4, S_3.

- **Diagnosis**

  All patients with hypertension should have urinalysis for protein, blood, potassium, creatinine, BUN, and an ECG for evidence of LV hypertrophy. Other testing is performed to exclude a suspected secondary cause.

- **Disease Severity**
  Evidence of end-organ damage including CNS, renal, and cardiac dysfunction.

CNS. Lacunar infarcts and stroke.

Renal. Elevated creatinine, BUN.

Cardiac. LV hypertrophy, cardiomegaly, CHF, MI, aortic enlargement, and aortic dissection. Natural history depends on the level of blood pressure and the extent and severity of organ involvement.

- **Concept and Application**
  The cause of essential hypertension remains unknown. Possible mechanisms include complex multifactorial genetic factors as well as abnormal responsiveness to sodium and calcium.

- **Management**
  In general, weight reduction in the obese patient and some restriction in salt are often very valuable in control. Step therapy has been evaluated over a 25-year period with evidence of improved life expectancy. Diuretics and β-blockers improve outcomes and are recommended as the initial choices. Other agents including ACE inhibitors and calcium antagonists are useful as secondary agents. As severity increases, anti-adrenergic drugs such as clonidine and vasodilators (eg, minoxidil) may be valuable.

B. Secondary Hypertension

A host of disease entities produce hypertension, including endocrine abnormalities, such as adrenal cortical hyperfunction (Cushing's disease), primary hyperaldosteronism, and pheochromocytoma; neurogenic, renal vascular, and parenchymal diseases; and entities associated with increasing stroke volume, eg, hyperthyroidism and aortic insufficiency.

- **H&P Keys**
  Wide-ranging disease process may be detected such as Cushingoid features, episodic marked elevation in blood pressure in pheochromocytoma, polyuria, polydipsia, and muscle weakness secondary to hypokalemia.

- **Diagnosis**
  BUN, creatinine level, thyroid-stimulating hormone (TSH) level, renal artery Doppler flow studies or angiography, urine and plasma catecholamine levels, plasma renin activity, serum and urine catecholamine levels.

- **Disease Severity**
  Depends on specific etiology and its natural history as well as response of blood pressure to therapy.

- **Concept and Application**
  Elevations of catecholamine levels, activation of the renin-angiotensin system with vasoconstriction, excessive sodium retention in primary and secondary aldosteronism, and excessive glucocorticoid production.

- **Management**
  Converting enzyme inhibitors may worsen renal functions in patients with bilateral renal artery stenosis, and renal function must be followed. Renal artery stenosis may respond to surgery, especially in patients with high renin from the affected kidney and suppression of renin production in the uninvolved kidney. Other secondary forms, eg, pheochromocytoma and Cushing's disease, can be cured with surgical removal of the tumor.

C. Malignant Hypertension

Sudden and severe elevation of blood pressure with evidence of acute end-organ damage. Includes hypertensive encephalopathy, rapidly deteriorating renal function, and acute CHF.

- **H&P Keys**
  Visual disturbances, severe headache, confusion, coma, seizures, edema, dyspnea, blood pressure greater than 200/115, papilledema, hemorrhage, and spasm on ophthalmoscopic exam, S_3 gallop, oliguria.

- **Diagnosis**
  BUN, creatinine levels, peripheral smear for microangiopathic hemolytic anemia, chest roentgenographic evidence of CHF.

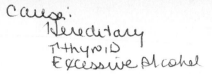

Cause:
Hereditary
↑thyroid
Excessive Alcohol

- **Disease Severity**
  Depends on the extent and severity of end-organ damage and may include stroke, refractory pulmonary edema, and progressive oliguric renal failure.

- **Concept and Application**
  The trigger for malignant hypertension is unknown. There is widespread fibrinoid necrosis of arterial walls. Cerebral autoregulation is impaired and cerebral blood flow is increased, which contributes to the encephalopathy.

- **Management**

  Nipride
  Labetalol

  Acute. Nitroprusside infusion in doses of 0.5 to 8 µg/kg/min can produce rapid, graded control of blood pressure and is recommended initial therapy. Also, continuous labetalol infusion in doses in the range of 2 mg/min have been effective.

  Long-Term. Other agents for long-term control are needed. Diuresis is useful to contract volume and decrease blood pressure and also to assist with CHF and encephalopathy. β-Blockers, ACE inhibitors, calcium antagonists are all effective. Renal function may deteriorate in the early phase, but persistent blood pressure control is needed to resolve the arterial lesions.

XII. LIPOPROTEINS AND ATHEROSCLEROSIS

A. Hyperlipoproteinemia

TG
Chylomicron
VLDL

Cholesterol
IDL
LDL
HDL

A wide array of disorders resulting from abnormalities in metabolism of the lipoproteins, which transport exogenously and endogenously produced cholesterol and triglycerides. The major lipoproteins are chylomicrons and very-low-density lipoproteins (VLDL), which transport triglycerides (TG), and intermediate-, low-, and high-density lipoproteins (IDL, LDL, HDL), which primarily transport cholesterol. Hyperlipoproteinemias occur as a result of a genetic defect in synthesis or degradation or secondary to diabetes, hyperthyroidism, and excessive alcohol ingestion. Classification is based on the recognized abnormality in lipoproteins and the type of lipid that accumulates in the serum (see table).

Type	Lipoprotein Abnormality	Lipid Accumulation
I	Chylomicrons	TG
IIA	LDL	Cholesterol
IIB	LDL and VLDL	Cholesterol and TG
III	Chylomicrons and IDL	TG and cholesterol
IV	VLDL	TG
V	VLDL and chylomicrons	TG and cholesterol

Most important are accumulations in LDL, which are associated with premature atherosclerosis.

- **H&P Keys**
  Cutaneous, tendinous, tuberous, and eruptive xanthomes, premature atherosclerosis, lipemia retinalis, and pancreatitis.

- **Diagnosis**
  Examination of serum for creamy, chylomicron layer, measurement of serum lipids, eg, cholesterol, TG, HDL, and LDL. High LDL is associated with an increased risk of atherosclerosis and MI. Occasionally, lipoprotein electrophoresis required for definitive characterization.

- **Disease Severity**
  The extent of atherosclerosis and its complications include MI, stroke, peripheral vascular disease. Patients with high level of TG frequently develop recurrent pancreatitis.

- **Concept and Application**
  In familial hypercholesterolemia, premature, accelerated atherosclerosis and MI occurs in the third or fourth decade. The hyperlipoproteinemias are genetically transmitted as a result of single or multiple gene disorders.

- **Management**

  General. Dietary restriction of fats and weight reduction control of secondary factors, eg, cessation of alcohol, optimum control of diabetes. Elimination of other risk factors for CAD.

Drug Therapy. Dependent on lipid abnormality, severity, and associated disease. In patients with known atherosclerosis or significant risk factors, lipid therapy should be considered when the LDL > 130 mg/dL. Available agents include:

1. Cholestyramine. Not absorbed. Binds bile acids in the gut, stimulating conversion of cholesterol to bile.
2. Nicotinic acid. Reduces production of VLDL by liver and lowers LDL, HDL, and TGs.
3. 3-Hydroxy-3-methylglutaryl coenzyme A (HMG CoA)-reductase-inhibitors. Lower LDL by blocking endogenous cholesterol biosynthesis.
4. Fibric acid derivatives gemfibrozil and clofibrate. Increase breakdown of VLDL and IDL, hence lower TGs and increase HDL cholesterol.

B. Atherosclerosis

Results as a response to injury of vascular endothelium with thrombus formation. Initially, isolated macrophages or foam cells infiltrate endothelium. Later, lipid-rich lesions with smooth muscle and fibrous collagen cap form mature atheromatous plaque. Acute coronary syndromes (unstable angina and MI) occur when there is acute plaque rupture and thrombus formation.

- **H&P Keys**
  Chest pain, neurologic deficits, including motor or sensory abnormalities, intermittent claudication, reduction in peripheral pulses and pressure.

- **Diagnosis**
  ECG, stress testing, and myocardial perfusion imaging, noninvasive vascular assessment, including carotids, arterial Doppler, cardiac catheterization, and angiography.

- **Disease Severity**
  Extent of motor and sensory deficit after stroke, impairment in cardiac function after MI, exercise limitation, claudication.

- **Concept and Application**
  The development of atherosclerosis is multifactorial and related to injury of the endothelium as well as the factors that enhance thrombosis. Endothelial cells produce a variety of substances that cause vasoconstriction and smooth-muscle proliferation. Acute plaque disruption occurs as a result of alterations of stress at plaque surface. Exposure of damaged vessel wall leads to the adherence of platelets, development of thrombus, and ultimately occlusion of the vessel.

- **Management**
  Prevention of atherosclerosis and plaque rupture with thrombosis is complex and requires multiple interventions. Major risk factors include cigarette smoking, hypertension, diabetes, and elevated cholesterol. Management is directed at eliminating these risk factors. Thrombosis is enhanced by catecholamines (stress), cigarette smoking, and familial predisposition. Aspirin therapy is effective in both primary and secondary prevention.

XIII. PERIPHERAL ARTERIAL VASCULAR DISEASE

A. Chronic Atherosclerotic Occlusion

Associated with generalized atherosclerosis and frequently coexists with CAD as well as cerebral vascular disease.

- **H&P Keys**
  Intermittent claudication (exertional calf, thigh, and buttocks discomfort), rest pain with more severe reduction in blood flow, subclavian steal syndrome, reduction in blood pressure in affected limb (or limbs), decreased or absent pulses, vascular bruits over subclavian aorta or femoral arteries. Elevational pallor, dependent rubor, and prolonged venous filling time of the legs. Ulcers and gangrene.

- **Diagnosis**
  Doppler pressure measurements before and after exercise and calculation of ankle-brachial index, pulse volume recordings (PVR), peripheral angiography.

- **Disease Severity**
Severe if ankle-brachial index less than 0.4. Resting ischemia, ulcerations, and gangrene. Recurrent neurologic symptoms with subclavian steal syndrome.

- **Concept and Application**
Progressive atherosclerotic lesions produce reduction in blood flow to the affected limbs. Associated with generalized atherosclerosis. Steal syndrome results from a lesion in left subclavian before the vertebral artery and exercise results in "steal" of blood from the cerebral circulation.

- **Management**

Medical. Control of atherosclerotic risk factors. Smoking cessation most important. Exercise may stimulate collateral blood flow. Vasodilators are ineffective. Pentoxifylline improves exercise ability in approximately one third of patients.

Surgical. Revascularization with bypass procedure or angioplasty for limiting symptoms or for limb salvage; sympathectomy for pain relief; amputation.

B. Acute Arterial Occlusion

Sudden cessation of blood flow as a result of an embolus, acute thrombosis, or vasospasm.

- **H&P Keys**
Appropriate setting with sudden onset of pain, then loss of sensation, paralysis and cool, cyanotic, mottled limb.

- **Diagnosis**
Doppler studies, angiography, two-dimensional echo to evaluate thrombolytic source.

- **Disease Severity**
Occlusion of an artery to an extremity leads to paralysis, cyanosis, and loss of viability with tissue necrosis, ulceration, and gangrene.

- **Concept and Application**
Majority of emboli are from cardiac sources. Intracardiac thrombosis occurs in MI and atrial fibrillation; also in valvular disease, especially MS and prosthetic valves. Acute and chronic bacterial endocarditis and vegetations may embolize. Large-vessel occlusion occurs with bulky vegetations, especially in fungal endocarditis. Acute thrombosis occurs in some infectious diseases, especially rickettsial, eg, Rocky Mountain spotted fever, connective tissue disease, and hypercoagulable states.

- **Management**
Heparin administration. Prompt evaluation with arteriography and embolectomy. After reperfusion, especially in the leg muscle compartments, fasciotomy may be necessary to relieve compressive symptoms. Additional therapy may be required after the source of embolus is identified, eg, valve replacement for mitral stenosis or acute endocarditis.

C. Vasculitis Syndromes

Encompasses a wide variety of conditions, characterized by inflammation of the blood vessel wall. The syndromes include:

1. Necrotizing vasculitis: polyarteritis nodosa
2. Hypersensitivity angitis
3. Giant cell arteritis: Takayasu's, temporal arteritis
4. Other: thromboangiitis obliterans; mucocutaneous lymph node syndrome

- **H&P Keys**
Wide-ranging because arterial thrombosis can affect any organ system. Systemic signs and symptoms include: fever, weight loss, arthritis, organ dysfunction from occlusion of cerebral vessel limb or digital arteries, absent or decreased pulses, differential blood pressures, vascular bruits. Also, elevated sedimentation rate, leukocytosis.

- **Diagnosis**
Arterial biopsy, eg, in temporal arteritis to confirm vessel inflammation. Arterial Doppler studies, PVR, and aortography.

- **Disease Severity**
Dependent on extent and severity of organ dysfunction or compromising blood flow

[handwritten margin note: Virchow — abn vascular wall / Blood stasis / hypercoagulable]

to the limbs. Patients may develop stroke, gangrenous bowel, MI, ischemia to limbs and digits.

- **Concept and Application**
  In general, vasculitis occurs because of immune injury. There is a deposition of immune complexes in the arterial wall, which initiates acute inflammatory response and leads to thrombosis. There also may be cell-mediated vascular injury.

- **Management**
  Many of these entities respond partially to treatment with systemic glucocorticoids, eg, temporal arteritis and Takayasu's disease. Occasionally responses are seen from other cytotoxic agents. Cessation of smoking in thromboangiitis. Sympathectomy is of value to relieve pain.

XIV. PERIPHERAL VENOUS VASCULAR DISEASES AND PULMONARY EMBOLISM

A. Venous Thrombosis

Occurs in a wide variety of settings. Predisposing factors include trauma or surgery, especially orthopedic, prolonged bed rest for any reason, pregnancy, and a variety of neoplasms. The disease commonly affects the lower extremities, although upper extremities can be involved.

- **H&P Keys**
  Recognition of the appropriate setting and predisposing factors. Calf swelling, tenderness, and warmth nonspecific.

  Superficial Venous Thrombosis. Hot, red, swollen visible vein.

  Chronic. Leg swelling and superficial varicosities.

- **Disease Severity**

  Acute. Pulmonary embolus is the primary risk; however recurrent deep venous thrombosis (DVT) can lead to a chronic state.

Chronic. Refractory edema, stasis ulceration with superimposed chronic cellulitis.

- **Diagnosis**
  Impedance plethysmography, Doppler ultrasonography, and ventilation perfusion lung scan.

- **Concepts and Application**
  Virchow described the triad of venous thrombosis: (1) abnormality of the vascular wall; (2) stasis of blood flow; and (3) hypercoagulable state. Thrombosis may occur because of deficiency of antithrombin III or fibrinolytic proteins C and S, a circulating lupus anticoagulant, and homocystinuria.

- **Management**

  Acute. Heparin in continuous infusion for 7 to 10 days, adjusted so partial thromboplastin time (PTT) is approximately two times control value.

  Chronic. Anticoagulation for 6 to 12 months with warfarin, longer (indefinite) if DVT recurs. Elevation of legs when possible, full waist-length, graduated compression stockings, meticulous skin care.

  Prophylaxis. With 5000 U heparin every 8 to 12 hours in high-risk clinical situations needs to be initiated prior to surgical procedure. Below-the-knee thrombosis can merely be followed if no proximal venous disease is detected; anticoagulation may not be required.

B. Pulmonary Embolism

A common event in hospitalized patients, frequently unrecognized, with high morbidity and mortality.

- **H&P Keys**
  Sudden dyspnea, pleuritic chest pain, hemoptysis, syncope, unexplained tachycardia, supraventricular dysrhythmias, pulmonary hypertension with a right ventricular lift, wide, persistent splitting and loud pulmonic component of the second heart sound.

- **Diagnosis**

  ECG. Nonspecific ST-T wave changes, right axis deviation.

Chest Roentgenogram. Dilatation of pulmonary artery, abrupt cutoff. Ventilation perfusion lung scan, pulmonary angiogram, detection of DVT.

- **Disease Severity**
  The size of the embolus and the resultant extent and severity of obstruction of the pulmonary arteries. Hemodynamic deterioration can occur with shock and peripheral hypoperfusion and is more severe with preexisting heart or lung disease. Impairment of gas exchange and arterial hypoxemia.

- **Concept and Application**
  The majority of pulmonary embolisms occur in the setting of DVT. Embolization of clot from below the calf is rare. The best approach to the disease is prophylaxis, prevention, early detection, and treatment of DVT.

- **Management**
  Heparin, with initial dose of 5000 U and continuous infusion to maintain PTT approximately two times control. Intermittent regimens can be employed. With recurrent embolization or contraindication to anticoagulant therapy, venal caval filter or plication is effective in prevention of further emboli. If severe hemodynamic compromise occurs, thrombolytic therapy with streptokinase (initial bolus of 250 000 U and 24-hour infusion) is favored over acute embolectomy.

XV. DISEASES OF THE AORTA

A. Aneurysms

Pathologic dilatation of a segment of blood vessel. A true aneurysm involves all three layers of the vessel wall and is distinguished from a *pseudoaneurysm,* which involves only the intima and media. Classified by their location and gross appearance: thoracic versus abdominal, and fusiform versus saccular.

- **H&P Keys**
  Most aneurysms are asymptomatic. Symptoms of pain may be produced by expanding aneurysms; often a harbinger of rupture and represents a medical emergency. Acute rupture may occur without warning and is always life-threatening. Compression of contiguous blood vessels may result in other symptoms, including stroke from systemic embolization or compression of carotid vessels in thoracic aortic aneurysms and impairment of lower-extremity blood flow in expanding abdominal aortic aneurysms.

Abdominal Aortic Aneurysms. Presence of palpable, pulsatile, and tender abdominal mass with abdominal bruit.

Thoracic Aortic Aneurysms. Tracheal deviation, hoarseness, and CHF because of aortic dilatation and resulting aortic regurgitation. Patients with abdominal aneurysms may also have distal arterial embolization and lower-extremity claudication. Most abdominal aneurysms occur distal to the renal arteries.

- **Diagnosis**
  Radiography including chest roentgenogram and abdominal films may demonstrate the enlarged aorta sometimes outlined by calcium. More definitive studies include thoracic and abdominal ultrasonography, CT scan, and MRI scan. Thoracic and abdominal aortography are often performed prior to surgery to outline the extent of aneurysm.

- **Disease Severity**
  Determined by location, size of aneurysm, and rate of dilatation. For abdominal aneurysms exceeding 6 cm in diameter, the 2-year mortality related to rupture is approximately 50%, and for those 4 to 6 cm in diameter, 25%.

- **Concept and Application**
  Atherosclerosis is the most common cause of aortic aneurysm. Abdominal aortic aneurysms are almost always due to atherosclerosis, whereas those of the ascending

[handwritten notes at top of page:]
Abd - Arthrosclerosis
Thoracic: Cystic medial necrosis
atherosclerosis
syphilis
bact inf or rheum.

thoracic aorta may be caused by cystic medial necrosis, atherosclerosis, syphilis, bacterial infections, or rheumatic aortitis. Aneurysms of the descending thoracic aorta that are contiguous with infradiaphragmatic aneurysms are usually due to atherosclerosis.

- **Management**
  Location and extent of the aneurysm using radiographic imaging techniques (CT scan, MRI, aortography) followed by operative excision of the aneurysm and replacement with graft. Reimplantation of branch vessels is often necessary.

B. Aortic Dissection   *[handwritten: (L) subclavian]*

Caused by a transverse or circumferential tear of the aortic intima in areas with high shear forces (left subclavian artery and right lateral ascending aortic wall).

- *Type 1.* Dissection in proximal aorta, may extend into the arch.
- *Type 2.* Dissection limited to aortic arch.
- *Type 3.* Dissection begins distal to left subclavian artery and extends for variable distance inferiorly.

- **H&P Keys**
  Acute dissection is characterized by a sudden onset of severe and tearing pain associated with diaphoresis. Pain usually from front of chest to interscapular area. May be associated with syncope, dyspnea, or weakness. Blood pressure may be high or low, differential pulses, pulmonary edema, neurologic symptoms (stroke or spinal cord compression), aortic regurgitation producing CHF. Abdominal aortic dissection may be accompanied by bowel ischemia and hematuria, whereas thoracic dissection may be accompanied by superior vena caval syndrome, hoarseness, airway compromise, dysphagia, inferior MI with hemopericardium and cardiac tamponade.

- **Diagnosis**
  Chest roentgenogram, ECG, CT scan, MRI, and aortography.

- **Disease Severity**
  Physical examination for involvement of brain, peripheral arteries, kidneys, spinal cord, heart. Continued pain or symptoms of compromise to major arterial branches indicate active propagation of dissection. Hypotension or shock, oliguria, mentation.

- **Concept and Application**
  Disruption of aortic intima, possibly related to medial hemorrhage at areas with high shear forces. Pulsatile flow dissects along elastic laminar plates of aorta, creating false lumen. Underlying condition may be related to cystic medial necrosis of aortic wall or collagen dysfunction (Marfan syndrome).

- **Management**   *[handwritten: B Blockers, ↓ load reducing]*
  Emergency operation is indicated for patients with symptoms indicating propagating dissection. Emergency operation carries a high operative mortality, but active propagation is often fatal if not stabilized. Stabilization with medical therapy including β-blockers and after-load reducing agents (nitroprusside) is preferred for ≥ 14 days if possible before surgical correction. For patients with stable and uncomplicated distal aortic dissection, medical therapy is preferred and includes long-term use of β-blockers and orally administered afterload-reducing agents.

C. Aortic Occlusion

Chronic occlusive disease that generally involves the distal abdominal aorta below the renal arteries.

- **H&P Keys**
  Claudication, impotence in males (Leriche's syndrome). Symptoms vary depending on presence and adequacy of collateral blood flow. Physical findings include absent or depressed femoral and distal pulses and presence of bruits over abdominal aorta and femoral arteries. Lower-extremity skin loss, atrophic skin changes, cool extremities, peripheral skin ulcerations.

- **Diagnosis**
Physical examination, noninvasive Doppler evaluation of arterial blood flow, ankle-brachial index (ABI) (sphygmomanometry). Abdominal aortography to define anatomy prior to revascularization.

- **Disease Severity**
Dependent on collateral blood flow.

- **Concept and Application**
Atherosclerotic; nonatheromatous disease may be associated with smoking (Buerger's disease, or thromboangiitis obliterans).

- **Management**
Preoperative assessment by aortography and surgical revascularization. Cessation of smoking and modification of diet are important in stabilizing this progressive disease.

D. Aortitis

Syphilitic, rheumatic, Takayasu's disease, giant cell aortitis.

1. Syphilitic Aortitis   *PRoximal*

Usually affecting the proximal aorta, resulting in aortic root dilatation and aneurysm formation.

- **H&P Keys**
Often asymptomatic. As it progresses, may cause compression and erosion into adjacent structures; rupture may occur.

- **Diagnosis**
Chest roentgenogram, two-dimensional echo, cardiac catheterization, immunologic screening, rapid plasma reagin (RPR), venereal disease research laboratory (VDRL).

- **Disease Severity**
Long latency period: 15 to 30 years after initial infection. Symptoms may occur from aortic regurgitation or narrowing of coronary ostia or from compression to adjacent structures (esophagus), or rupture. Serologic tests confirm diagnosis. Evaluation includes chest roentgenogram, ultrasonography, CT scan, MRI, and aortography.

- **Concept and Application**
Destruction of collagen elastic tissue, leading to dilatation of aorta with scar formation and calcification, is due to obliterative endarteritis of the vasa vasorum in the adventitia. This is an inflammatory response to invasion of the adventitia by spirochetes.

- **Management**
Antibiotic treatment (penicillin) and surgical excision and repair.

2. Rheumatic Aortitis

Includes rheumatoid arthritis, ankylosing spondylitis, psoriatic arthritis, Reiter's syndrome, Behçet's syndrome, relapsing polychondritis, and inflammatory bowel disorders.

3. Takayasu's Aortitis   *Asian descent*

An inflammatory disease of the aortic arch resulting in obstruction of the aorta and its major branches. Also termed *pulseless disease*, a panarteritis with marked intimal hyperplasia. Usually found in young females of Asian descent and associated with fever, malaise, weight loss, and other systemic symptoms. ESR is elevated. Symptoms chronically include upper-extremity claudication, syncope, cerebral ischemia. No definitive therapy; the disease is progressive. Surgical bypass of stenotic arteries may be necessary, and anticoagulation to prevent thrombosis may be advisable.

4. Giant Cell Aortitis

An inflammatory disorder infecting large and medium-size arteries and resulting in focal granulomatous lesions. It may be associated with polymyalgia rheumatica. Obstruction of medium-sized arteries, including the temporal and ophthalmic arteries, may occur.

- **H&P Keys**
Fever, malaise, myalgias, headache, jaw pain, scalp tenderness, visual changes.

- **Diagnosis**
Elevated ESR, anemia. Biopsy of arterial wall.

- **Disease Severity**
  Symptoms related to involvement of branch vessels.

- **Concept and Application**
  Inflammation, poorly understood.

- **Management**
  Long-term corticosteroids.

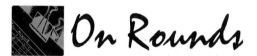

Cardiology at a Glance

Myocardial Infarction   *CAL*
- Chest Pain, diaphoresis, 20% without pain
- Transmural or Q wave has ST segment elevation and T wave inversions
- Non-transmural has ST depression, T wave inversion
- CK-MB peaks at 24 hours
- AST or SGOT peaks at 48–72 hours
- LHD peaks at 3–5 days

Prinzmetal's or Variant Angina
- Angina at rest
- Younger patients
- ECG positive for ST elevation during symptoms
- Gold standard diagnostic test: Spasm on angiography when ergonovine is given

MR → APICAL SM → AXILLA

VSD → SM LLSB

- Treatment: Nitrates, calcium channel blockers, stop smoking, avoid cocaine

Signs of Heart Failure
Left Side, Low Output:
- Fatigue, dyspnea, PND, orthopnea
- S3 or S4, displaced cardiac impulse, CXR, echo

Left Side, High Output:
- Brisk pulse, dyspnea, orthopnea, hyperdynamic circulation

Right Side:
- Fatigue, RV heave, JVD, hepatomegaly, atrial arrhythmias
- ECG may show RV or RA hypertrophy
- Echo may show RV dilation and hypokinesis

Mural thrombi common ī ANT MI

ANT MI - DAMAGE EXCLUSIVELY L vent.
INF MI - DAMAGE BOTH ventricle
inferior MI better prognosis then ant

BIBLIOGRAPHY

ACC/AHA Task Force. ACC/AHA guidelines for the early management of patients with acute myocardial infarction. *Circulation.* 82:664–707.

Benotti JR, Grossman W. Restrictive cardiomyopathy. *Ann Rev Med.* 1984;35:113–25.

24th Bethesda Conference. Cardiac transplantation. *J Am Coll Cardiol.* 1993;22:1–64.

Braunwald E. Heart Disease: *A Textbook of Cardiovascular Medicine.* 2nd ed. Philadelphia: WB Saunders Co; 1984.

Hurst JW, Schlant RC, Rackley CE, et al, eds. *The Heart.* 7th ed. New York: McGraw-Hill Information Services Co; 1990.

Wilson JD, Braunwald E, Isselbacher KJ, et al, eds. *Harrison's Principles of Internal Medicine.* 12th ed. New York: McGraw-Hill, Inc; 1991.

Zipes DP, Jalife J. *Cardiac Electrophysiology: From Cell to Bedside.* Philadelphia: WB Saunders Co; 1990.

MR Assoc ī papillary muscle dysf.

Syndrome X (Microvascular Angina)

nl coronary angiogram ; no coronary spasm

PT - CP similar angina ; (+) STRESS TEST

Defective endothelium dependant DILATION

in coronary microcirculation.

Angina Due AS ; IHSS

CI to stress testing

AS

IHSS

Unstable angina

Malignant PVC's

EKG suggest ischemia

severe COPD

CHF.

Don't use Persentine c̄ ASTHMATIC/COPD - N̄ Bronchospasm

MI: NITRATES

BBlocker

Ca̅ channel

ASA

Heparin

MINC Syndrome - MI c̄ nl coronaries

associated c̄ younger PT; cocaine usage

S/P MI TDA follow by ~~Streptokinase~~ Heparin

Heparin no benefit c̄ APSAC

Careful use nitrates inferior MI - very sensitive
to preload Δ

2

Dermatology

Gary R. Kantor, MD, and Richard L. Spielvogel, MD

I. ACUTE EXANTHEMS

A. Varicella (Chickenpox) *[FACE/SCALP ↓ TRUNK]*

- **H&P Keys**
  Rash begins on face and scalp and rapidly spreads to trunk with relative sparing of extremities. Typical lesions are vesicles with a pink base, but lesions at all stages of development (macules, papules, vesicles, pustules, crusted lesions) are characteristic. Fever, chills, malaise, and headache may accompany. Mucous membranes may be affected.

- **Diagnosis**
  Positive Tzanck smear demonstrating multinucleated giant cells, viral culture.

- **Disease Severity**
  Mildest cases in infants and most severe cases in adults. Fever correlates with disease severity. Prolonged fever may be associated with complications such as pneumonia. Scarring is more severe in adults.

- **Concept and Application**
  Viral entry through mucosa of upper respiratory tract and oropharynx, primary (incubation) and secondary (infection) viremia, humoral and cellular immune response terminate viremia; immunity is complex and antibody alone does not guarantee total immunity; varicella-zoster immune globulin can be used in immunocompromised patients (lymphoma, leukemia, HIV positive) up to 3 days after exposure. *[VZIG 3DAYS]*

- **Management**

Topical. Cool compresses, calamine lotion, antibiotics for secondary bacterial infection.

Systemic. Antihistamines, acetaminophen, acyclovir.

B. Herpes Zoster (Shingles)

- **H&P Keys**
  Prodrome of pain and paresthesia in involved dermatome (may simulate pleurisy, myocardial infarction, ulcer, renal colic); typical rash is localized, unilateral, does not cross midline, grouped vesicles on a pink base, which form pustules and crusts (Fig. 2–1).

- **Diagnosis**
  Same as varicella.

- **Disease Severity**
  Pain is more severe in elderly patients; disease is more severe in immunocompromised (skin necrosis and scarring, postherpetic neuralgia, dissemination).

- **Concept and Application**
  Infection is a recrudescence of latent infection with varicella-zoster infection, passed to the skin and mucosa by sensory nerves from dorsal ganglia; cellular immunity is more important in host resistance (increased incidence of infection in patients with HIV or defects in cellular immunity).

- **Management**

Topical. Same as varicella.

Systemic. Acyclovir 800 mg 5 times/d for 1 week, famciclovir 500 mg 3 times/d, analgesics.

For Postherpetic Neuralgia. Topical capsaicin cream (Zostrix).

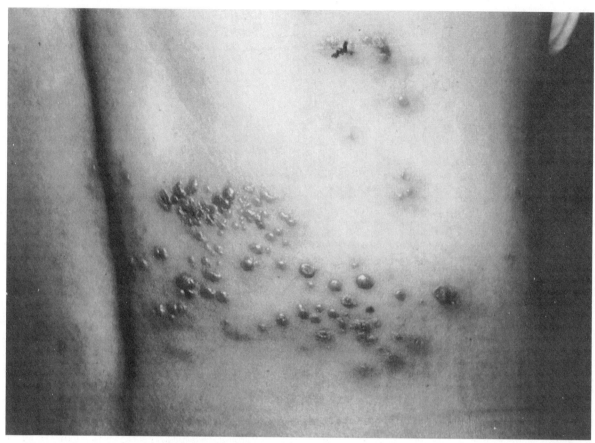

Figure 2–1. Herpes zoster. Some lesions in this example are hemorrhagic.

II. OTHER SKIN INFECTIONS

A. Mycoses, Dermatophytosis

Red scaly patch central clearing

- **H&P Keys**
  Contact with infected person or animals, typical annular reddish scaly plaques with central clearing, hair loss with scalp involvement (tinea capitis); fissuring, scaling, or blisters with foot involvement (tinea pedis).

- **Diagnosis**
  Potassium hydroxide (KOH) preparation, fungal culture, Wood's light (some cases of tinea capitis).

- **Disease Severity**
  Toenails involved (onychomycosis) usually with tinea pedis; hand infection usually accompanied by tinea pedis; extensive or chronic involvement in immunodeficiency states (HIV infection, lymphomas) and endocrine disorders (Cushing's, diabetes).

- **Concept and Application**
  Infection dependent on climatic conditions (tinea pedis more common where occlusive footwear is used; tinea corporis more common in hot, humid climates under occlusive garments), host factors (men are more susceptible), virulence of organisms.

- **Management**
  Topical antifungals for most limited infections, oral agents (eg, griseofulvin) for extensive disease and tinea capitis. Onicomycosis can be treated with itraconazole.

B. Candidiasis, Mouth (Thrush)

- **H&P Keys**
  Asymptomatic, white patches resembling milk curds or cottage cheese on tongue or

oral mucosa; fissuring and redness at corners of mouth (perlèche).

- **Diagnosis**
  KOH preparation, culture.

- **Disease Severity**
  Associated with broad-spectrum antibiotics, diabetes, malignant neoplasms, and HIV infection.

- **Concept and Application**
  Candida albicans is a saprophyte that colonizes the oropharynx, gastrointestinal (GI) tract, and vagina in most individuals. Infection develops from diminished host defenses.

- **Management**
  Nystatin suspension, clotrimazole troches.

C. Candidiasis, Cutaneous

[handwritten: ↓ Thyroid hypoadrenalism hypoparathyroid]

- **H&P Keys**

Acute. Inflammatory plaques with satellite pustules in moist, macerated folds of skin (eg, axillae, submammary).

Chronic. Same as acute, but also may develop heavily crusted lesions on skin and thickened nail plate.

- **Diagnosis**
  KOH preparation, culture, pathologic studies.

- **Disease Severity**

Acute. Increased predisposition in obesity, diabetes, and occupations (wet work: waitresses, dishwashers, housecleaners).

Chronic. Associated with endocrinopathies (hypoparathyroidism, hypoadrenalism, hypothyroidism), circulating autoantibodies, chronic active hepatitis, thymoma.

- **Concept and Application**
  See candidiasis, mouth (above). In chronic types, cell-mediated immune defect selective for *Candida*.

- **Management**

Topical. Nystatin powder, imidazole cream or lotion (clotrimazole, econazole).

Systemic. Ketoconazole, fluconazole.

D. Cellulitis, Abscess of Finger or Toe (Paronychia)

- **H&P Keys**
  Redness, swelling, local pus collection in nail fold.

- **Diagnosis**
  Gram's stain of pus, bacterial and fungal culture (*Staphylococcus* or *Candida* usually causative).

- **Disease Severity**
  May cause nail-plate deformity.

- **Concept and Application**
  Barrier function of nail fold (cuticle) altered by trauma and moisture.

- **Management**
  Antiseptic soaks (Burow's solution), β-lactamase penicillins, ketoconazole.

E. Cellulitis, Abscess of Other Local Infections

- **H&P Keys**

Cellulitis. Local area of redness, tenderness, warmth, and edema; may be accompanied by constitutional symptoms.

Abscess. Local pus collection with tenderness and fluctuation.

- **Diagnosis**
  Culture, Gram's stain.

- **Disease Severity**
  Systemic toxicity suggests bacteremia.

- **Concept and Application**

Cellulitis. Breaks in skin allow entry of organism; beta-hemolytic strep common in adults (erysipelas); hemophilus in children.

Abscess. Most often arises from an infected hair follicle (furuncle); staph most common.

- **Management**

Cellulitis. Oral penicillin or β-lactamase penicillin; IV antibiotics in severe cases.

Abscess. Incision and drainage, β-lactamase penicillin.

F. Impetigo

Bullous STAPH

- **H&P Keys**
  Golden-yellow, crusted lesions on face, nose, or around mouth (beta-hemolytic strep, staph); may be bullous (staph) (Fig. 2–2).

- **Diagnosis**
  Bacterial culture, Gram's stain.

- **Disease Severity**
  May be spread by close contacts. Secondary infection of preexisting skin lesions (insect bites, abrasions, herpes simplex, eczema) is common.

- **Concept and Application**
  Highly communicable infection in which the organism produces a superficial skin blister that rapidly ruptures, forming a crust. Crowding, poor hygiene, neglected wounds, and minor trauma contribute to spread. Bullous variant caused by phage group II type 71 staph.

- **Management**
  Topical mupirocin (Bactroban) ointment. β-Lactamase antibiotics for bullous type.

III. SKIN ERUPTIONS

A. Scabies

- **H&P Keys**
  Marked itching (especially in the evening); papules, vesicles, and burrows in typical sites (interdigital web spaces, volar wrists, axillae, areolae, umbilicus, genitals, knees, ankles) (Fig. 2–3).

- **Diagnosis**
  Skin scraping with a drop of mineral oil on slide will demonstrate mites or their products.

- **Disease Severity**
  Itching may interfere with sleep and daily activities. Variant (Norwegian scabies) produces crusted, scaly lesions and is found in elderly, mentally retarded, or immunocompromised patients.

- **Concept and Application**
  May be sexually transmitted.

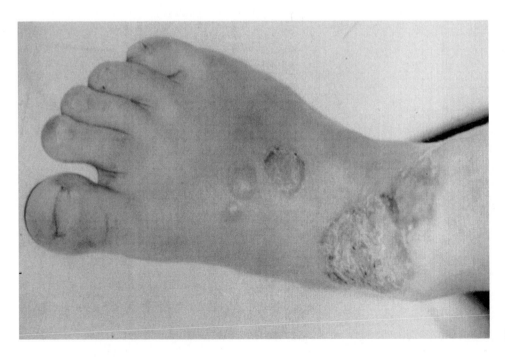

Figure 2–2. Bullous impetigo.

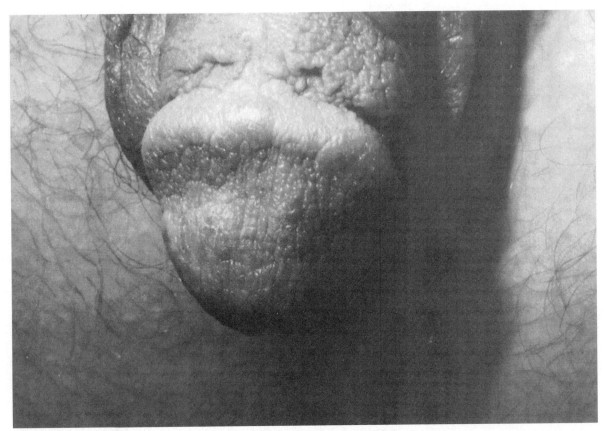

Figure 2–3. Nodules on glans penis typical of scabies.

GUTTATE PSORASIS - TRIGGER
STREP PHARYNGITIS

• **Management**
Lindane (Kwell), permethrin cream (Elimite). Antihistamines and topical steroids for itching.

B. Other Inflammatory Conditions of Skin

1. Psoriasis

• **H&P Keys**
Well-demarcated reddish plaques with adherent silvery scale (Fig. 2–4). Typically chronic, symmetric, and familial. Variable itching, shows Koebner's phenomenon (lesions occur after trauma). *Sites:* elbows, knees, scalp, buttocks, nails. *Variants:* pustular, erythrodermic, guttate, palmoplantar.

• **Diagnosis**
Clinical lesions are characteristic; biopsy to confirm.

• **Disease Severity**
Arthritis may be associated. Pustular and erythrodermic variants associated with systemic toxicity. Guttate psoriasis triggered by strep pharyngitis. Some drugs (β-blockers, lithium, systemic steroids) cause flare.

• **Concept and Application**
Hyperproliferation of epidermis. Multiple mediators involved, including cyclic nucleotides, polyamines, proteases, and leukotrienes. Topical corticosteroids normalize hyperproliferation. Benoxaprofen (Oraflex) inhibits leukotrienes.

• **Management**

Topical. Tars, corticosteroids, anthralin, calcipotriene (Dovonex) ointment.

Phototherapy. UVB, psoralen plus UVA (PUVA).

Systemic. Methotrexate, etretinate (Tegison).

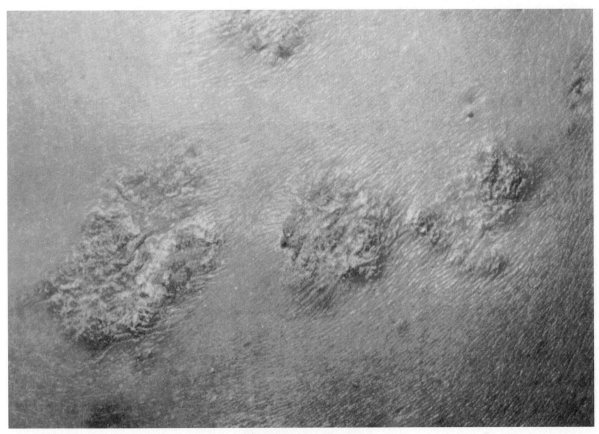

Figure 2–4. Plaques of psoriasis.

2. Seborrheic Dermatitis

- **H&P Keys**
  The mildest form is flaking of scalp (dandruff). Scale is yellowish and greasy. Variable erythema. Also affects external ear canal, eyebrows, nasal crease. Occasionally involves presternal area, axillae, umbilicus, and groin. In infant, referred to as cradle cap.

- **Diagnosis**
  Clinical exam. Biopsy excludes other disorders.

- **Disease Severity**
  May be severe and treatment-resistant in HIV patients. More frequent and severe in neurologic disorders (eg, Parkinson's disease).

- **Concept and Application**
  Oily skin is a predisposing factor, but the disorder is not a disease of sebaceous glands. Worse in fall and winter. *Pityrosporum* yeast is abundant in lesions and may be trigger factor.

- **Management**
  Shampoos with selenium sulfide (Selsun), zinc pyrithione (Head and Shoulders), tar. Low-potency corticosteroid lotions or creams.

3. Contact Dermatitis

- **H&P Keys**
  Linear, itchy, erythematous plaques with or without blisters. Rhus plants (poison ivy, oak, sumac) most common cause. Nickel (costume jewelry) (Fig. 2–5), neomycin (Neosporin), and fragrances (perfumes) are frequent causes. Has 24- to 28-hour delay from contact to development of rash.

- **Diagnosis**
  History and physical exam, biopsy, patch tests.

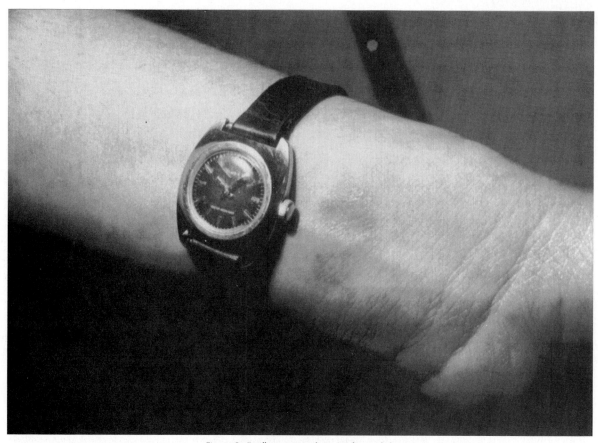

Figure 2–5. Allergic contact dermatitis from nickel.

- **Disease Severity**
  May be generalized. Itching can be severe. Can become chronic if precipitating cause not eliminated. Frequent cause for work disability.

- **Concept and Application**
  Type IV delayed hypersensitivity. Occasionally type I hypersensitivity (contact urticaria to foods, latex).

- **Management**
  Avoidance of precipitating antigen. *Mild cases:* topical corticosteroids. *Severe cases:* systemic corticosteroids, antihistamines.

4. Atopic Dermatitis

- **H&P Keys**
  Personal or family history of atopy. Marked itching. May begin in infancy. Excoriations and erythematous plaques in antecubital and popliteal fossae, posterior neck. Redundant eyelid fold, hyperlinear palmar creases, dry skin, and cataracts are associated findings.

- **Diagnosis**
  History and physical exam, biopsy, blood eosinophilia, IgE levels.

- **Disease Severity**
  May generalize (erythroderma). *Staphylococcus aureus* is a frequent colonizer and may trigger flares. Increased suspectibility to herpes infection (Kaposi's varicelliform eruption) and fungal infection.

- **Concept and Application**
  Unknown cause. In some patients, allergens (eg, foods) may provoke itching, dermatitis, and bronchospasm.

- **Management**
  Avoidance of irritants, moisturizers, oral antihistamines, topical corticosteroids. β-Lactamase antibiotics if flare by staph organisms suspected.

5. Dermatitis (Eczema)

- **H&P Keys**

  Contact dermatitis and atopic dermatitis are subtypes. Lesions are erythematous plaques with variable minute blisters, scale, excoriation, and crust. Round configuration resembling ringworm (nummular dermatitis) (Fig. 2–6). When present on legs with venous stasis and varicosities (stasis dermatitis), associated with hyperpigmentation and ulcers. Type related to severe dry skin (asteatotic dermatitis, eczema craquelé).

- **Diagnosis**

  History and physical exam, biopsy.

- **Disease Severity**

  May generalize (autoeczematization). Itching may be severe and interfere with daily living and sleep.

- **Concept and Application**

  Unknown. Dry skin exacerbates all forms of eczema.

- **Management**

  Moisturizers, oral antihistamines, topical or systemic corticosteroids. For stasis dermatitis, leg elevation, support stockings, edema reduction, and treatment of infection.

6. Urticaria (Hives)   *Ho VASculitis*

- **H&P Keys**

  Acute or chronic (greater than 6 weeks). Lesions are fleeting (usually hours) in duration. Mildly itchy, pink swellings (wheals). Precipitating cause may be known to patient.

- **Diagnosis**

  History and physical. Biopsy in chronic cases to rule out vasculitis. To be differenti-

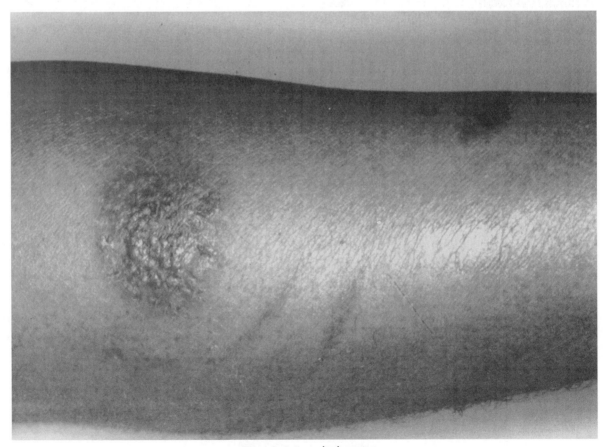

Figure 2–6. Nummular dermatitis.

ated from dermographism (hives occurring after scratching).

- **Disease Severity**
  May be associated with laryngeal spasm or bronchospasm. Angioedema (deep swelling in skin) may be associated (if prominent feature, rule out hereditary angioedema associated with C1 esterase inhibitor deficiency).

- **Concept and Application**
  Numerous causes. Both type I and II mechanisms implicated. Mast cell degranulation leads to edema and vascular permeability.

- **Management**
  Elimination of cause if known (drugs, foods, bites most common). Antihistamines. Avoidance of systemic corticosteroids.

7. Drug Reactions

- **H&P Keys**
  Variable presentation. Disseminated itchy pink macules and papules (morbilliform) are typical (eg, mononucleosis patient given amoxicillin). Time course of rash usually corresponds to offending medication. Other presentations: urticaria, erythema multiforme (targetoid lesions), photosensitivity, vasculitis, fixed (lesions recur in same spot with rechallenge).

- **Diagnosis**
  History and physical exam. Biopsy. Some drugs are more frequent offenders (trimethoprim-sulfamethoxazole, phenytoin, thiazides, penicillins).

- **Disease Severity**
  May generalize (erythroderma). Itching may be severe. Erythema multiforme (Stevens-Johnson syndrome, toxic epidermal necrolysis) may be life-threatening. Systemic vasculitis may be associated with cutaneous lesions (palpable purpura).

- **Concept and Application**
  Immunologic (types I to IV) and nonimmunologic mechanisms.

- **Management**
  Cessation of offending medication. Antihistamines, soothing topical emollient lotions

(Sarna). Systemic corticosteroids should be used with caution.

C. Other Diseases of Skin and Subcutaneous Tissue

1. Bullous Pemphigoid

- **H&P Keys**
  Elderly patients; itching; large, tense blisters and urticarial plaques; negative Nikolsky's sign (cannot induce blister with blunt pressure).

- **Diagnosis**
  Biopsy for routine studies and immunofluorescence, serum for indirect immunofluorescence (to detect circulating autoantibody).

- **Disease Severity**
  Blisters may be large and leave large denuded areas, mucosal lesions are painful, itching can be marked.

- **Concept and Application**
  Autoimmune mechanisms with IgG and complement infiltrating skin; immunosuppressives used for treatment. Rarely may be caused by drugs (Lasix).

- **Management**
  Local skin care; topical superpotent corticosteroids for limited disease; systemic steroids or other immunosuppressives for generalized disease.

2. Herpes Gestationis

- **H&P Keys**
  Clinical presentation identical to bullous pemphigoid except occurs in second or third trimester of pregnancy.

- **Diagnosis**
  History and physical exam, skin biopsy and immunofluorescence (differentiate from pruritic urticarial papules and plaques of pregnancy [PUPPP], which begins on abdomen [usually striae] and occurs late in pregnancy).

- **Disease Severity**
  May increase fetal mortality or premature delivery; fetus may be born with skin lesions.

- **Concept and Application**
Autoimmune mechanism. Not related to herpes virus. Oral contraceptives may exacerbate disease in patients with documented disease.

- **Management**
Some cases of mild disease can be managed with antihistamines and topical steroid creams. Most patients require systemic steroids.

3. Pemphigus *ASSOCIATED c̄ MALIGNANT neoplasm*

- **H&P Keys**
Two types: superficial (foliaceus) and common (vulgaris). Vulgaris type shows fragile blisters and Nikolsky's sign. Oral lesions are common and often presenting feature. Lesions usually tender or painful, not itchy. Increased frequency in people of Jewish or Mediterranean origin (Fig. 2–7).

1) superficial (foliaceus)
common (vulgaris)

- **Diagnosis**
History and physical exam, skin biopsy for histology and immunofluorescence, serum for indirect immunofluorescence.

- **Disease Severity**
Oral lesions may interfere with intake of solid foods; large denuded raw surfaces may occur; can be fatal if diagnosis and treatment are not established.

- **Concept and Application**
Autoimmune mechanism with antibodies to intercellular substrate of epithelium (skin and mucosae). Immunosuppressives mainstay of treatment. Pemphigus associated with malignant neoplasms (paraneoplastic pemphigus) recently described resembles erythema multiforme.

- **Management**
Local skin care; antibiotics for secondary infection; high-dose systemic steroids; "steroid-

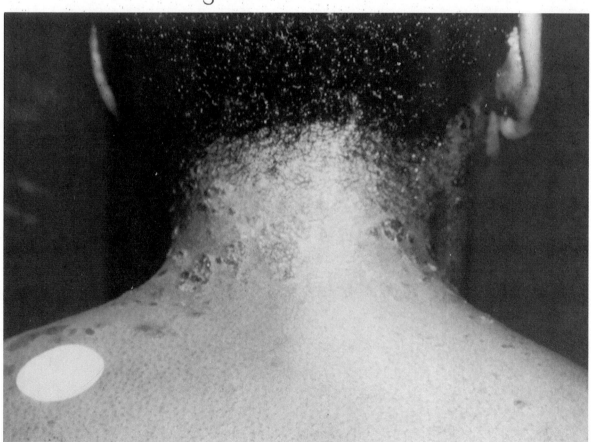

Figure 2–7. Fragile blisters and erosions in pemphigus vulgaris.

sparing" agents such as dapsone and azathioprine may be used.

4. Dermatitis Herpetiformis

- **H&P Keys**
Markedly itchy dermatosis characterized by symmetric grouped blisters (often excoriated) on extensor surfaces of skin (elbows, knees, scalp, back). Associated with gluten-sensitive enteropathy (usually asymptomatic).

- **Diagnosis**
History and physical exam; skin biopsy for histology and immunofluorescence.

- **Disease Severity**
Itching usually severe. Associated steatorrhea, anemia.

- **Concept and Application**
High occurrence of HLA-B8. Gluten plays a critical role (gluten-free diet used for treatment). IgA in skin probably has gut origin.

- **Management**
Gluten-free diet, dapsone, sulfapyridine.

5. Erythema Multiforme

- **H&P Keys**
Target lesions (irislike) are typical. Lesions often on palms and soles as well as remainder of skin. May show central blister. Two forms: minor and major (Stevens-Johnson syndrome). Major form involves two or more mucosal surfaces (Fig. 2–8).

- **Diagnosis**
Physical examination, skin biopsy.

- **Disease Severity**
Major form associated with significant morbidity. Toxic epidermal necrolysis (which resembles major form in early stages) produces widespread denudation resembling a

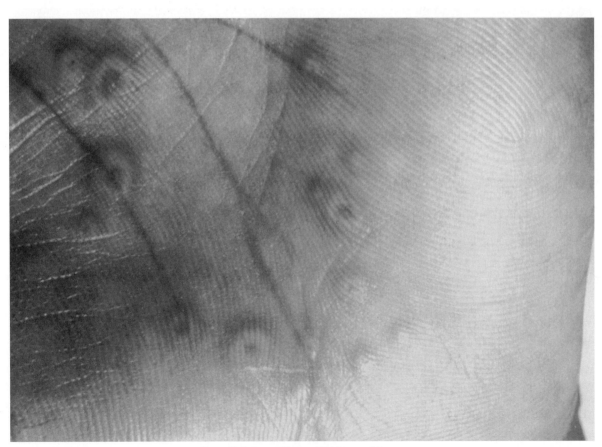

Figure 2–8. Targetoid lesions of erythema multiforme.

burn, and it is associated with mortality from fluid loss and infection.

- **Concept and Application**
Minor form often associated with herpes infection (immune complexes found in skin). Major form associated with drugs and *Mycoplasma.*

- **Management**
Local skin care, antihistamines, systemic steroids in severe cases.

6. Erythema Nodosum

Strep
SARCOID
TB

- **H&P Keys**
Tender, red, warm nodules on legs; may show bruising; nonulcerating; heal without scarring.

- **Diagnosis**
Incisional biopsy for confirmation in atypical cases. To search for underlying cause antistreptolysin-o (ASO) titer, throat culture (strep), chest roentgenogram (sarcoidosis), purified protein derivative (PPD) (tuberculosis).

- **Disease Severity**
Extratibial sites occasionally involved. Associated fever, chills, malaise, arthralgias.

- **Concept and Application**
Immunologic.

- **Management**
Bed rest, nonsteroidal anti-inflammatory drugs (NSAIDS), potassium iodide, steroids.

D. Symptoms Involving the Skin

1. Pruritus (Itching), Generalized

- **H&P Keys**
Excoriations (no primary lesions) in accessible areas. No rash in nonreachable areas (eg, mid back, "butterfly sign"). Examine for lymphadenopathy and signs for systemic cause.

- **Diagnosis**
History most helpful in determining cause. When unaccompanied by rash, drugs or systemic causes are possible. If systemic cause considered, rule out uremia, hepato-

biliary obstruction, polycythemia vera, hyperthyroidism, and Hodgkin's disease.

- **Disease Severity**
Severe itching interferes with quality of life and sleep. Secondary psychiatric disease (eg, depression) may be present.

- **Concept and Application**
Cause undetermined in many cases.

- **Management**
Treatment of cause if known. For unknown causes, antihistamines (hydroxyzine, doxepin), soothing emollient lotions (Sarna). UV light helpful in refractory cases.

2. Pruritus Ani

- **H&P Keys**
Itching around rectum with excoriations.

- **Diagnosis**
History and physical exam. Cellophane tape applied to area may show pinworms.

- **Disease Severity**
Bleeding and fissures.

- **Concept and Application**
Irritation from stool (possibly related to diet) on skin and mucosae. Improved with meticulous anal hygiene.

- **Management**
Avoid external irritants (soaps, medication). Good anal hygiene. Soothing lotions (Balneol).

3. Pruritus, Localized

- **H&P Keys**

Acute. Excoriations.

Chronic. Nodules (prurigo nodularis) or scaly plaques (lichen simplex chronicus).

- **Diagnosis**
History and physical exam, biopsy will confirm.

- **Disease Severity**
Disfiguring scars. In factitial dermatitis (self-inflicted) bizarre configuration of lesion is characteristic. Those patients often have psychologic problems.

- **Concept and Application**
  In some cases an inciting event (insect bite, rash) leads to self-perpetuating itch–scratch cycle. In other cases no such event is apparent.

- **Management**
  Breaking itch–scratch cycle. Corticosteroids (triamcinolone acetonide [Kenalog 10]) injected into nodules. Superpotent topical corticosteroids for lichen simplex chronicus. Psychologic counseling in severe cases.

E. Insect Bites, Nonvenomous

4. Pediculosis

- **H&P Keys**
  Itching, excoriation, and secondary infection of affected sites. Head lice (pediculosis capitis), pubic lice (pediculosis pubis) (Fig. 2–9), body lice (pediculosis corporis). Nits on hair. Adult lice can be seen with hand lens.

- **Diagnosis**
  Presence of nits or adult lice on physical examination.

- **Disease Severity**
  Lice can transmit some rickettsial diseases.

- **Concept and Application**
  Transmitted by casual or sexual contact. Often epidemic in schools (head lice).

- **Management**
  Lindane (Kwell), permethrin cream (Elimite).

5. Mosquitoes and Flies

- **H&P Keys**
  Itchy and edematous papules on exposed sites.

- **Diagnosis**
  History and physical exam, skin biopsy for atypical lesions.

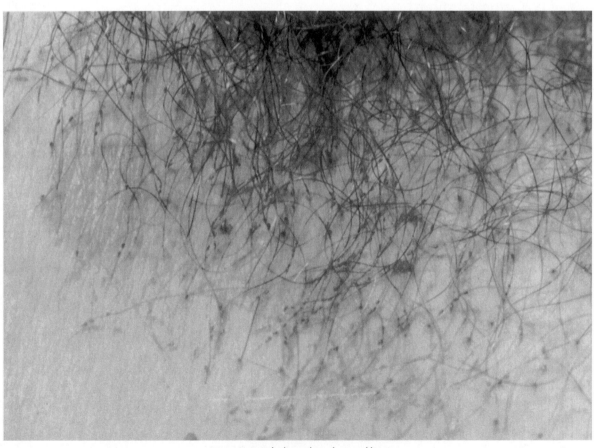

Figure 2–9. Pediculosis pubis with nits and lice.

- **Disease Severity**
  Spectrum of cutaneous findings dependent on host sensitivity. Organisms largely responsible for transmission of disease (malaria, yellow fever, encephalitis, dengue).

- **Concept and Application**
  Female inserts blood tube through skin and injects anticoagulant. Mosquitoes attracted to scents and bright colors. Diethyltoluamide (Off) is an effective repellent.

- **Management**
  Local care, antihistamines, topical steroids.

6. Fleas

- **H&P Keys**
  Pets (cats, dogs, birds) in household. Characteristic pattern of lesions grouped in threes ("breakfast, lunch, dinner"). Blisters in severely allergic individuals.

- **Diagnosis**
  History and physical exam.

- **Disease Severity**
  May have generalized reaction in some individuals (papular urticaria).

- **Concept and Application**
  Survival of adult fleas for months in the absence of an animal host makes fleaborne epidemics difficult to eradicate.

- **Management**
  Veterinary care of pet, good housecleaning, symptomatic treatment with antihistamines, and topical steroids.

IV. NAILS AND HAIR

A. Ingrowing Nails

- **H&P Keys**
  Great toe most common; painful inflammatory soft-tissue swellings; ill-fitting footwear and improper nail care.

- **Diagnosis**
  History and physical exam.

- **Disease Severity**
  Interferes with ambulation; secondary cellulitis.

- **Concept and Application**
  Overcurvature or developmental abnormality of nail plate with trauma and improper nail care causes nail plate to embed into soft tissue and inflammation and infection to ensue.

- **Management**
  Antiseptic soaks, analgesics, rest, antibiotics, elevating corner of nail plate with cotton.

B. Other Disease of Hair and Hair Follicle

1. Acne Vulgaris

- **H&P Keys**
  Onset in adolescence; comedones (whiteheads and blackheads), papules, pustules, cysts; face, chest, and back.

- **Diagnosis**
  History and physical exam; presence of comedones differentiates from other similar disorders.

- **Disease Severity**
  Cosmetic disfigurement; scarring.

- **Concept and Application**
  Multiple factors: plugging of hair follicle, increased sebum, bacterial infection, genetics. Retin-A causes unplugging of follicles, benzoyl peroxide and antibiotics decrease bacterial population.

- **Management**
  Benzoyl peroxide, topical and oral antibiotics, tretinoin (Retin-A), isotretinoin (Accutane) (for nodulocystic type).

2. Rosacea

- **H&P Keys**
  Adult onset, women predominate, associated with flushing; telangiectasia (dilated blood vessels), papules, pustules symmetrically distributed on face (Fig. 2–10); no comedones.

- **Diagnosis**
  History and physical exam; may resemble malar erythema of lupus erythematosus.

- **Disease Severity**
  Keratitis may be associated.

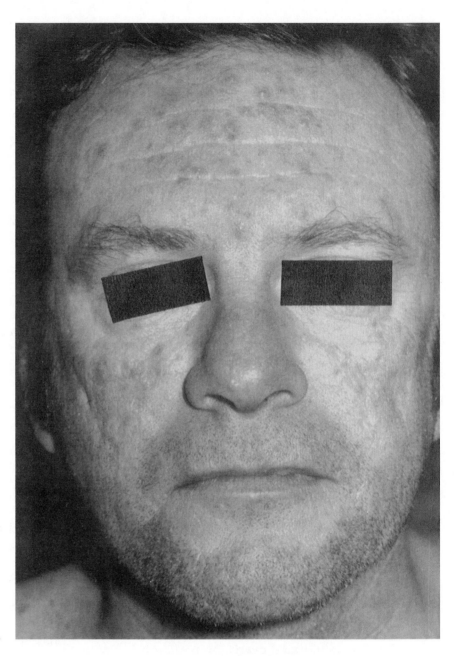

Figure 2–10. Rosacea.

- **Concept and Application**
  Flushing with increase in skin temperature provoked by hot liquids, spicy foods, and alcohol.

- **Management**
  Reduction or elimination of provoking factors, metronidazole (MetroGel), oral tetracycline.

3. Alopecia Areata

- **H&P Keys**
  Localized round or oval patches of hair loss without visible skin inflammation; children or adults; any hair-bearing area may be affected; may be stress-provoked.

- **Diagnosis**
  History and physical exam, biopsy.

- **Disease Severity**
  May involve entire scalp (alopecia totalis) or entire body (alopecia universalis); associated with other autoimmune disorders (vitiligo, Hashimoto's thyroiditis).

- **Concept and Application**
  Autoimmune lymphocytes react against hair follicles.

- **Management**
  Intralesional corticosteroids, minoxidil (avoidance of systemic corticosteroids), anthralin.

V. LUMPS AND TUMORS OF THE SKIN

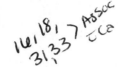

A. Viral Warts (Verrucae)

- **H&P Keys**
  Common wart (verruca vulgaris), palmoplantar wart (verruca palmaris/plantaris), flat wart (verruca plana), genital wart (condyloma acuminatum); latter is sexually transmitted; spread by trauma.

- **Diagnosis**
  History and physical exam; biopsy.

- **Disease Severity**
  Numerous lesions associated with immunodeficiency; certain viral types (16, 18, 31, 33) associated with cancer.

- **Concept and Application**
  Papillomavirus infection.

- **Management**
  Destructive modalities: topical acids (salicylic and lactic [Duofilm]), liquid nitrogen, excision, laser vaporization.

B. Molluscum Contagiosum

- **H&P Keys**
  Discrete umbilicated pearly papules in children and adults; may be transmitted sexually.

- **Diagnosis**
  History and physical exam, biopsy.

- **Disease Severity**
  Numerous, large, and disfiguring in AIDS patients.

- **Concept and Application**
  DNA poxvirus infection.

- **Management**
  Electrodesiccation and curettage, liquid nitrogen.

C. Secondary Syphilis

- **H&P Keys**
  Lesions appear 6 to 12 weeks after onset of chancre. Associated lymphadenopathy. Great imitator—many cutaneous expressions. Macules, brownish-red papules, variable scale. Often involve palms and soles (ham colored) (Fig. 2–11).

- **Diagnosis**
  History and physical exam, darkfield microscopy, serology, biopsy.

- **Disease Severity**
  Associated findings: mucous patches, condyloma lata, pharyngitis, iritis, periostitis, arthralgias, hepatosplenomegaly.

- **Concept and Application**
  Sexually transmitted spirochetal infection. Untreated may progress to tertiary phase (granulomas, gummas).

- **Management**
  Benzathine penicillin (tetracycline or erythromycin in penicillin-allergic). Beware of Jarisch-Herxheimer reaction (acute exacerbation of disease with treatment).

D. Premalignant and Malignant Neoplasm of Skin

1. Actinic Keratosis (Solar Keratosis)

- **H&P Keys**
  Sign of chronic sun damage; light-complected individuals (Northern European); multiple discrete, rough, adherent scaly red patches on sun-exposed areas.

- **Diagnosis**
  History and physical (other signs of sun damage: wrinkling, lentigines, etc); biopsy.

- **Disease Severity**
  May be associated with frank skin cancer (basal or squamous cell carcinoma).

- **Concept and Application**
  Chronic sun exposure causes malignant keratinocyte transformation confined to lower layers of the epidermis. Sunscreens are protective.

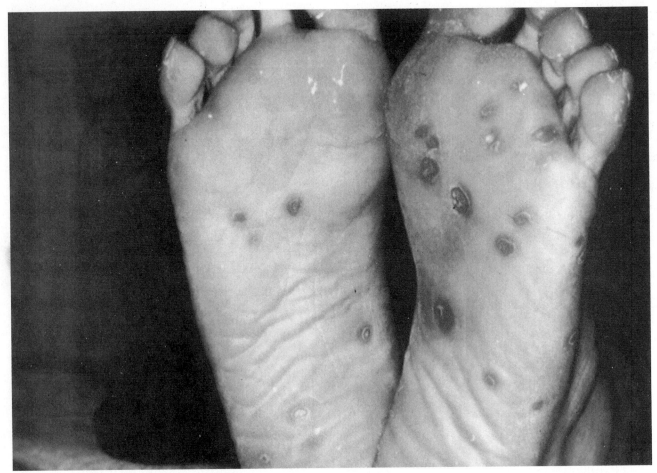

Figure 2–11. Secondary syphilis.

- **Management**
  Liquid nitrogen, topical 5-fluorouracil, excision.

2. Bowen's Disease (Squamous Cell Carcinoma in Situ)

- **H&P Keys**
  Sun-exposed or protected skin; may arise from preexisting actinic keratosis or de novo; more infiltrated and less scaly than actinic keratosis.

- **Diagnosis**
  History and physical exam, biopsy.

- **Disease Severity**
  Previously associated with arsenic exposure; no increased risk of underlying malignant neoplasm. Lesion on penis called erythroplasia of Queyrat.

- **Concept and Application**
  Malignant keratinocyte transformation of full thickness of epidermis.

- **Management**
  Excision.

3. Basal Cell Carcinoma

- **H&P Keys**
  Slowly growing, pearly papule or nodule on sun-exposed skin (Fig. 2–12A); most common form of skin cancer; lesions often ulcerate (rodent ulcer) and have rolled borders; infiltrate locally and very rarely metastasize.

- **Diagnosis**
  History and physical exam, biopsy.

- **Disease Severity**
  A sign of chronic sun injury. Variants: pigmented (resembles nodular melanoma),

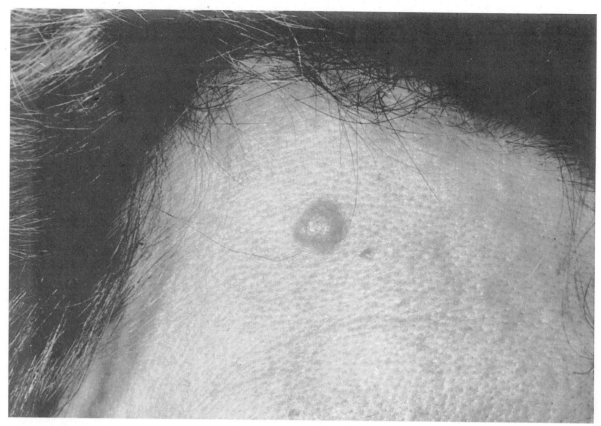

Figure 2–12. A. Basal cell carcinoma.

morpheaform (most locally aggressive type), superficial (typically on trunk, may resemble eczema), infiltrative (may recur after treatment).

- **Concept and Application**
  Malignant tumor of skin related to chronic sun injury.

- **Management**
  Excision, destruction (electrical, freezing).

4. Squamous Cell Carcinoma

- **H&P Keys**
  Enlarging indurated papule or nodule with variable adherent scale on sun-exposed sites (skin and mucosa) in older people.

- **Diagnosis**
  History and physical exam, biopsy.

- **Disease Severity**
  May arise from preexisting actinic keratosis (low incidence of metastasis). When occurs

de novo, higher rate of metastasis. Tumors on lower lip, particularly, have prevalence of metastasis (Fig. 2–12B).

- **Concept and Application**
  Numerous factors: sunlight, x-rays, arsenic ingestion, immunosuppression, chronic ulcers, burns, smoking.

- **Management**
  Excision.

5. Malignant Melanoma

- **H&P Keys**
  Enlarging, asymmetric, irregularly bordered, variably colored, large (over 6 mm) pigmented patch. Black color is suspicious. First is flat (radial growth), then becomes nodular (vertical growth) (Fig. 2–13). May bleed and ulcerate.

- **Diagnosis**
  Excisional biopsy.

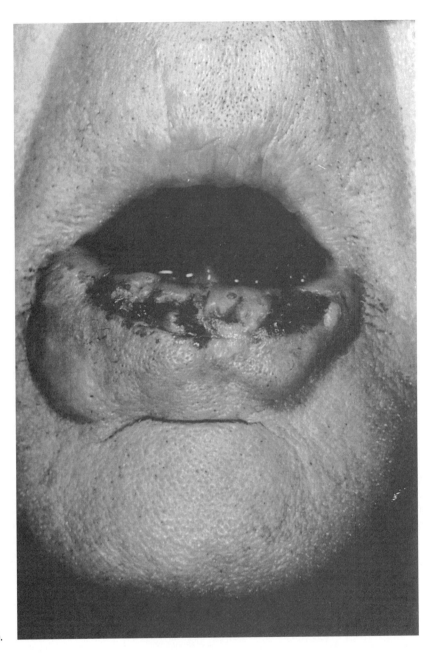

Figure 2–12. B. Squamous cell carcinoma of lower lip.

- **Disease Severity**
  Aggressive tumor with high propensity to metastasize widely. Prognosis related to depth of skin invasion (Clark's and Breslow's levels). Lesions less than 1 mm have good prognosis, greater than 3 mm have guarded prognosis.

- **Concept and Application**
  Related to intermittent intense sun exposure (blistering sunburns). Higher incidence in white-collar professionals. May develop from congenital moles or chronic sun exposure (lentigo maligna). Superficial spreading is most common; nodular is worst prognostically; acrolentiginous (hands, feet, mucosae) is most common in blacks.

- **Management**
  Excision, with surgical margins determined by depth of tumor invasion. Lymph node dissection controversial. Examination and lab screening for metastasis. Treatment for metastatic disease unsatisfactory.

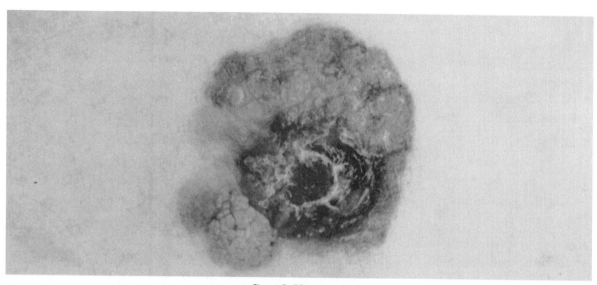

Figure 2-13. Melanoma.

E. Lipoma

- **H&P Keys**
  Single or multiple, rubbery or compressible subcutaneous masses, most often on trunk, posterior neck, or forearms. Angiolipomas are often multiple and painful.

- **Diagnosis**
  Physical exam, excisional biopsy.

- **Disease Severity**
  Rarely, infiltrates into skeletal muscle. May occur in Gardner's syndrome.

- **Concept and Application**
  Benign tumor of adipose tissue.

- **Management**
  None if asymptomatic, excision.

F. Benign Neoplasms of Skin

1. Melanocytic Nevus

- **H&P Keys**
  Pigmented, well-demarcated, symmetric macule (junctional nevus), papule (compound nevus), or flesh-colored papule (intradermal nevus).

- **Diagnosis**
  History and physical exam, biopsy.

- **Disease Severity**
  Number of nevi correlate with life risk of melanoma; congenital (at birth) nevi often have hair; large type (bathing trunk nevi) have increased risk of malignant transformation.

- **Concept and Application**
  A proliferation of altered melanocytes in skin.

- **Management**
  None unless melanoma is considered in differential diagnosis. Congenital nevi should be excised at a young age.

2. Atypical (Dysplastic) Nevus

- **H&P Keys**
  Familial or sporadic, large, irregularly bordered, pigmented macules and papules.

- **Diagnosis**
  History and physical exam; biopsy.

- **Disease Severity**
  Multiple familial atypical nevi associated with increased risk of melanoma. Lesions are not necessarily precursors.

- **Concept and Application**
  Proliferation of melanocytes with varying cytologic atypia.

- **Management**
  Excision if melanoma is a diagnostic consideration; sun precaution and sunscreens; semiannual complete skin exams.

3. Dermatofibroma (Histiocytoma)

- **H&P Keys**
Firm, pigmented macule or papule that depresses centrally when palpated ("dimpling sign"). Often on lower leg and preceded by trauma (eg, bite).

- **Diagnosis**
History and physical exam, biopsy.

- **Disease Severity**
Multiple lesions may be associated with lupus erythematosus.

- **Concept and Application**
Proliferation of fibrohistiocytes after trauma.

- **Management**
Excision if desired.

4. Hemangioma

- **H&P Keys**
Capillary or strawberry nevus (congenital), cavernous (bluish-purple-subcutaneous), senile (red papules on trunk of elderly people).

- **Diagnosis**
History and physical exam.

- **Disease Severity**
Multiple cutaneous lesions may be associated with internal organ involvement (central nervous system [CNS], liver, GI tract). Large cavernous lesions may be associated with consumption of clotting factors. Kasabach-Merritt syndrome: hemangiomas and thrombocytopenia.

- **Concept and Application**
Localized proliferation and dilatation of capillaries.

- **Management**
Capillary hemangiomas may self-involute. Laser treatment for cosmetically disfiguring or deep lesions.

5. Pyogenic Granuloma

- **H&P Keys**
Rapidly developing, bleeding, bright-red pedunculated papule or nodule (Fig. 2–14). Usually in young people. Preceding trauma.

- **Diagnosis**
History and physical exam, biopsy.

- **Disease Severity**
None; differentiate from other tumors (melanoma, carcinoma).

- **Concept and Application**
Overproliferation of granulation tissue in response to injury.

- **Management**
Excision, laser.

6. Blue Nevus

- **H&P Keys**
Blue-black macule or papule; more common on extremity.

- **Diagnosis**
Clinical examination, biopsy.

- **Disease Severity**
None; differentiate from thrombosed hemangioma, tattoo, and melanoma.

- **Concept and Application**
Proliferation of dendritic melanocytes in dermis.

- **Management**
Excision.

7. Seborrheic Keratosis

- **H&P Keys**
Most common benign skin lesion. Warty, light to dark brown stuck-on plaques. Multiple in various stages of development (Fig. 2–15).

- **Diagnosis**
History and physical exam, biopsy.

- **Disease Severity**
Multiple itchy, eruptive seborrheic keratoses may be sign of internal malignant neoplasm ("sign of Leser-Trélat").

- **Concept and Application**
Proliferation of keratinocytes.

- **Management**
None unless irritated or suspicion of melanoma or nonmelanoma skin cancer.

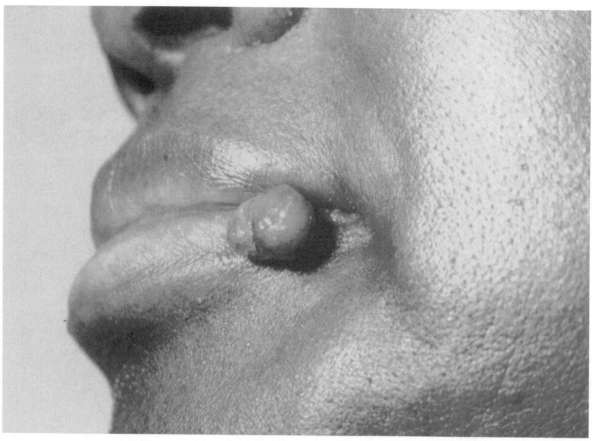

Figure 2–14. Pyogenic granuloma.

G. Acquired Keratoderma (Tylosis)

- **H&P Keys**
  Localized or diffuse thickening of skin on palms and soles.

- **Diagnosis**
  History and physical exam.

- **Disease Severity**
  May be sign of internal malignant neoplasm (esophagus). May appear at menopause (keratoderma climacterium).

- **Concept and Application**
  Unknown.

- **Management**
  Keratolytic agents (salicylic acid, urea), lubrication.

H. Follicular Cyst (Epidermal Cyst, Sebaceous Cyst)

- **H&P Keys**
  Slowly enlarging, soft, movable mass. May show punctum. Most common on face or trunk.

- **Diagnosis**
  History and physical exam.

- **Disease Severity**
  May rupture or become infected and cause pain.

- **Concept and Application**
  Follicular occlusion leads to cystic dilatation of follicle.

- **Management**
  Excision. (Note: cyst contains keratin, not sebum.)

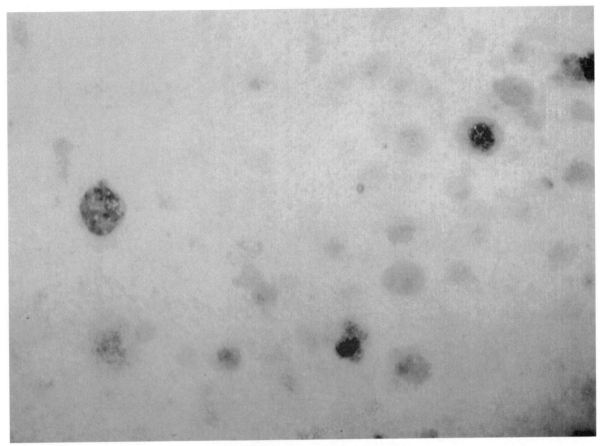

Figure 2–15. Numerous seborrheic keratoses.

VI. OTHER CONDITIONS

A. Decubitus Ulcer

- **H&P Keys**
  Four grades, depending on depth of ischemia; most common over bony prominences (sacrum, greater trochanter, ischium, calcaneus, malleolus). Nutritional deficiency, spasticity, loss of cutaneous sensation are contributory factors.

- **Diagnosis**
  Clinical exam, roentgenography, culture, biopsy.

- **Disease Severity**
  Grades III (into subcutaneous fat) and IV (into underlying muscle) may be associated with osteomyelitis and severe morbidity.

- **Concept and Application**
  Prolonged pressure leads to ischemia and cutaneous necrosis.

- **Management**
  Treatment of secondary infection, relief of pressure, saline or acetic acid dressings, debridement, skin graft.

B. Ulcer of Lower Limbs

1. Stasis Ulceration   *medial side*

- **H&P Keys**
  Minimally painful, superficial, well-demarcated ulcer with red base and variable crust (Fig. 2–16). Typically on medial side of ankle. Associated stasis dermatitis, pigmentation, and varicose veins.

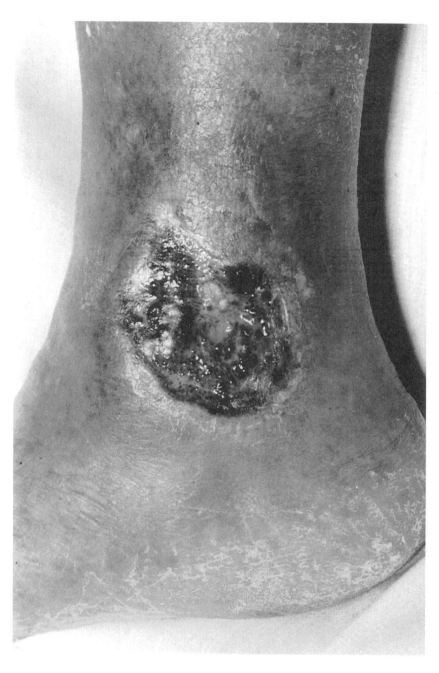

Figure 2–16. Stesis ulcer.

- **Diagnosis**
  Clinical exam; biopsy in atypical lesions.

- **Disease Severity**
  Multiple or large ulcers may occur; secondary cellulitis.

- **Concept and Application**
  Ischemia from venous back pressure, preventing capillary flow.

- **Management**
  Bed rest, leg elevation, hydrocolloid dressings (Duoderm), compression bandage (Unna boot), compression stockings (Jobst), surgery of varicose veins.

2. Arteriosclerotic Ulcer

- **H&P Keys**
  Markedly painful, dry, shallow necrotic ulcer on foot or lateral leg. Foot is cold and

hypoesthetic. Rest pain and claudication. Other signs and symptoms of atherosclerosis.

- **Diagnosis**
Palpation of peripheral pulses, Doppler studies, arteriography.

- **Disease Severity**
Significant associated large and small arterial disease.

- **Concept and Application**
Chronic obstruction of small and large vessels by atheromas.

- **Management**
Address of underlying disease, stopping smoking, antiplatelet agents, pentoxifylline (Trental).

3. Pyoderma Gangrenosum   *ulc colitis Chrohns*

- **H&P Keys**
Painful nodule or pustule that rapidly ulcerates, with a tender, undermined border. Associated with ulcerative colitis, Crohn's disease, arthritis, paraproteinemia, and leukemia.

- **Diagnosis**
Look for underlying diseases in previously undiagnosed cases.

- **Disease Severity**
Lesions may be large and involve other sites than legs. Ulcers usually indicate activity of bowel disease.

- **Concept and Application**
Disturbance in immunoregulation.

- **Management**
Systemic steroids, dapsone.

C. Cutaneous Manifestations of Systemic Disease

1. Lupus Erythematosus   *ANA SMA Ro SSA La SSB*

- **H&P Keys**
Three types: acute (systemic), subacute (antinuclear antibody [ANA] negative), chronic (discoid) (Fig. 2–17).

Vascular Connective tissue

Acute. Malar erythema (butterfly rash), Raynaud's phenomenon, mouth ulcers, alopecia, vasculitis.

Subacute. Annular or polycyclic (resembling tinea or psoriasis), photosensitivity.

Chronic. Scarring, red, scaling plaques, primarily on sun-exposed areas. Review of systems check.

- **Diagnosis**
History and physical exam; laboratory studies may include: complete blood count, ANA, urinalysis, SMA, Ro (SS-A), La (SS-B); skin biopsy, immunofluorescence.

- **Disease Severity**
Acute may have serious renal or CNS manifestations. Subacute is associated with a low risk of CNS or renal disease. Chronic is usually limited to the skin only.

- **Concept and Application**
Autoimmune disease involving vasculature and connective tissue.

- **Management**
Sunscreens, topical and systemic corticosteroids, antimalarials.

2. Dermatomyositis   *✓ internal malignancy*

- **H&P Keys**
Proximal muscle weakness, heliotrope rash (eyelid erythema), Gottron's papules (purple papules on knees and knuckles).

- **Diagnosis**
History and physical exam, creatine phosphokinase (CPK), Aldolase, skin and muscle biopsy, electromyogram (EMG).

- **Disease Severity**
In adults may herald internal malignant neoplasms.

- **Concept and Application**
Multisystem disorder with autoantibodies.

- **Management**
Topical and systemic steroids, rest, cytotoxic agents.

CREST
Calcinosis
Raynaud
Esoph. dysftn
Scleroderma
telangiectasia

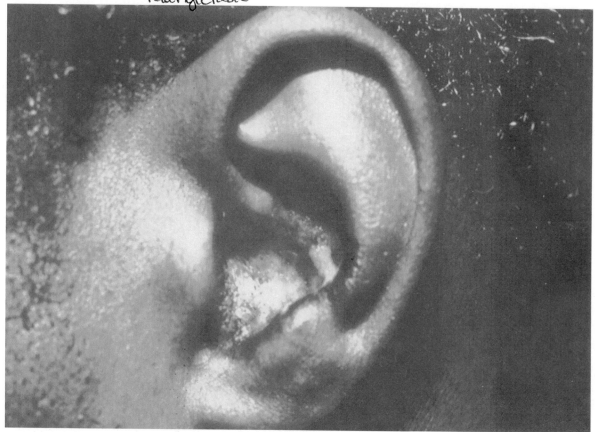

Figure 2–17. Discoid lupus erythematosus of the external auditory canal.

Scl 70

Localized morphea
Diffuse. progressive
systemic

3. Scleroderma

- **H&P Keys**
  Localized: morphea. *Diffuse:* progressive systemic sclerosis. Latter also associated with Raynaud's phenomenon, dysphagia, masklike face. Skin is tight, woody, bound down.

- **Diagnosis**
  History and physical exam, skin biopsy, ANA, anticentromere antibody, Scl-70 (antitopoisomerase).

- **Disease Severity**
  Progressive systemic sclerosis associated with multisystem involvement: renal, lung, esophagus. Variant: CREST = calcinosis, Raynaud's, esophageal dysfunction, sclerodactyly, telangiectasia; better prognosis; associated with anticentromere antibody.

- **Concept and Application**
  Unknown etiology. Excessive collagen deposition in skin and other organs.

- **Management**
  Symptomatic, physical therapy, penicillamine.

4. Livedo Reticularis

- **H&P Keys**
  Mottled, netlike vascular erythema; aggravated by cold exposure; most common in women under 40.

- **Diagnosis**
  History and physical exam.

- **Disease Severity**
  Associated disease: arteriosclerosis, collagen vascular disease, endocrine disorders, drugs (amantadine).

- **Concept and Application**
  Vasospasm of arterioles.

- **Management**
  Avoidance of cold exposure, treatment of associated medical conditions.

5. Amyloidosis, Systemic

- **H&P Keys**

Specific. Waxy papules or nodules on face, macroglossia.

Nonspecific. Purpura (most common), especially after proctoscopy, alopecia.

- **Diagnosis**
  Exam, biopsy (Congo red stain demonstrates amyloid in tissue).

- **Disease Severity**
  Systemic organ involvement, associated myeloma.

- **Concept and Application**
  Immunoglobulin-related amyloid deposited in skin and other organs.

- **Management**
  Symptomatic, possibly colchicine, possibly melphalan or prednisone.

6. Behçet's Disease

- **H&P Keys**

Triad. Aphthous ulcers, genital ulcers, uveitis.

Skin lesions. Erythema nodosum, ulcers.

- **Diagnosis**
  Clinical exam.

- **Disease Severity**
  Associated findings: arthritis, retinal vasculitis, cardiovascular and neurologic effects.

- **Concept and Application**
  No known etiology; more frequent in men.

- **Management**
  Systemic steroids, colchicine, azathioprine, chlorambucil, cyclophosphamide.

7. Tuberous Sclerosis

- **H&P Keys**
  Autosomal dominant, seizures, retardation. Skin lesions: white spots (ash-leaf macule, earliest lesion), adenoma sebaceum (Fig. 2–18), connective tissue nevi (shagreen patch), periungual fibrous tumors.

- **Diagnosis**
  History and physical exam, biopsy of adenoma sebaceum.

- **Disease Severity**
  Variable expression. Some patients may show cutaneous features only.

- **Concept and Application**
  Genetic multisystem disease.

- **Management**
  Control seizures, supportive management.

8. Necrobiosis Lipoidica

- **H&P Keys**
  Yellow-brown atrophic plaques on shins, may ulcerate.

- **Diagnosis**
  History and physical exam, biopsy.

- **Disease Severity**
  Most causes associated with diabetes.

- **Concept and Application**
  Necrosis of the lower dermis, with granulomatous inflammation and vasculitis.

- **Management**
  Topical and intralesional corticosteroids, antiplatelet agents.

9. Porphyria Cutanea Tarda

- **H&P Keys**
  Photosensitivity, blisters on backs of hands, scars, increased hair growth ("werewolf"), hyperpigmentation.

- **Diagnosis**
  Urine will fluoresce under Wood's light; blood, urine, stool studies for porphyrins; skin biopsy.

- **Disease Severity**
  May be hereditary, but induced by ethanol, estrogens, chloroquine, chlorinated phenols, iron. Diabetes in 25%.

- **Concept and Application**
  Uroporphyrinogen decarboxylase deficiency.

- **Management**
  Stop provoking drugs or chemicals, phlebotomy.

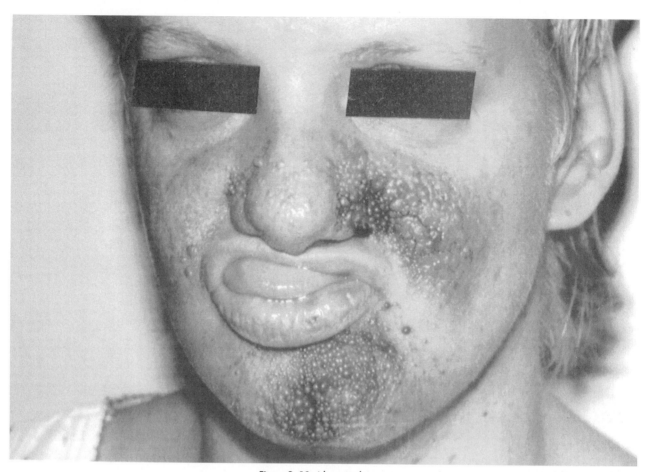

Figure 2–18. Adenoma sebaceum.

D. Cutaneous Signs of Internal Malignant Neoplasms

1. See dermatomyositis, sign of Leser-Trélat (seborrheic keratoses), keratoderma (tylosis).
2. Acanthosis nigricans (Fig. 2–19). Velvety brown patches on axillae and neck; associated with GI carcinomas (stomach), lung cancer, as well as obesity, endocrine disease.
3. Sweet's syndrome. Tender, vesicular papules and plaques on face, extremities, and upper trunk; may be associated with leukemia.
4. Cowden's syndrome (multiple hamartoma syndrome). Warty lesions on face (trichilemmomas), gums, hands, and feet; associated with breast cancer, thyroid tumors.
5. Gardner's syndrome (see lipomas). Large epidermal cysts, fibromas, lipomas, osteomas; autosomal dominant; polyps and carcinoma of GI tract.
6. Peutz-Jeghers syndrome. Frecklelike pigmented spots on lips, nose, fingertips; autosomal dominant; hamartomatous GI polyps; low frequency of malignancy.
7. Torres's syndrome. Benign and malignant sebaceous tumors of skin; high incidence of colon cancer; possibly autosomal dominant.
8. Multiple mucosal neuroma syndrome. Multiple neuromas (whitish nodules) on lips and anterior tip of tongue; medullary carcinoma of thyroid, pheochromocytoma, parathyroid adenomas (multiple endocrine neoplasia [MEN] type III); autosomal dominant.
9. Glucagonoma syndrome. Necrolytic migratory erythema (erosive, annular, intense erythema) around orifices, abdomen, thighs, and distal extremities; alpha cell tumor of pancreas.

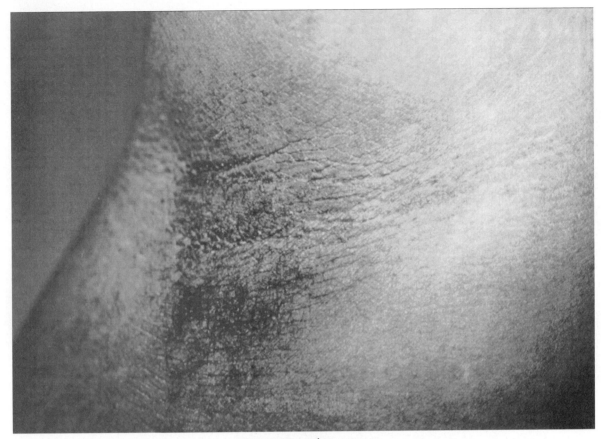

Figure 2–19. Acanthosis nigricans.

E. Nail Signs and Disease

1. Onycholysis. Nail plate lifts off nail bed; associated with trauma, psoriasis, hyperthyroidism.
2. Terry's nails. Proximal two thirds of nail is white; associated with low serum albumin, cirrhosis, congestive heart failure.
3. Splinter hemorrhages. Streaks of blood under distal portion of nail plate; associated with trauma, subacute bacterial endocarditis (SBE).
4. Beau's lines. Horizontal nail depressions (Fig. 2–20); associated with temporary arrest of nail growth from severe illness.
5. Clubbed nails. Overcurvature of nail plate and loss of nail-digit angle; associated with cardiopulmonary disease, cancer.
6. Muehrcke's nails. Two horizontal white stripes; associated with low albumin, nephrosis.
7. Yellow nails. Yellow discoloration of nail plate, no cuticles, associated with lymphedema, pulmonary effusion.
8. Half-and-half nails. White proximal half, distal brown nail; associated with chronic renal failure.

F. Diseases and Disorders of Newborns

1. Erythema toxicum neonatorum. Pinkish macules, papules, and pustules; self-limited.
2. Port-wine stain (nevus flammeus). Most often facial or neck (stork bite), flat vascular patch; associated with Sturge-Weber syndrome, particularly if it involves the upper eyelid; treatment with laser.
3. Café-au-lait macules. More than five are associated with neurofibromatosis.
4. Mongolian spot. Blue discoloration of sacrum; common in black races; no clinical significance or treatment.

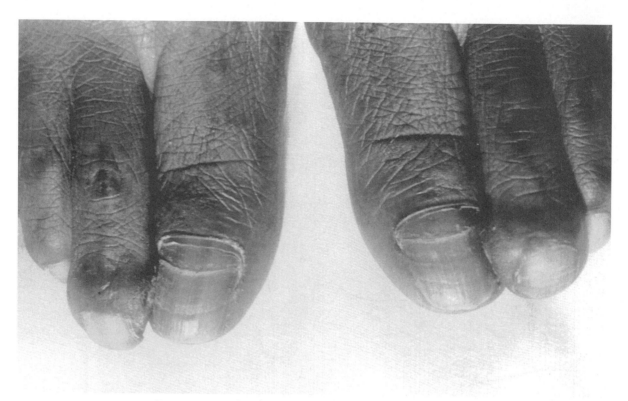

Figure 2–20. Beau's lines (patient had ruptured berry aneurysm 6 months previously).

5. Miliaria. Itchy red papules from blockage of sweat duct; aeration is critical; mild topical steroids.
6. Ataxia-telangiectasia. Telangiectasia of bulbar conjunctiva and skin; ataxia, bronchiectasis, IgA deficiency; autosomal recessive.

BIBLIOGRAPHY

Arnold HL, Odom RB, James WD. *Andrews' Diseases of the Skin, Clinical Dermatology.* 8th ed. Philadelphia: WB Saunders Co; 1990.

Fitzpatrick TB, et al. *Color Atlas and Synopsis of Clinical Dermatology.* New York: McGraw-Hill Book Co Inc; 1982.

Fitzpatrick TB, et al. *Dermatology in General Medicine.* 3rd ed. New York: McGraw-Hill Book Co Inc; 1987.

Portwine - Sturge Weber

3

Endocrinology

Doris G. Bartuska, MD, FACP, Joan Lit, MD, and Kurt S. Kodroff, MD

I. THYROID GLAND DISORDERS

A. Hyperthyroidism

1. Usually Autoimmune Graves' Disease

- **H&P Keys**

  Family history of thyroid disease, weight loss, palpitations, nervousness, muscle weakness, hot perspiration, dyspnea, increased bowel movements, change in menstrual pattern, eye symptoms (burning, tearing, diplopia, proptosis).

  Thyroid enlargement with a bruit, hyperactive reflexes, systolic hypertension, pretibial myxedema, onycholysis, proximal myopathy, systolic hypertension, ophthalmopathy.

  Hyperthyroidism in the elderly is seen in a toxic nodular goiter or single hyperfunctioning nodule. Cardiac manifestations are common (atrial fibrillation, congestive failure) and patient is apathetic rather than hyperkinetic.

- **Diagnosis**

  Levels of total or free thyroxine (T_4) (elevated), triiodothyronine (T_3) uptake (elevated), and thyrotropin (thyroid-stimulating hormone [TSH]) (suppressed). Estrogen in pills or pregnancy increases T_4-binding globulin; in this situation, the T_4 is increased and the T_3 uptake is decreased. Assay of thyroid antibodies may be performed to rule out Hashimoto's thyroiditis. An iodine (I) 123 thyroid uptake and scan can be performed if the diagnosis is not secure or if radioactive iodine therapy is planned.

- **Disease Severity**

  Tachyarrhythmia, atrial fibrillation, severe weight loss, mental status change, and fever, as in thyroid storm.

- **Concept and Application**

  Hypermetabolism and hyperkinesis resulting from autonomous thyroid hormone secretion. Decreased thyroid hormone production with antithyroid drugs and decreased autonomic nervous system hyperactivity with β-blocking drugs.

- **Management**

  Antithyroid drugs: methimazole or propylthiouracil. Beta-blockade with propranolol, metoprolol, atenolol, or radioactive iodine. Rarely, thyroid surgery after becoming euthyroid. Increased calories and vitamin intake.

B. Hypothyroidism

- **H&P Keys**

  Usually secondary to chronic autoimmune (Hashimoto's) thyroiditis, radioactive iodine treatment, or thyroid surgery. History of thyroid disease in the family, fatigue, weakness, cold intolerance, sleepiness, dry skin, hoarseness, constipation, depression, slow mentation, menstrual irregularities, infertility, weight gain.

  On physical examination, a firm goiter with multiple nodular (Hashimoto's disease) or a nonpalpable gland; bradycardia; myxedema; slow, hoarse speech; cool, dry, thick skin; delayed relaxation of deep-tendon reflexes; yellow skin (carotenemia); loss of scalp hair and eyebrows.

- **Diagnosis**

  Assay of TSH (elevated), total or free T_4 (low), thyroid antibodies, antimicrosomal antibodies (now called antithyroid peroxidase [TPO]), or antithyroglobulin to confirm Hashimoto's disease. If positive, these patients and their families have an increased incidence of other autoimmune diseases, such as Graves', pernicious anemia, rheumatoid arthritis, adrenal insufficiency, and premature menopause.

- **Disease Severity**

  Mental status: confusion, dementia, stupor, or coma; decreased ventilation and abnormal blood gases, hypothermia, cardiomyopathy, ataxia.

- **Concept and Application**

  Hypometabolic state caused by decrease or lack of thyroid hormone.

- **Management**

  Levothyroxine sodium (L-thyroxine [T_4]) is the treatment of choice. The dose is titrated according to the supersensitive TSH assay.

Adults usually need 0.1 to 0.125 mg PO/d. Older patients need 0.05 to 0.075 mg PO/d. If there is a history of cardiac disease, a lower initial dose is indicated (0.025). Drugs such as cholestyramine, antacids, and iron supplements interfere with T_4 absorption in the gastrointestinal (GI) tract. If dosages are readjusted, the patient should have a repeat T_4 and TSH in 6 weeks to assess the therapeutic response.

C. Neoplasms of the Thyroid Gland

- **H&P Keys**

Most thyroid nodules are benign. The most common cancer is papillary, followed by follicular, medullary with amyloid, and the most aggressive is anaplastic, which is more common in the elderly.

Family history, thyroid disease, head or neck irradiation as a child. May be single thyroid nodule or a large nodule in a multinodular gland. New-onset hoarseness: indirect laryngoscopy needed to rule out recurrent laryngeal nerve involvement.

- **Diagnosis**

Fine-needle aspiration for histocytopathologic examination. If specimen inadequate, repeat the aspiration. Assay of T_4, TSH, and thyroid antibodies to determine if patient has Hashimoto's thyroiditis with a lumpy thyroid. Baseline thyroid ultrasonogram to check nodule size and rule out a cyst. I 123 thyroid uptake and scan will reveal if the nodule is cold (more likely to be malignant) or hot. A thyroglobulin level is occasionally helpful as a tumor marker. If elevated, it can be rechecked after surgery and followed for recurrence of the tumor.

- **Disease Severity**

Size of thyroid nodule, nodes, hoarseness, metastases, or lung roentgenogram. Past history of head or neck irradiation.

- **Concept and Application**

None.

- **Management**

If frozen-section pathology specimen is benign at time of surgery, a subtotal thyroidectomy is performed. If the specimen is carcinoma, a total thyroidectomy and regional lymph node exploration is performed. I 131 ablation of any remaining thyroid tissue or metastases follows.

L-thyroxine is given for TSH suppression (less than 0.3 in the new supersensitive TSH assay) usually 0.125 to 0.175 mg PO/d.

II. PARATHYROID GLANDS

A. Hypercalcemia

- **H&P Keys**

Family history of hypercalcemia or renal stones and multiple endocrine neoplasia (MEN) types I or II. Many are asymptomatic or have fatigue, lethargy, nocturia, weakness, constipation, depression, or renal colic from renal stones.

- **Diagnosis**

Levels of calcium, phosphorus, intact parathyroid hormone. If a smoker, chest roentgenogram and assessment of parathyroid-hormone–related peptide and 1-25 hydroxy vitamin D for hypercalcemia resulting from granulomatosis diseases (eg, tuberculosis [TB] or sarcoid). Humoral hypercalcemia of malignancy, hyperparathyroidism, granulomatosis disease. Drugs: (calcium, vitamin A and D) thiazide, lithium. Rule out familial hypocalciuric hypercalcemia and renal failure.

- **Disease Severity**

Kidney stones, muscle weakness, peptic ulcer, pancreatitis, lethargy, confusion, stupor, or coma.

- **Concept and Application**

Tumors, such as lung carcinoma, producing humoral bone-resorbing factors or causing bone destruction, such as breast carcinoma, myeloma.

Primary hyperparathyroidism (adenoma or hyperplasia of all four glands) may be familial (autosomal dominant) as part of MEN I, which includes tumors of the pituitary and pancreas (insulinoma, gastrinoma), or MEN II, which includes hyperparathyroidism, pheochromocytoma, and medullary thyroid carcinoma.

- **Management**
Hydration (IV isotonic saline), diuresis (IV furosemide), plicamycin, calcitonin, glucocorticoids, or bisphosphonates. When the diagnosis is established, if surgery is indicated remove the neoplasm or neck exploration directed at the parathyroids. There may be postoperative hypocalcemia after parathyroid surgery, which should be treated with IV and PO calcium. Vitamin D may be needed.

III. PITUITARY GLAND

A. Anterior Pituitary

- **H&P Keys**
Galactorrhea, amenorrhea, infertility, visual changes (prolactinomas); enlargement of hands, jaw, feet (acromegaly); signs of Cushing's. May be a nonfunctioning adenoma presenting with visual changes, hypogonadism, fatigue, loss of axillary and pubic hair.

- **Diagnosis**
Assays of T_4, TSH (rule out hypothyroidism, which elevates prolactin levels). Prolactin level (rule out drugs acting on the central nervous system that elevate prolactin, eg, phenothiazines).

   Obtain a growth hormone and somatomedin C level. To rule out a corticotropin (previously adrenocorticotropic hormone [ACTH])-producing tumor, do an overnight dexamethasone suppression test (AM cortisol level should be less than four). May need a 24-hour urine-free cortisol test. Perform a magnetic resonance imaging test (MRI) with gadolinium of the pituitary and hypothalamus to find lesion, eg, neoplasm, vascular (infarction), infiltration (TB or sarcoid).

- **Concept and Application**
Tumors may be functioning, producing prolactin, growth hormone, ACTH, or TSH.

Some tumors (suprasellar craniopharyngioma, see calcifications) cause hypopituitarism by pressure necrosis of the pituitary or infiltration with a granulomatous disease.

- **Management**
Depends on the etiology. Bromocriptine for prolactinoma; the drug and transphenoidal surgery for macroprolactinoma with visual changes. Surgery for other adenomas, with possible addition of radiation therapy. Replacement therapy with hydrocortisone, T_4, sex steroids for hypopituitarism. Increased glucocorticoids for stress (infections, other surgery, anesthesia).

B. Posterior Pituitary

1. Diabetes Insipidus

- **H&P Keys**
Failure to concentrate urine, hypernatremia with thirst, polydipsia, polyuria.

- **Diagnosis**
Check intake of fluids and output of urine, urine and serum osmolality, and perform water deprivation test.

- **Concept and Application**
Caused by brain trauma, neurosurgery, sarcoid, brain tumors (pinealoma, craniopharyngioma), histiocytoses. Nephrogenic diabetes insipidus (no response to vasopressin) should be ruled out.

- **Management**
Hydration, depending on intake and output. Aqueous vasopressin injections and nasal spray desmopressin (DDAVP).

2. Syndrome of Inappropriate Vasopressin Secretion (SIADH), Hyponatremia

- **H&P Keys**
Inability to dilute urine, extracellular fluid expanded without edema, mental confusion, urine hypertonic to plasma. Rule out adrenal insufficiency, diuretic therapy, nephrosis cirrhosis, hypothyroidism, compulsive water drinking.

- **Management**
  Fluid restriction (less than 1 L/d) may need sodium chloride IV; for longer term, demeclocycline.

IV. ADRENAL GLAND

A. Adrenal Insufficiency

- **H&P Keys**
  Fatigue, weight loss, anorexia, nausea, vomiting, abdominal pain, hyperpigmentation, volume depletion.

- **Diagnosis**
  Electrolyte determination for hyponatremia, hyperkalemia, hypoglycemia. Low morning cortisol level. Cosyntropin (Cortrosyn) stimulation test.

- **Disease Severity**
  Hypotension or circulatory collapse, hypoglycemia, hyperkalemia, fever.

- **Concept and Application**
  Destruction of adrenal gland by autoimmune, infiltrative, or infectious etiology.

- **Management**

  Acute. Hydrocortisone 100 mg IV, followed by 100 mg IV every 8 hours, IV 5% dextrose, and normal saline solution (D5 NSS) or NSS to reverse hypotension and dehydration. Dexamethasone 4 mg (if diagnosis has not been established) or hydrocortisone 100 mg IV initially, followed by 100 mg IV every 6 hours (if known adrenal insufficiency).

  Chronic. Hydrocortisone in split dose morning and evening or long-acting glucocorticoids (prednisone, dexamethasone) at bedtime. Fludrocortisone 0.1 to 0.2 mg/d titrated to electrolytes and plasma renin activity. Instructions for additional medication during times of stress, febrile illness.

B. Cushing's Syndrome

- **H&P Keys**
  Centripetal obesity, violaceous striae > 1 cm wide, general and proximal muscle weakness, easy bruising, dorsocervical and supraclavicular fatty deposition, moon facies, plethora, menstrual irregularities, hirsutism, sexual dysfunction, hyperpigmentation.

- **Diagnosis**
  Elevated late afternoon cortisol levels. Baseline 24-hour urinary free-cortisol elevation. Elevated ACTH level. Dexamethasone suppression tests: overnight: 1 mg at 11 PM, serum cortisol at 8 AM; low-dose: 0.5 mg every 6 hours for 48 hours, with 24-hour urine collection for cortisol and 17-hydroxysteroids; high-dose: 2 mg every 6 hours for 48 hours, with 24-hour urine collection for cortisol and 17-hydroxysteroids. Computed tomographic scan (CT) or MRI of pituitary. CT of chest and abdomen. Petrosal sinus sampling.

- **Disease Severity**
  Rapidity of symptom onset, hypokalemia, congestive heart failure, paper-thin skin, osteoporosis.

- **Concept and Application**
  Overproduction of cortisol; ACTH-producing pituitary or carcinoid tumor, cortisol-producing adrenal adenoma, exogenous steroid use.

- **Management**

  Acute. Removal of source of excess hormone (transsphenoidal hyposphysectomy, adrenal adenectomy, removal of carcinoid tumor), pituitary irradiation. Postsurgical replacement dose of steroids until adrenal-pituitary axis resumes function.

  Chronic. Ketoconazole, aminoglutethimide, metyrapone, or mitotane for nonoperative cases.

C. Hirsutism

- **H&P Keys**
  Age of onset, rate of progression, family history. Terminal hair growth in central location (upper lip, chin, neck, chest), clitoromegaly, male-patterned baldness, menstrual irregularities, male body habitus.

- **Diagnosis**
  17-hydroxy Progesterone, dehydroepiandrosterone (DHEA-S), testosterone, cortisol levels. Thyroid function tests. CT of abdomen.

- **Disease Severity**
  Rapid onset of hair growth, menstrual irregularities, virilization, prepubertal or older age of onset.

- **Concept and Application**
  Overproduction of androgens of adrenal or gonadal origin (hyperplasia, tumor, exogenous); hypersensitivity of hair follicles to normal levels of androgens.

- **Management**

Acute. Removal of source of excess androgen.

Chronic. Electrolysis, bleaching. Spironolactone twice a day. Replacement hydrocortisone for cases of congenital adrenal hyperplasia.

D. Pheochromocytoma

- **H&P Keys**
  Episodes of pallor, palpitations, and headaches, orthostatic hypotension, tachycardia, labile hypertension, panic attacks. Personal or family history of medullary carcinoma of the thyroid, hyperparathyroidism, or other endocrine tumors.

- **Diagnosis**
  Supine and standing blood pressures, 24-hour urine collection for catecholamines, metanephrines, and vanillylmandelic acid (VMA), serum catecholamines, clonidine suppression testing, CT of adrenals or MRI of abdomen, methyliodobenzylguanidine imaging.

- **Disease Severity**
  Persistent severe hypertension, frequent episodes, increased duration of episodes.

- **Concept and Application**
  Tumor of enterochromaffin cells, which produce excessive amounts of catecholamines.

- **Management**

Acute. Alpha-blockade, phenoxybenzamine (dose adjusted to cessation of paroxysms and hypertension) for 10 to 14 days, followed by surgery to remove tumor; phentolamine or nitroprusside for acute hypertensive crisis. β-Blockade added only after establishment of α-blockade.

Chronic. Phenoxybenzamine, β-blockers, metyrosine (catecholamine synthesis inhibitor).

E. Congenital Adrenal Hyperplasia

- **H&P Keys**
  Family history of congenital adrenal hyperplasia, dehydration, hypotension, and salt wasting in infants; hirsutism; virilization; ambiguous genitalia; hypertension.

- **Diagnosis**
  Elevated levels of adrenal androgens, cortisol precursors, or mineralocorticoid precursors, depending on the specific enzyme abnormality.

- **Disease Severity**
  Hypotension, salt wasting, failure to thrive in infants; severe genital ambiguity.

- **Concept and Application**
  Complete or partial dysfunction of one of the enzymes utilized in the production of cortisol from cholesterol (21-hydroxylase, 11β-hydroxylase, 17α-hydroxylase, 3β-hydroxysteroid dehydrogenase, cholesterol side-chain cleavage enzyme). May be due to an absolute or relative absence of the enzyme or abnormal enzyme structure or function. Backup of enzyme substrates causes the clinical sequelae associated with each specific enzyme abnormality.

- **Management**

Acute. Aggressive fluid repletion, hydrocortisone IV every 6 hours.

Chronic. Infants and children: assignment of gender. Replacement dose steroids, with lowest possible dose to ensure adequate hormone concentrations and minimize growth-retarding potential of steroid therapy. Surgical reconstruction of genitalia toward assigned gender.

Adults (partial enzyme blockages): Treatment of hirsutism with electrolysis, spironolactone. Replacement dose glucocorticoids if menstrual irregularities interfere with desired fertility.

V. CLINICAL LIPOPROTEIN DISORDERS

A. Type I Familial Chylomicronemia

- **H&P Keys**
  Childhood presentation with abdominal pain or acute pancreatitis; eruptive xanthoma, hepatosplenomegaly.

- **Diagnosis**
  Increased triglycerides (>1000), cloudy plasma, lipoprotein electrophoresis.

- **Disease Severity**
  Development of diabetes mellitus.

- **Concept and Application**
  Deficiency of lipoprotein lipase or its cofactor (apo C-II).

- **Management**
  Very-low-fat diet (<20 g/d), supplemental medium-chain triglycerides, alcohol avoidance.

B. Type II Hyperlipoproteinemia

- **H&P Keys**
  Premature coronary artery disease (CAD), tuberous and tendinous xanthomas, corneal arcus.

- **Diagnosis**
  Lipoprotein measurements with elevated low-density lipoprotein (LDL) alone (type IIa pattern) or elevated LDL and triglycerides (type IIb.)

- **Disease Severity**
  Family history, age of onset of CAD, degree of lipid elevation.

- **Concept and Application**
  Three distinct diseases: familial hypercholesterolemia (defect in LDL receptor), familial combined hyperlipidemia (overproduction of apoprotein B100), polygenic hypercholesterolemia.

- **Management**
  Low-fat and low-cholesterol diet, drug therapy with niacin, cholestyramine, HMG-CoA reductase inhibitors alone or in combination; gemfibrozil may be used but not in combination with HMG-CoA (hydroxymethylglutaryl coenzyme A) reductase inhibitors.

C. Type III Dysbetalipoproteinemia

- **H&P Keys**
  Obesity, palmar xanthomas, premature CAD.

- **Diagnosis**
  Elevated cholesterol and triglycerides; lipoprotein analysis shows elevated very-low-density lipoprotein (VLDL) and intermediate-density lipoprotein (IDL), VLDL-cholesterol and plasma triglyceride ratio below 0.30.

- **Disease Severity**
  Presence of premature CAD.

- **Concept and Application**
  Abnormality in apolipoprotein E.

- **Management**
  Weight loss, screening for hypothyroidism, niacin, or gemfibrozil, alcohol avoidance.

D. Type IV Hyperlipoproteinemia

- **H&P Keys**
  May be obese, presence of CAD, gallstones.

- **Diagnosis**
  Elevated triglycerides, elevated VLDL, decreased high-density lipoproteins (HDL); rule out renal disease, diabetes with appropriate tests.

- **Disease Severity**
  Premature CAD.

- **Concept and Application**
  Autosomal dominant inheritance as familial hypertriglyceridemia or familial combined hyperlipidemia.

- **Management**
  Weight loss, diet low in cholesterol and saturated fat, alcohol and estrogen avoidance; niacin or gemfibrozil.

E. Type V Hyperlipoproteinemia

- **H&P Keys**
  Obesity, history of pancreatitis; eruptive xanthomas, hepatosplenomegaly.

- **Diagnosis**
  Elevated triglycerides, cloudy plasma, increased chylomicrons and VLDL.

- **Disease Severity**
  History of recurrent pancreatitis, diabetes.

- **Concept and Application**
  Multiple molecular defects.

- **Management**
  Weight reduction, low-fat diet, gemfibrozil, niacin.

F. Decreased High-Density Lipoprotein

- **H&P Keys**
  Often associated with states of increased triglycerides.

- **Diagnosis**
  Lipid profile, electrophoresis with low alpha region.

- **Disease Severity**
  Presence of premature CAD.

- **Concept and Application**
  Multiple defects.

- **Management**
  Risk factor modification, possible drug therapy.

G. Elevated Lp(a) Lipoprotein

- **H&P Keys**
  None.

- **Diagnosis**
  Electrophoresis.

- **Disease Severity**
  Premature CAD, stroke.

- **Concept and Application**
  LDL-like particle but with apo B-100 linked to a glycoprotein (apo [a]), which is structurally similar to plasminogen; may be prothrombotic.

- **Management**
  Risk factor modification; efficacy of drug therapy undetermined.

VI. DIABETES MELLITUS

A. Type I

Insulin-dependent, juvenile-onset.

- **H&P Keys**
  Younger patients, before age 20, Type I diabetes includes 10% of all patients with diabetes. Weight loss, polyphagia, polydypsia, polyuria, nausea, abdominal pain, and recent infection. Diabetic ketoacidosis (DKA) 30% to 50% concordance rate in identical twins.

- **Diagnosis**
  Blood sugars >140 mg/dL on two occasions, glucose can be as high as 1000 with ketoacidosis (low bicarbonate, low Pco_2, K^+ may be high, serum and urine ketones are positive, and glycosylated hemoglobin is high).

- **Disease Severity**
  DKA, tachycardia, fever, poor skin turgor, lethargy, Kussmaul's respirations (deep, regular, frequent), stupor, coma. Presence of retinopathy, cardiomyopathy, atherosclerosis, nephropathy, neuropathy, angina, or previous myocardial infarction.

- **Concept and Application**
  Insulin lack, increased lypolysis, free fatty acids, and ketones. Glucagon excess, decreased malonyl CoA, and increased ketones. HLA types on chromosome 6 increase risk (HLA-DR3 and HLA-DR4). Viral infection of the pancreas with mumps, coxsackie, rubella. Autoimmune destruction of the B cells with lymphocytic infiltration. Antibodies to the islet cells are found. Can be associated with other autoimmune diseases such as Hashimoto's thyroiditis.

- **Management**
  American Diabetes Association (ADA) diet: carbohydrates, 55% to 60%; protein, 15% to

20%; fat <30%. Tight control to normalize blood sugar and lipids. The Diabetes Control and Complications Trial (DCCT) has shown that near normalization of blood sugar prevents the microvascular complications and neuropathy and nephropathy.

Insulin (split-mixed regimen) before breakfast and dinner, regular and intermediate (2/3 AM, 1/3 before dinner). Glycosylated hemoglobin (HbA1c) 7% with home glucose monitoring (before food 90 to 100 mg/dL and after meals less than 180). Regular insulin in addition to normalize blood sugar. Some patients prefer the insulin pump instead of multiple injections.

Exercise for weight reduction, increasing insulin sensitivity, and improving cardiovascular health (DKA); regular insulin (insulin pump or multiple dose); hydration; K^+ replacement; treatment of any infection.

B. Type II

Non–insulin-dependent, non–ketosis-prone, mature onset; includes 90% of patients with diabetes mellitus.

• **H&P Keys**
Family history, obesity, limited exercise, polyuria, polyphagia, polydipsia, weakness. Consider other causes of hyperglycemia, eg, Cushing's syndrome, hyperthyroidism, growth hormone excess, steroid drugs, chronic pancreatitis, cystic fibrosis.

• **Diagnosis**
Fasting blood sugar >140 mg/dL, 2 hours after eating >200. Consider pregnancy and steroid use. Glycosylated hemoglobin over 7%.

• **Disease Severity**
Similar to those in type I but less severe retinopathy, neuropathy, nephropathy (use angiotensin-converting enzyme [ACE] inhibitors in patients with hypertension and/or microalbuminuria). Vascular disease; because of high incidence of heart disease, treat all risk factors (hyperlipidemia, hypertension, obesity, smoking, lack of exercise).

• **Concept and Application**
Multiple defects. Patients overweight; impaired insulin secretion and insulin resistance, with increased glucose production in the liver and decreased glucose uptake in muscle and adipose tissue.

• **Management**
ADA diet (weight reduction as needed), exercise, low-fat diet or lipid-lowering agent, oral agents (glipizide, metformis, acarbose, glyburide, glimepiride). Intensive diabetes education and home glucose monitoring, and insulin with or without the oral sulfonylureas. Antihypertensive drugs, foot care, and regular urine testing for microalbuminuria, ophthalmologic exam. Prevention by maintaining ideal body weight and exercise.

C. Hyperosmolar Hypercalcemic Nonketotic Coma (HHNK)

• **H&P Keys**
Usually an elderly patient has an infection or cardiovascular accident and water intake is decreased, resulting in severe dehydration from an osmotic diuresis, which increases the hyperglycemia and causes prerenal azotemia. Other causes include high-protein tube feedings, peritoneal dialysis, high carbohydrate intake. Blood sugars are high, with low bicarbonate and normal plasma ketones (lactic acidosis). Serum osmolality is high. The average fluid deficit is 10 L.

• **Management**
Hydrations with isotonic saline, then half-strength saline. When plasma glucose approaches normal, 5% dextrose to increase free water is given. Insulin (low dose) to control hyperglycemia.

D. Hypoglycemia

• **H&P Keys**
In patients who do not eat or after eating (reactive) develop anxiety, sweating, hunger, headache, palpitations, blurred vision, irritability, pallor, nausea, diminished mental acuity, convulsions, syncope. Past history of gastrointestinal surgery, malab-

sorption, or use of insulin or an oral hypoglycemic agent.

- **Diagnosis**
Simultaneous measurement of glucose, insulin, C peptide, and urine sulfonylurea metabolites during an episode of hypoglycemia; may need hospitalization for a 72-hour fast. Insulin antibodies can be determined.

    Causes include drugs (insulin, sulfonylureas, ethanol, pentamidine, etc). Liver disease, renal failure, adrenal or pituitary insufficiency, insulinoma, malnutrition, cancers that make an insulinlike growth factor.

    Blood sugars less than 45 mg/dL in men and less than 35 in women with symptoms, which improve with an increase of plasma glucose (Whipple's triad).

- **Disease Severity**
Lethargy, coma, seizures, syncope. In diabetes, symptoms may be masked if autonomic neuropathy is present or if the patient is on β-blockers.

- **Concept and Application**
Imbalances between hepatic production and glucose utilization. Increased utilization (insulinoma, exogenous insulin, sulfonylureas). Glucose overutilization by other tumors (sarcoma, fibroma, hepatoma, etc). Diminished glucose production from alcoholism, liver disease, adrenal or pituitary deficiency.

- **Management**
Depends on the level of blood sugar and symptoms. If mild, frequent meals and snacks. Treatment of the underlying cause. Decreased dose of insulin or sulfonylurea. When severe, 50 mL of 50% glucose in water IV, then infusion of 10% glucose to keep plasma glucose >100 mg/dL. Glucagon injection (1 mg) not effective if hepatic glycogen stores are depleted. Surgery for an insulinoma or a nonpancreatic carcinoma. Diazoxide and octreotide have been used.

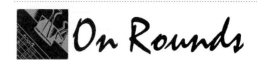
On Rounds

Adrenal Disorders

Adrenal Insufficiency
- Symptoms include fatigue, weight loss, anorexia, hyperpigmentation
- Diagnosis by electrolytes (hyponatremia, hyperkalemia) and Cortrosyn stimulation test
- Caused by autoimmune, infiltrative or infectious disorders
- Treatment includes hydrocortisone

Cushing's Syndrome
- Symptoms include centripetal obesity, violaceous striae, proximal muscle weakness, moon facies, fatty deposits on back
- Diagnosis by elevated late afternoon cortisol, dexamethasone suppression test, CT/MRI of the pituitary
- Treatment includes removal of source of excess hormone (surgery or irradiation)

Congenital Adrenal Hyperplasia
- Symptoms include hirsutism, virilization, ambiguous genitalia, hypertension, hypotension
- Diagnosis by elevated adrenal androgens, cortisol precursors or mineralocorticoid precursors
- Treatment includes fluids, hydrocortisone

BIBLIOGRAPHY

Bierman EL, Glomset JA, eds. Disorders of lipid metabolism. In: Wilson J, Foster I, eds. *Williams Textbook of Endocrinology.* 8th ed. Philadelphia: WB Saunders Co; 1992.

Brewer AB. Lipids. In: *A Review of Endocrinology: Diagnosis and Treatment.* Endocrine Fellows Foundation; 1993.

DeGroot LJ. *Endocrinology.* Philadelphia: WB Saunders Co; 1995; 1, 2, 3.

Felig P. *Endocrinology and Metabolism.* 3rd ed. New York: McGraw-Hill; 1995.

Greenspan FS. *Basic and Clinical Endocrinology.* 2nd ed. East Norwalk, CT: Appleton-Century-Crofts; 1986.

Ingbar SH. *The Thyroid: A Fundamental and Clinical Text.* 6th ed. Philadelphia: JB Lippincott; 1991.

Layon JA. *Fluids and Electrolytes.* In: *Critical Care.* Philadelphia: JB Lippincott; 1988.

Lebovitz H. *Therapy for Diabetes Mellitus and Related Disorders.* 2nd ed. Alexandria, VA: American Diabetes Association Inc; 1994.

Mahley RW, Weisgraber KH, Innerarity TL, et al. Genetic defects in lipoprotein metabolism. *JAMA.* 1991; 265: 78–83.

Scanu AM, Lawn RM, Berg K. Lipoprotein (a) and atherosclerosis. *Ann Intern Med.* 1991;115:209–218.

Scriver CR. *The Metabolic Basis of Inherited Disease.* 7th ed. New York: McGraw-Hill; 1995.

Speroff L. *Clinical Gynecologic Endocrinology and Infertility.* 5th ed. Baltimore, MD: Williams & Wilkins; 1995.

Thompson JS. *Genetics in Medicine.* Philadelphia: WB Saunders Co; 1986.

Williams *Textbook of Endocrinology* Wilson J, Foster D, eds.. 8th ed. Philadelphia: WB Saunders Co; 1992.

4

Diseases and Disorders of the Digestive System

Margaret R. Khouri, MD, FACP

I. ESOPHAGUS

[handwritten: Alcohol/tob - sp cell / Barretts - esoph adeno]

A. Malignant Neoplasms of the Esophagus

- **H&P Keys**
  Progressive dysphagia, substernal pain, odynophagia, anorexia, and weight loss, cough caused by aspiration or tracheoesophageal fistula, guaiac-positive stool, and iron-deficiency anemia.

- **Diagnosis**
  By combining endoscopic brush cytology with multiple endoscopic biopsies, the diagnostic yield is 90% to 99%. Endoscopic fine-needle aspiration cytology for cancers of the intra-abdominal esophagus.

- **Disease Severity**
  Endosonography is superior to computed tomography (CT) for assessing esophageal wall penetration and regional node involvement. CT scanning to assess distant organ involvement of liver and lungs.

- **Concept and Application**
  Predisposing conditions: Achalasia, lye stricture, head and neck squamous carcinoma. Use of alcohol and tobacco increases the risk of squamous cell carcinoma. Barrett's esophagus (columnar epithelium arising in an esophagus damaged by reflux esophagitis) is a major risk for developing esophageal adenocarcinoma.

- **Management**
  Survival correlates best with TMW staging. Most patients present with metastasized disease, a poor prognosis. Surgical treatment offers best chance for cure and good quality of swallowing. Radiation and/or chemotherapy may improve survival. Only half the patients have resectable disease,

Chemoradiation - Sq cell.

and in up to 75% the resection is palliative. Combined chemotherapy and radiation therapy may be efficacious for squamous cell cancer. Therapeutic endoscopic procedures are best for advanced esophageal cancer. Endoscopic intubation with self-expandable metallic stents, laser and bipolar coagulation may be tried.

B. Esophagitis   *MUSE*

- **H&P Keys**
  Heartburn and regurgitation of sour material into the throat, water brash, dysphagia, odynophagia, chest pain, cough, laryngitis, asthma, bronchitis, pneumonitis.

Hyper reflux
Hyper secretins

- **Diagnosis**
  No single test can assess all aspects of disease: Endoscopy to assess tissue damage and presence of Barrett's metaplasia, prolonged ambulatory pH monitoring to show reflux, correlate symptoms and atypical manifestations (laryngitis, asthma, noncardiac chest pain) with reflux episodes, and monitor response to therapy, manometry to assess peristalsis and lower esophageal sphincter function.

- **Disease Severity**
  Endoscopy establishes the presence and severity of esophagitis and its complications. Metaplasia, ulcers, strictures, erosions (MUSE). Ambulatory pH monitoring assesses extent of acid exposure (% of time pH <4).

- **Concept and Application**
  Transient relaxations of the lower esophageal sphincter (LES) are the dominant mechanism responsible for gastroesophageal reflux. Gastric acid is the major factor leading to esophageal mucosal damage. Most individuals with reflux are "hyperrefluxers" rather than "hypersecretors" of acid.

- **Management**
  Symptoms rarely remit spontaneously. H$_2$-antagonists (cimetidine, ranitidine, famotidine, nizatidine) have been the cornerstone of treatment. The proton pump inhibitors, lansoprazole and omeprazole will produce more complete acid suppression and heal-

ing. Patients with gastroesophageal reflux disease have a high relapse rate (60% to 80% within 1 year) unless therapy is continued. Proton pump inhibitors with or without the prokinetic cisapride are more effective than H$_2$-antagonists with or without cisapride in preventing recurrence.

C. Motor Disorders of the Esophagus: Achalasia, Scleroderma Esophagus, and Diffuse Esophageal Spasm

- **H&P Keys**
  A history of dysphagia is the most frequent complaint when ingesting solids and liquids simultaneously or when ingesting liquids alone. Chest pain, heartburn, pulmonary symptoms, chronic cough, hoarsness, and globus sensation.

- **Diagnosis**
  Esophageal manometry to characterize (1) peristaltic performance, (2) contractile force, (3) LES basal pressure, and (4) LES relaxation. Upper endoscopy or barium esophagram excludes strictures, obstruction.

- **Disease Severity**
  Secondary weight loss, anemia, nutritional compromise, and pulmonary problems.

- **Concept and Application**

  Achalasia. Failure of relaxation of LES resulting in functional obstruction to passage of food and fluid.

  Scleroderma. Aperistaltic esophagus, absent LES tone, and free reflux. If untreated may lead to complications of reflux disease.

  Diffuse Esophageal Spasm. Some peristalsis, diffuse and simultaneous nonperistaltic contractions with up to 30% of swallows.

- **Management**
  Achalasia responds to pneumatic dilatation, local botulinum toxin injection or surgery (myotomy). Scleroderma responds to aggressive management of gastroesopha-

geal reflux; diffuse esophageal spasm may respond to dietary changes and therapy with calcium channel blockers. Diffuse esophageal spasm is managed with dietary changes, and calcium channel blockers.

II. STOMACH

A. Gastric Cancer

- **H&P Keys**
  Paucity of early symptoms; advanced disease: epigastric pain, early satiety, abdominal bloating, meal-induced dyspepsia.

- **Diagnosis**
  Endoscopic biopsy and brush cytology give a positive diagnostic yield in 97% to 100% of cases.

- **Disease Severity**
  Physical exam of abdomen, rectum, vagina, and lymph nodes. Endosonography for preoperative T and N staging. CT scanning of chest, abdomen, and pelvis to assess distant organ involvement.

- **Concept and Application**
  Increased risk with adenomatous gastric polyps, atrophic gastritis, autoimmune gastritis, pernicious anemia, hypertrophic gastropathy (Ménétrier's disease), or primary immunodeficiency. Patients with gastric cancer are more likely to have had *Helicobacter pylori* infection within 20 years.

- **Management**
  Surgery for cure for early gastric cancer. Palliative surgery, with adjuvant or neoadjuvant chemotherapy (5-fluorouracil alone, or cisplatin, etoposide, and doxorubicin) for advanced or disseminated disease.

B. Gastric Ulcer

- **H&P Keys**
  Two major etiologic factors: chronic nonerosive (type B) gastritis caused by *H. pylori* infection and nonsteroidal anti-inflammatory drugs (NSAIDs). Nonradiating abdominal pain localized to epigastrium and relieved by food is classic. Some patients present with perforation or acute hemorrhage without antecedent pain.

- **Diagnosis**
  Evaluate with upper endoscopy with brush cytology and at least six biopsies to exclude a small (1% to 3%), but definite, risk of gastric cancer. Endoscopic biopsy is the definitive test for *H. pylori*. Histologic examination or culture may also be used.

- **Disease Severity**
  Complications include hemorrhage, perforation, penetration, obstruction, and intractability.

- **Concept and Application**
  Peptic ulcer disease (gastric or duodenal) usually is associated with *H. pylori* infection. Patients with peptic ulcer disease without *H. pylori* infection were probably using NSAIDs.

- **Management**
  Discontinue NSAIDs. If NSAIDs are required ulcers will heal with standard acid suppression therapy. Prophylactic misophyostil 200 mg BID will reduce recurrence if chronic NSAIDs fail. Treatment regimens for *H. pylori* involve antimicrobial drugs combined with acid-suppressing agents. Traditional "triple therapy" was the first therapeutic regime that proved to be effective in promoting healing and eradicating the infection. Problems with "triple therapy" included metronidazole resistance, frequent side effects, and poor patient compliance. Newer and less complicated regimens have emerged. See Table 4–1 for triple therapy regime and alternative emergent regimens.

C. Duodenal Ulcer

- **H&P Keys**
  Epigastric pain, nonradiating, relieved by food. Pain that awakens patient from sleep, usually between 12 and 3 AM.

- **Diagnosis**
  Upper gastrointestinal (GI) endoscopy and biopsy to document *H. pylori* infection by

TABLE 4–1. TREATMENT OF *H. PYLORI* IN PEPTIC ULCER DISEASE (DUODENAL AND GASTRIC ULCER)

Drug	Dosage (mg/tabs)	Frequency	Weeks	Success Rate (%)
Traditional "triple therapy"				
Metronidazole	250	TID	2	85–98
Tetracycline	500	QID	2	
Bismuth subsalicylate	2 tabs	QID	2	
Ranitidine	300	Once	6	
Emerging therapies				
Metronidazole	500	BID	1 or 2	>90
Clarithromycin	250	BID	1 or 2	
Omeprazole*	20	BID	1 or 2	
Amoxicillin	750	TID	2	80–95
Omeprazole*	40	TID	2	
Clarithromycin	500	BID	2	80–95
Lansoprazole	30	BID	2	
Amoxicillin	1 g	BID	2	

* lansoprazole can be substituted for omeprazole.

urease test or upper GI radiography. Serologic tests for *H. pylori* if biopsy not performed. Serologic tests alone may be misleading by failing to distinguish patients with nonulcer dyspepsia, GE reflux, irritable bowel syndrome (IBS), and coincidental *H. pylori* infection from ulcer patients.

- **Disease Severity**
  Complications include hemorrhage, perforation, penetration, and obstruction. Refractory ulcers in three settings: noncompliance, continued heavy smoking, and unsuspected hypersecretory disorders, such as gastrinoma (Zollinger-Ellison [Z-E] syndrome).

- **Concept and Application**
  H. pylori infection is strongly associated in 90% to 95% of cases. *H. pylori* is an essential cofactor. *H. pylori*–negative duodenal ulcer is rare (<2%–5%) and may be due to Crohn's disease, Z-E syndrome, and aspirin or NSAID use.

- **Management**
  1. Eradicate *H. pylori* (see Table 4–1).
  2. Document clearance at 6 weeks by en-

doscopic biopsy for urease test or histology.

Serology is not helpful to document clearance as antibody remains present for several months (serologic scar). Maintenance therapy with H_2-receptor antagonist may be indicated for: those over 65, with previous complications (hemorrhage or perforation), with known aggressive ulcer disease, with history of frequent recurrences, who are heavy smokers, with concomitant serious disease that increase the hazards of complications or surgical procedures (eg, cardiac, renal, respiratory, or hepatic failure), or with coincident therapy with drugs that damage the duodenal mucosa, such as NSAIDs and potassium chloride.

D. Gastritis and Duodenitis

- **H&P Keys**
  Epigastric pain, nausea, and vomiting upper GI bleeding; however, most cases are asymptomatic.

- **Diagnosis**
  Endoscopy and biopsy are more sensitive than double-contrast radiology for all forms of gastritis and duodenitis. Schilling test to assess vitamin B_{12} absorption in patients with chronic atrophic gastritis.

- **Disease Severity**
  Endoscopy.

- **Concept and Application**
  H. pylori is the leading cause of gastric and duodenal mucosal inflammation. Acute erosive injury to gastroduodenal mucosa is caused by noxious agents such as NSAIDs, alcohol, potassium chloride, chemotherapy drugs. Autoimmune gastritis and pernicious anemia cause malabsorption of vitamin B_{12}. Less common causes of gastroduodenal inflammation are Crohn's disease, tuberculosis (TB), idiopathic granulomatous gastritis, and cytomegastovirus (CMV) in HIV patients.

- **Management**
  Avoidance of conditions and agents that cause noxious injury to the mucosa. Indi-

cations for eradication of *H. pylori* are currently limited to the coexistence of peptic ulcer and gastric lymphoma (primary B-cell lymphoma).

E. Delayed Gastric Emptying

- **H&P Keys**
  Typical symptoms are: Postprandial fullness, bloating, distention, nausea, late postprandial vomiting of undigested food.

- **Diagnosis**
  Exclude mechanical obstruction with endoscopy or barium radiography. Solid-phase radionuclide gastric emptying scan is the standard test.

- **Disease Severity**
  By physical examination. Look for dehydration, metabolite and electrolyte abnormalities, malnutrition, vomiting, lab (complete blood count [CBC], albumin, total protein, electrolytes and others).

- **Concept and Application**
  Regulation of gastric emptying is a complex and multifactorial phenomenon. Common in diabetics, postsurgical states, and many acute illnesses.

- **Management**
  Avoid medications that inhibit gastric emptying. Modify diet (small meals), treat underlying disorder, and prokinetic drugs (cisapride, metaclopramide, bethenecol).

III. SMALL INTESTINE

A. Acute Enteric Infections

- **H&P Keys**
  Most acute watery diarrheas are caused by infectious agents acquired by fecal-oral transmission. *Recognize epidemiologic clues:* Classical relationships between vehicle and disease, certain unusual foods represent greater risk, high-risk groups: travelers to developing nations, vacationers in the United States, especially campers, homosexuals, prostitutes, intravenous drug abusers. Other than infectious agents, the differential diagnosis of acute watery diarrhea includes accidental ingestion of toxins such as organophosphates, Paraquat, poisonous mushrooms, and medications.

Correlate Signs and Symptoms with Pathophysiology. Patients with acute diarrhea of small bowel origin complain of nausea, vomiting, abdominal pain that is generally mild, crampy, and diffuse; watery diarrhea is of large volume (>1 L). Other symptoms include headache, malaise, anorexia, arthralgias, myalgias, vomiting, chills, and rarely low-grade fever. Dehydration tends to be severe only in the very young and very old.

- **Diagnosis**
  Organisms that typically cause acute watery diarrheal disorders, such as enteropathogenic and enterotoxigenic *Escherichia coli* are not routinely sought by stool culture. Illness is typically mild and self-limited, requiring only symptomatic therapy in most individuals. Diagnostic evaluation may be indicated in the setting of community outbreak and when the illness is severe.

- **Disease Severity**
  Parameters of severity include: prolonged duration (>3 days), severe volume depletion; or impaired host.

- **Concept and Application**
  Watery diarrhea is caused by toxin-producing organisms, either via a preformed toxin or from a toxin elaborated after adherence. Preformed toxins cause vomiting within 4 hours of ingestion, another useful clue to the diagnosis. Both the invasive organisms that cause minimal inflammation, such as the enteric and the organisms that adhere, infect, or colonize, such as the enteropathogenic and enteroadherent *E. coli*, protozoa, such as *Giardia*, cryptosporidia, and helminths.

- **Management**
  Assess the degree of dehydration and replace fluid and electrolyte deficits. Alert patients are given oral rehydration solutions: Infants and children: 50–100 mL/kg over 4

Dermatitis Herpetiformis [handwritten annotation]

to 6 hours; adults require up to 1000 mL per hour. Replace stool loss plus insensible losses until diarrhea stops. Bismuth subsalicylate (Pepto-Bismol) is safe and efficacious for acute bacterial diarrhea. Opiates and anticholinergics impair motility and may prolong the elimination of microbes and are not indicated.

Antibiotic Therapy. Indicated for traveler's diarrhea, cholera, pseudomembranous colitis, parasites, and sexually transmitted infections; also immunosuppressed patients, debilitated patients with malignancy, patients with valvular or vascular prostheses, hemolytic anemia, and those with prolonged or relapsing course.

Also usually indicated for: Camplobacteriosis, *Aeromonas, Plesiomonas,* noncholera vibrios, protracted *Yersinia,* and in nursery school outbreaks of enteropathogenic *E. coli.*

B. Celiac Disease (Gluten Sensitivity)

[handwritten annotation: IgG antigliadin (AGA); IgA antiendomyial antibody]

- **H&P Keys**
  Bulky, pale, foul-smelling stools, abdominal distention, borborygmi, flatus, cramps, weight loss, fatigue, weakness, anemia. Children present with failure to thrive. The majority of patients (approximately 60%) have latent disease. IgG antigliadin antibody (AGA) and IgA antiendomyial antibody are the most sensitive and specific screening tests. Use of these tests is justifiable in screening populations at increased risk. Elevated levels of antireticulin antibody (ARA) is the most sensitive predictor for disease latency, especially in asymptomatic relatives of probands and in screening patients with insulin-dependent diabetes mellitus (IDDM). Higher risk in persons with affected first-degree relative, patients with IDDM, connective tissue disorders, Sjögren's syndrome, and autoimmune thyroid diseases.

- **Diagnosis**
  Low serum carotene level, increased qualitative fecal fat excretion as indicated by Sudan III stain, low D-Xylose absorption test, small-intestine mucosal biopsy. Patients with dermatitis herpetiformis may also have gluten sensitivity.

- **Disease Severity**
  Weight loss, malnutrition, osteogenic bone disease, anemia, hemorrhage caused by malabsorption of vitamin K, neurologic and neuropsychiatric manifestations. Complications include malignant disease, especially lymphoma, refractory sprue, ulcerative jejunoileitis, hyposplenism with splenic atrophy and neuropathy.

- **Concept and Application**
  Ingestion of wheat gluten and similar proteins in rye, barley, and oats in genetically susceptible individuals leads to damage to small intestine mucosa and malabsorption of most nutrients. Environmental factors (nutrient deficiency, metabolic stress, infection, tumor) may precipitate symptoms. Ingestion of milk products may aggravate symptoms as a secondary lactase deficiency develops with extensive intestinal disease.

- **Management**
  Gluten-free diet, lifelong. Improvement usually noted within 48 hours, although may take weeks or months to achieve full remission. Clinical symptoms improve before histologic return to normal mucosal architecture. Supplemental iron, folate, zinc, vitamin D. Lack of improvement within 6 to 8 weeks prompts search for inadvertent ingestion of gluten.

IV. COLON

A. Invasive Diarrhea

- **H&P Keys**
  Crampy lower abdominal pain, tenesmus, stool bloody or mucoid, volume <1 L/d; fecal leukocytes are usually seen. History of prior administration of antibiotics suggests *Clostridium difficile* as causative agent. Systemic symptoms may provide a clue to the diagnosis: Hemolytic uremic syndrome

(hemolytic anemia, uremia, renal failure and differentiated intravascular coagulation [DIC]) occurs with both *Shigella* and enterohemorrhagic *E. coli*. Reiter's syndrome (arthritis, urethritis, and uveitis) occurs after *Salmonella*, *Shigella*, *Campylobacter*, and *Yersinia* infections. Guillain-Barré sydrome occurs after *Campylobacter jejuni* infection.

- **Diagnosis**
Stool studies for bacterial pathogens, ova, and parasites, stool cytotoxin assay for *C. difficile*. Proctosigmoidoscopy may show erythema, ulceration, hemorrhage, or pseudomembranes, yellow-white, raised plaques characteristic of pseudomembranous colitis associated with *C. difficile*.

- **Disease Severity**
Fever, tachycardia, volume depletion, leukocytosis, abdominal distention, guarding, tenderness, decreased bowel signs, signs of toxemia; development of peritoneal signs suggests progression to toxic megacolon.

- **Concept and Application**
Invasive organisms cause histologic damage and may also produce signs and symptoms of systemic infection. Species of *Shigella*, *Salmonella*, *Campylobacter*, *Yersinia*, *Clostridium*, and *Entamoeba histolytica* produce invasive diarrhea.

  - **Management**
Barium enema can make symptoms worse and should be avoided. Oral rehydration in mild disease, intravenous hydration for the more severely ill. Antibiotic therapy with vancomycin or metronidazole for *C. difficile*, ciprofloxacin or trimethoprim sulfamethoxazole for *Shigella*. Other enteric infections, such as *Campylobacter* and intestinal *Salmonella*, are self-limited and usually don't require antibiotics. Antidiarrheals, which may delay clearance of the pathogen, should be avoided.

B. Irritable Bowel Syndrome (IBS)

- **H&P Keys**
Abdominal pain and altered bowel habits with symptoms continuous or intermittent for at least 3 months. Six symptoms more commonly associated with IBS than other GI disorders are: abdominal distention, pain with bowel action, more frequent stools with the onset of pain, passage of mucus, and the sensation of incomplete evacuation. Obtain a dietary history, review medications, exclude symptoms that are suggestive of organic disease, such as: weight loss, fever, blood in stool.

- **Diagnosis**
No abnormalities on standard laboratory tests (CBC, chemistry panel, erythrocyte sedimentation rate), normal flexible sigmoidoscopy and normal histology on mucosal biopsy. If diarrhea is predominant symptom: consider lactose deficiency, examine stool for ova and parasites, fecal leukocyte, and fat by Sudan stain; assess thyroid function. Symptoms suggestive of upper GI or biliary tract disease should be evaluated with appropriate endoscopic, radiographic, or ultrasonographic studies.

- **Disease Severity**
Symptom severity, restriction of daily activities.

- **Concept and Application**
A chronic disorder considered functional with identifiable structural or biochemical abnormalities. Related disorders include noncardiac chest pain, nonulcer dyspepsia, and biliary dyskinesia.

- **Management**
Establish a therapeutic physician–patient relationship. Educate patient about the benign nature of the illness and excellent long-term prognosis. Physical exercise, avoidance of foods that exacerbate symptoms, fiber supplements, and mild anticholinergic drugs to control crampy pain, opiate-type drugs (diphenoxylate hydrochloride with atropine sulfate or loperamide hydrochloride) to control diarrhea. If pain is the predominant symptom low-dose tricyclic antidepressants may be helpful.

C. Colorectal Carcinoma

- **H&P Keys**
  Abdominal pain, change of bowel habits, iron-deficiency anemia, rectal bleeding, fecal occult blood test.

  Assessment of Risk. Increased risk of colorectal cancer in persons with affected first-degree relative, multiple affected relatives, and younger age of diagnosis. Risk also is increased if first-degree relative has breast, uterine, prostate, or ovarian cancer and in families with adenomatous polyposis of the colon and rectum (APC) mutations and polyposis typical of familial adenomatous polyposis. Increased risk in patients with previous adenomas or cancer and in patients with IBS, especially ulcerative colitis with pan colitis >7 years or left-sided colitis >10 years. Increased risk also in hereditary nonpolyposis colorectal carcinoma (Lynch syndromes I and II).

- **Diagnosis**
  Yearly rectal examination and testing evacuated stool for occult blood. Flexible sigmoidoscopy every 3 to 5 years in asymptomatic patients beginning at 50 years. Screening colonoscopy for patients at increased risk every 1 to 3 years. APC patients also require DNA testing, ophthalmoscopy, and search for other extracolonic manifestations.

- **Disease Severity**
  Full colonoscopy if adenoma is found on flexible sigmoidoscopy. Once colon cancer is diagnosed, curative therapy requires resection. Preoperative evaluation includes full colonoscopy to exclude a second primary cancer, CT scan of the abdomen and pelvis, and CBC. Tumor-associated antigens (carcinoembryonic antigen [CEA]), tissue plasminogen activator (TPA), and carcinomatous antigen 19-9 (CA 19-9) are tumor markers.

- **Concept and Application**
  Colorectal cancer is second most frequent cause of death from cancer in the United States. Most carcinomas arise from adenomatous polyps (adenoma-carcinoma sequence). Adenomatous polyps are considered premalignant, whereas hyperplastic polyps are not.

- **Management**
  Preoperative radiation for rectal cancers, resection of isolated pulmonary and hepatic metastases. Adjuvant chemotherapy after surgery for patients with stage C disease (regional lymph node involvement with no distant metastasis).

D. Appendicitis

- **H&P Keys**
  Abdominal pain, typically midabdominal at onset, anorexia, onset of nausea and vomiting, followed by the relocation of pain to right lower quadrant, elevated temperature. On physical examination, localized or diffuse tenderness, signs of peritonitis.

- **Diagnosis**
  CBC with white blood cell count with differential, urinalysis, serum beta human chorionic gonadotropin (hCG) if female. Abdominal roentgenogram is occasionally helpful; ultrasonography of the right lower quadrant for periappendiceal fluid, edema, or abscess.

- **Disease Severity**
  Onset of peritoneal signs indicates surgical intervention required.

- **Concept and Application**
  Acute inflammation, obstruction with abscess formation and possible rupture. A significant cause for morbidity and mortality particularly in children and the elderly. Mortality significantly increased with free perforation.

- **Management**
  Appendectomy.

E. Inflammatory Bowel Disease (IBD): Ulcerative Colitis (UC) and Crohn's Disease (CD)

- **H&P Keys**
  Dominant symptom in UC is diarrhea, usually bloody, and tenesmus. In CD of

the small intestine, colicky pain, bloating, weight loss, fever, perianal disease (fissures, fistulas, and perirectal abscesses); less commonly, hematochezia. Risk of second case in first-degree relatives is >15%. Extra-intestinal manifestations include sclerosing cholangitis, ankylosing spondylitis, colitic arthritis, pyoderma gangrenosum, erythema nodosum, uveitis, and episcleritis.

- **Diagnosis**
Exclude acute enteric infections (*Clostridium difficile, Shigella, Salmonella, E. coli*) and chronic enteric infections (*Campylobacter, Yersinia*, amebiasis, and TB), acute venereal infections (gonorrhea, syphilis, lymphogranuloma venereum, and chlamydia). Endoscopic examination at initial presentation to establish diagnosis and define extent of disease. Differentiation of UC from CD based on clinical presentation, roentgenographic, endoscopic, and histologic findings.

- **Disease Severity**
Frequency and severity of diarrhea, systemic signs and symptoms (fever, hypotension, tachycardia), anemia. Complications: Perforation, stricture, toxic megacolon, abscesses and fistulas, obstruction, perianal disease.

- **Concept and Application**
Pathogenesis is unknown, but genetic and environmental factors play a role. Increased risk for cancer of the bowel in patients with IBD. Most observations have concerned cancer complicating UC; more and more data support a similar risk in CD.

- **Management**
Determined by extent and severity of disease. Sulfasalazine for mild to moderate acute and chronic colitis; for sulfa-intolerant, 5-amino salicyclic acid (ASA) preparations: 5-ASA linked via azo linkage (olsalazine [Dipentum]); pH-dependent release of 5-ASA–coated granules (Pentasa, Asacol); Rowasa enemas. Corticosteroids for acute management of moderate to severe UC and CD. Fulminant colitis requires addition of broad-spectrum antibiotics (in-

corporating metronidazole). Metronidazole for perianal disease. Immunosuppressives (azothiaprine, 6-mercaptopurine) for fistulas and disease poorly controlled by corticosteroids. Nutritional support. Colectomy for UC unresponsive to medical therapy cures UC. Other indications for colectomy: high-grade dysplasia found at multiple sites or low-grade dysplasia found on three or more consecutive examinations. Surgery in CD for complications: fistulas, obstruction, abscess, toxic megacolon, since risk of recurrence is high. Surveillance colonoscopy at 1- to 2-year intervals after 7 years of symptoms and extensive colitis in patients with UC and after 13 years with left-sided colitis.

F. Ischemic Bowel Disease

- **H&P Keys**   PAIN OUT DROP TO EXAM Thumbprinting
Typically in patients over age 60 with significant cardiac disease; may have history of "intestinal angina," arrhythmias, recent myocardial infarction, previous arterial emboli; rheumatic heart disease, atherosclerotic heart disease predispose. In early occlusive mesenteric ischemia, acute crampy abdominal pain out of proportion to physical findings, spontaneous evacuation. Pain with absence of defecatory urge in nonocclusive ischemia. Other signs: Vomiting, diarrhea, abdominal distention, hyperperistalsis, tenderness, hematochezia. For thrombotic disease of mesenteric veins, predisposing conditions include peritonitis, abdominal inflammation, trauma, portal hypertension, intra-abdominal tumors, coagulopathy, oral contraceptives.

- **Diagnosis**
Hemoconcentration, leukocytosis, elevated amylase levels; abdominal roentgenograms may show "thumbprinting caused by submucosal hemorrhage and edema; visceral arteriography to exclude acute thromboses.

- **Disease Severity**
Abdominal tenderness, distention, leukocytosis, hemoconcentration, bloody peritoneal transudate, metabolic acidosis (late).

- **Concept and Application**
Four syndromes: Acute mesenteric infarction, ischemic colitis, focal ischemia, and intestinal angina. Infarction results from abrupt arterial occlusion. Nonocclusive ischemia results from poor perfusion. Venous thrombosis has a more insidious course.

- **Management**
Early intervention for acute occlusive disease of arteries or veins. Treatment for nonocclusive ischemia: bowel rest, fluids, antibiotic therapy resulting in complete resolution in 50%, healing with stricture in 30%, and gangrenous gut requiring resection in 20%.

G. Intestinal Obstruction

- **H&P Keys**
Crampy, spasmodic abdominal pain, vomiting, borborygmi, abdominal distention, obstipation; can develop slowly (months or years) or acutely (over hours). With mechanical obstruction, distress is apparent by extreme restlessness. With ileus, pain is usually less severe. Careful inspection of skin; palpation of umbilicus, lower-trunk inguinal, and femoral areas to detect hernias, intra-abdominal masses, hepatosplenomegaly; rectal and vaginal exam for masses and occult blood. Bowel sounds are infrequent and hypoactive in ileus. In obstruction, bowel sounds become loud, high-pitched, and hyperactive.

- **Diagnosis**
Biochemical and hematologic tests including CBC; levels of amylase, alkaline phosphatase, aspartate aminotransferase, alanine aminotransferase, lactate dehydrogenase; acid–base balance; roentgenographic obstruction series, including plain films of the abdomen to localize the level of obstruction, upright chest film in the lateral and posteroanterior views to detect pneumonia, free air, air-fluid levels. Use barium for retrograde studies but avoid barium if perforation is a possibility. CT scan may be helpful. Endoscopy to visualize and obtain tissue for biopsy from obstructing lesions

in the esophagus, stomach, duodenum, rectum, and large intestine.

- **Disease Severity**
Fever, rebound tenderness, leukocytosis, unexplained hyperamylasemia.

- **Concept and Application**
Most common causes of obstruction in adults are adhesions and hernias in the small bowel and cancer in the colon.

- **Management**
Decompression via nasogastric tube for either obstruction or ileus. Complete obstruction requires urgent surgery to detect strangulation, resect necrotic bowel, and preserve viability of adjacent bowel as soon as preoperative fluid and electrolyte resuscitation and nasogastric decompression are established.

H. Diverticulitis

- **H&P Keys**
Acute onset of left lower quadrant pain, fever; palpable sigmoid mass on physical examination.

- **Diagnosis**
Leukocytosis, roentgenographic obstruction series, ultrasonographic or CT imaging. As the process resolves, endoscopic studies or barium studies to exclude sigmoid carcinoma.

- **Disease Severity**
Persistent fever, rebound tenderness, leukocytosis, abdominal distention suggests peritonitis or bowel obstruction.

- **Concept and Application**
Colonic diverticula are herniations of mucosa and submucosa through the colonic muscle at sites where arteries penetrate the muscle. High prevalence (over one third of Americans over 60) attributed to lack of dietary fiber. When diverticulitis occurs, a diverticulum perforates, causing inflammation and abscess of pericolonic tissue. Fistulas to bladder or bowel can occur.

- **Management**
In absence of peritonitis, initial treatment is bowel rest and parenteral antibiotics; 70%

respond with no further episodes. Abscess, fistulas, or bowel obstruction require surgery in 20% to 30%.

I. Constipation

- **H&P Keys**
Onset and duration of complaint: constipation present from birth or neonatal period suggests congenital disorder; recent onset demands a workup for organic disorders. Frequency of defecation, defecatory difficulties such as excessive straining, discomfort, sense of incomplete evacuation. Drug history. Careful physical examination with abdominal palpation for distention, retained stool, prior surgical procedures, autonomic dysfunction; anorectal and perineal examination.

- **Diagnosis**
Flexible sigmoidoscopy and barium enema; exclude metabolic and endocrine disorders such as diabetes mellitus, hypothyroidism, hypercalcemia, hypokalemia; exclude muscular collagen vascular and neurogenic disorders. Anal manometry and full-thickness rectal biopsies when Hirschsprung's disease is suspected.

- **Disease Severity**
Colonic transit studies, defecography and anal manometry for patients with severe constipation who have not responded to simple dietary measures.

- **Concept and Application**
Impairment in large-bowel transit can be a primary motor disorder, in association with a large number of diseases and a side effect of many drugs.

- **Management**
Adequate dietary fiber, behavioral approaches, biofeedback, discouragement of routine use of laxatives except bulk-forming agents.

J. Peritonitis

- **H&P Keys**
Severe abdominal pain and rigidity, intercostal breathing, fever, tachycardia, hypovolemia, tenderness on direct and referred palpation, voluntary guarding, tenderness on rectal and pelvic exams, tenderness on percussion, loss of liver dullness, decrease or absence of bowel sounds.

- **Diagnosis**
Leukocytosis with left shift or leukopenia, hemoconcentration, metabolic acidosis, hyperkalemia, paralytic ileus or free air.

- **Disease Severity**
Suppurative peritonitis has abrupt onset and relatively short course with rapid progression. Mortality from fluid shifts, hypovolemia, and septic shock with resultant renal, respiratory, cardiac, and hepatic failure.

- **Concept and Application**
Common causes are intra-abdominal organ disease such as appendicitis, diverticulitis, perforating carcinoma, perforating ulcer, and trauma. Mortality results from fluid shifts and endotoxin that may cause hypovolemia and septic shock.

- **Management**
Fluid and electrolyte resuscitation, surgical repair of primary process and removal of debris, systemic antibiotics with careful monitoring of cardiac reserve via Swan-Ganz catheter, blood pressure, arterial blood gas determination, Foley catheter for recording urine volume, nasogastric intubation to decompress stomach, supplemental oxygen.

K. Familial Mediterranean Fever (Recurrent Polyserositis)

- **H&P Keys**
Autosomal recessive genetic disorder affects Armenians, Arabs, and Sephardic Jews. Most common manifestation is peritonitis. In 90% the first manifestation occurs at the end of the second decade.

- **Diagnosis**
No specific test. Six diagnostic features: fever, serositis, amyloidosis, ethnic background, family history, and exclusion of other causes. Unless a strong family history is obtained, the diagnosis is often made at laparotomy, where diffuse inflammation of serosal surfaces without other intra-

(handwritten margin notes at top:)
(1) Bulge but do not protrude
(2) prolapse strain/def - return spon
(3) Gut def - ...... digital reduct
(4) Irreducible

abdominal pathology are seen. No bacteria are cultured. Appendectomy is indicated so that future episodes can be differentiated from acute appendicitis.

- **Disease Severity**
  In most patients, the disease is relatively benign. Attacks precipitated by a variety of factors. Complications include amyloidosis, degenerative arthritis, renal vein thrombosis, narcotic addiction.

- **Concept and Application**
  Recurring inflammation of any serosal surface including peritoneum, pleura, pericardium, meninges, and synovial membranes.

- **Management**
  Colchicine treatment may prevent and ameliorate acute attacks and prevent amyloidosis.

V. RECTUM

A. Malignant Neoplasm of Rectum

See Colorectal Carcinoma

B. Hemorrhoids

- **H&P Keys**
  Anal discomfort, pruritus ani, fecal soiling, prolapse, bleeding, pain.

- **Diagnosis**
  Flexible sigmoidoscopy or colonoscopy. Occult bleeding in the stool requires a complete colonic evaluation, regardless of the presence of hemorrhoids. Hemorrhoids are classified according to their degree of protrusion or prolapse. First-degree bulge into the lumen of the anorectal canal on anoscopy but do not protrude out of the anus. Second-degree hemorrhoids prolapse out of the anus with defecation or straining but reduce to normal anatomic position spontaneously. Third-degree hemorrhoids prolapse out of the anus with defecation or straining and require digital reduction. Fourth-degree are irreducible and are at risk for strangulation.

- **Disease Severity**
  Acute, severe bleeding may require transfusion; chronic bleeding can cause iron-deficiency anemia. External hemorrhoid thrombosis can be extremely painful and must be distinguished from strangulated hemorrhoids, which are larger and more circumferential. Strangulated hemorrhoids cause significant pain and usually have an external and internal component and occur secondary to prolapse, with subsequent lack of blood supply. Progression to gangrene with resultant infection is life-threatening.

- **Concept and Application**
  Hemorrhoids result from dilatation of the superior and inferior hemorrhoidal veins. Internal hemorrhoids are lined with rectal mucosa and arise from the superior hemorrhoidal cushion above the mucocutaneous junction (dentate line). External hemorrhoids arise from the inferior hemorrhoidal venous plexus below the mucocutaneous junction and are lined by perianal squamous epithelium.

- **Management**
  Thrombosis of external hemorrhoids and mild bleeding of internal hemorrhoids: Treat with sitz baths, two to three per day. Bed rest to minimize additional thrombosis and swelling, stool-softening agents, topical therapy with anesthetic ointments and witch hazel–impregnated pads. Strangulated hemorrhoids require immediate surgical therapy. Other treatment options include rubber band ligation for third- and fourth-degree hemorrhoids and hemorrhoidectomy for strangulated hemorrhoids.

C. Anal Fissure

- **H&P Keys**
  Severe pain during or after defecation associated with scant, bright red rectal bleeding. Most commonly found in young and middle-aged adults.

- **Diagnosis**
  Inspection after spreading the buttocks; anoscopy difficult without topical anesthe-

sia. Linear tears perpendicular to dentate line.

- **Disease Severity**
Can progress to chronic fissure.

- **Concept and Application**
Because elliptical anal sphincteric fibers offer less muscular support posteriorly, 90% occur posterior midline. Lateral tears suggest underlying disease (IBD, proctitis, leukemia, carcinoma).

- **Management**
High-fiber diet and adequate fluid intake. Topical anesthetic preparations for symptomatic relief. Warm sitz baths to relax the anal sphincter. Chronic fissures (>6 weeks) usually require surgical therapy.

D. Anorectal Abscess

- **H&P Keys**
Acute pain and swelling. Pain in absence of swelling with small intersphincteric or pelvorectal abscesses. Sitting, movement, defecation increase pain. Antecedent history of constipation, diarrhea, trauma. Fever; malaise; purulent, foul-smelling drainage. Associated medical diseases include diabetes, hypertension, heart disease, IBD, neutropenic state as a result of hematologic malignancy.

- **Diagnosis**
Inspection of the perineum reveals redness, heat, swelling and tenderness, drainage from infected crypt orifice. Rectal examination is difficult without anesthesia.

- **Disease Severity**
Delay in making the diagnosis can lead to necrotizing anorectal infection and increases risk of overwhelming sepsis.

- **Concept and Application**
Obstruction, stasis, and infection of anal glands is most common cause. Obstruction may occur as a result of trauma, eroticism, diarrhea, hard stools, foreign bodies.

- **Management**
Abscesses require drainage; superficial abscesses can be drained under local anesthetic in outpatient setting. All others re-

quire drainage in operating room with anesthesia and surgical instrumentation. Antibiotics not necessary for otherwise healthy patients. Perioperative antibiotics for patients with underlying disease such as acute leukemia, valvular heart disease, diabetes. Postoperative management: Inspection to ensure proper healing, sitz baths, analgesia, bulk-forming agents to soften stool.

E. Anorectal Fistula

- **H&P Keys**
Chronic purulent drainage. Prior history of anorectal abscess. Pain with defecation but not as severe as with anorectal abscess or anal fissure. Perianal skin may be excoriated.

- **Diagnosis**
Inspection of the perineum usually reveals a red, granular papule from which pus is expressed. Anoscopy and sigmoidoscopy to identify primary orifice and proctocolitis.

- **Disease Severity**
Multiple secondary openings suggest either Crohn's disease or hidradenitis suppurativa.

- **Concept and Application**
Primary orifice is at level of dentate line. Secondary orifice is anywhere else on the perineum.

- **Management**
Anorectal fistula is approached surgically, with postoperative care similar to anorectal abscess. Anorectal disease as a manifestation of Crohn's disease requires special consideration. Metronidazole will heal perineal Crohn's disease. Discontinuation of therapy is associated with flaring of disease.

F. Pilonidal Disease

- **H&P Keys**
Pain, swelling, drainage midline skin lesion of internatal or gluteal cleft seen most commonly in young men.

- **Diagnosis**
Inspection: characteristic midline location. Appearance and lack of communication

with anorectum distinguish pilonidal disease from anorectal fistula and hidradenitis suppurativa.

- **Disease Severity**
Acute abscess versus chronic drainage.

- **Concept and Application**
Common acquired lesion of coccygeal skin, possibly induced by local stretching forces. Small skin pits secondarily invaded by hair precede development of draining sinus or abscess.

- **Management**
Acute pilonidal abscess requires incision, drainage, and hair removal. Chronic draining pilonidal lesions require surgical closure.

VI. GALLBLADDER

A. Acute Cholecystitis

- **H&P Keys**
Pain in epigastrium, shifting to right upper quadrant after 3 hours, may radiate to back; tenderness; guarding and a Murphy's sign (inspiratory arrest elicited when palpating the right upper quadrant); nausea, vomiting; fever, usually low-grade.

- **Diagnosis**
Mild leukocytosis (WBC ~ 12 000–16 000 cells/mm^3), serum bilirubin, alkaline phosphatase, and amylase may be elevated, usually less than twice the normal range.

    Ultrasound is the preferred initial screening study for acute cholecylitis. Cholescintigraphy is reserved for patients with normal ultrasonography but strong clinical suspicion of acute cholecystitis.

- **Disease Severity**
Secondary bacterial infection can progress to empyema, gangrene, perforation.

- **Concept and Application**
Most common cause of acute cholecystitis is obstruction of a distended gallbladder with concentrated bile. Acalculus (5% to 10%) occurs in setting of major surgery, critical illness, extensive trauma, and burns.

- **Management**
Standard treatment is cholecystectomy after resuscitation, stabilization and initiation of appropriate antibiotic regime.

B. Cholelithiasis

- **H&P Keys**
Biliary pain, nausea, vomiting. Predisposing factors include obesity, oral contraceptives, pregnancy, clofibrate, ileal disease or resection, and genetic factors.

- **Diagnosis**
Ultrasonography has more than 90% sensitivity in diagnosing gallstones.

- **Disease Severity**
Biliary pain lasting for more than 3 hours indicates progression to cholecystitis.

- **Concept and Application**
Cholesterol gallstones constitute 85% of all gallstones. Bile that is supersaturated with cholesterol can lead to formation of cholesterol gallstones.

- **Management**
Asymptomatic stones require no treatment. Symptomatic gallbladder stones are treated with cholecystectomy. Oral bile acid therapy (Ursodiol) is a treatment option for mildly symptomatic patients with small (<10 mm) cholesterol stones within a functioning gallbladder. Common bile duct stones, particularly in the elderly and those with comorbid disease are best treated via endoscopic retrograde cholangiopancreatography (ERCP).

C. Choledocholithiasis and Acute Suppurative Cholangitis

- **H&P Keys**
Biliary pain, involving the central upper abdomen, jaundice, chills and rigors (Charcot's triad), mild hepatomegaly, occasional rebound.

- **Diagnosis**
Leukocytosis with a left shift, mild elevation of serum transaminases and alkaline

phosphatase, hyperbilirubinemia, serum amylase level. Ductal dilatation documented by ultrasonography or CT. Lack of dilatation does not exclude obstruction. Gold standard is ERCP for diagnosis and management. Magnetic resonance cholangiopancreatogram (MRCP) and spiral CT provide excellent images of common duct stones and are among available noninvasive alternatives to diagnostic ERCP.

- **Disease Severity**
  Progression to ascending cholangitis and endotoxemia with shock, liver abscess.

- **Concept and Application**
  Gallstones passing into the common duct can lead to acute obstruction, bile stasis, bacterial infection.

- **Management**
  Initial resuscitation and stabilization, systemic antibiotics to cover *E. coli*, *Klebsiella*, *Pseudomonas*, and enterococci. Removal of obstruction via ERCP, and possible papillotomy, followed by active instrumentation for ductal clearance. If multiple large common-duct stones cannot be removed in one session, temporary drainage must be established via placement of stent or nasobiliary catheter to control biliary sepsis.

[handwritten margin note: E coli Klebsiella Pseud Enterococci]

VII. LIVER

A. Hepatitis

- **H&P Keys**
  Pertinent information: Age, gender, race, preceding episodes, history of chronic liver disease or cirrhosis, alcohol consumption (Table 4–2), drug and toxin exposure (include herbal as well as "traditional" medications), occupation and work environment, sexual history, immunologic and nutritional status, immunizations, travel history, and family history.

  Hepatitis may present with a flu-like or serum sickness syndrome, anorexia, malaise, fever, arthralgia, arthritis, rash, and/or angionecrotic edema, with or without

TABLE 4–2. CAGE QUESTIONNAIRE

1. Have you tried to *C*ut down on your drinking?
2. Are you *A*nnoyed by criticism of your drinking?
3. Do you fell *G*uilty about your drinking?
4. Do you need an *E*ye opener each morning?

Scoring: 1 point for each yes answer. A total of 2 or more indicates a likelihood of underlying alcoholism.

jaundice, dark urine, light stools, abdominal discomfort. Nonspecific constitutional symptoms may be present for a short or protracted time.

Physical findings may be subtle or nonexistent. Findings are often reflective of the duration and severity of liver disease and are common to all forms of hepatitis and include jaundice, hepatomegaly (typically mild), lymphadenopathy, ascites, splenomegaly, encephalopathy. Some findings are typically associated with alcoholic liver disease: palmar erythema, Muehrcke's lines and white nails, Dupuytren's contracture, parotid and lacrimal gland enlargement.

- **Diagnosis**
  The diagnosis requires hepatocellular necrosis, as reflected in the serum aminotransferase levels, aspartate aminotransferase (AST), and alanine aminotransferase (ALT), which are the most sensitive indicators of liver injury. In acute hepatitis, the ALT and AST are the first of the routine biochemical tests to become abnormal and the last to return to normal. Normal ALT and AST exclude the diagnosis of acute hepatitis.

  Although no features unequivocally distinguish one form of hepatitis from another, the pattern of aminotransferase elevations may provide a clue. In alcoholic hepatitis, the AST is typically two to three times greater than the ALT, and neither level is greater than 400 IU/L or eight times normal. In acute viral hepatitis, the aminotransferases are usually greater than 400 IU/L but less than 3000 to 4000 IU/L. Values greater than 4000 IU/L almost al-

[handwritten margin note: EtOH AST 2:3X > ALT]

ways indicate toxic or vascular injury to the liver.

[handwritten margin note: IgM]

Acute Viral Hepatitis. When suspected, virus-specific serologic tests for HBV (HBsAg, Hbc IgM), HAV (HAV IgM), HCV (anti-HCV IgM) are useful for differentiating among potential viral etiologies (Table 4–3).

Alcoholic Hepatitis. When suspected: Fever, anorexia, malaise, tender hepatomegaly, splenomegaly, encephalopathy, AST > ALT, increased gamma-glutamyl transpeptidase (GGTP), MCV, leukocytosis, electrolyte abnormalities.

Drug-Induced Hepatotoxicity. Always Suspect. Any drug is a potential culprit. However, the likelihood that a drug is responsible is greatest when the liver injury begins beween 5 and 90 days of taking the first dose and within 15 days of taking the last dose. A 50% or greater decline in the ALT within 8 days of stopping the drug without a further rise within 30 days also is suggestive of drug-induced hepatitis. Certain drugs have a well-documented association with the development of liver injury (Table 4–4).

[handwritten margin note: 10g/d — TAG/ Alcohol 2g/d]

Acute acetaminophen hepatotoxicity follows the ingestion of massive amounts of the drug for either suicidal or therapeutic intent (usually greater than 10 g/d). Chronic use of ethanol increases an individual's susceptability to acetaminophen hepatotoxicity at standard therapeutic doses (<2 g/d).

Other important causes of hepatotoxicity include drugs, mushroom poisoning, industrial chemicals, and environmental toxins (Table 4–5).

TABLE 4–3. DIAGNOSTIC SEROLOGY FOR ACUTE VIRAL HEPATITIS

Serology		
Preliminary	Confirmatory	Diagnosis
+Anti-HAV	+IgM anti-HAV	Acute hepatitis A
+HbsAg	+IgM anti-HBc	Acute hepatitis B*
+Anti-HCV	+RIBA, HCV RNA	Hepatitis C (acute or chronic)

* Get Anti-HDV if risk factors.

TABLE 4–4. PATTERNS OF HEPATOTOXICITY

Type of Reaction	Examples
Direct reaction	Acetamiophen, carbontetrachloride, mushrooms, phosphorus
Idiosyncratic reaction	Isoniazid, disulfiram, propylthiouracil
Toxic-allergic reaction	Halothane, isoflurane, ticrynafen
Allergic hepatitis	Phenytoin, amoxicillin-clavulanate, sulfonamides
Chronic hepatitis	Nitrofurantoin, methyldopa
Alcoholic hepatitis-like	Amiodarone, valproic acid

• **Concept and Application**

Hepatitis, a necroinflammatory process of the liver parenchyma, can be either acute (<6-month duration) or chronic (>6-month durations). Acute hepatitis can resolve, progress to hepatic failure, or continue as chronic hepatitis leading to cirrhosis and hepatocellular carcinoma.

A variety of pathogenic mechanisms may cause hepatitis, including viral infection, toxic injury, autoimmune and hereditary disorders.

Viral Hepatitis. Can be caused by infection with the hepatotropic hepatitis viruses A–E (HAV, HBV, HCV, HDV, HEV) and the non-A–E viruses. HAV and HEV can cause only acute viral hepatitis. HBV, HCV, HDV causes both acute and chronic viral hepatitis, cirrhosis, and hepatocellular cancer. HDV is dependent on HBV for both survival and replication. HDV induces illness only in the presence of HBV, either by coinfection or superinfection. HEV, an RNA virus, reported in developing nations in areas of poor sanitation after flooding, is similar to HAV but car-

TABLE 4–5. SOME IMPORTANT INDUSTRIAL AND ENVIRONMENTAL TOXIC CAUSES OF HEPATITIS

Chemical	Uses
Arsenic	Pesticides and in production of ceramics, drugs, dyes, fireworks, paint, petroleum, ink, and semiconductors
Carbon tetrachloride	Degreasers, fat processors, fire extinguishers, fumigant, insecticides, refrigerants, lacquer, ink propellants, rubber and wax
Tetrachloroethylene	Dry-cleaning agent, fumigant, solvent, degreaser
Yellow phosphorus	Munitions, explosives, fertilizers, rodenticides, semiconductors, luminescent coatings

ries a higher mortality, particularly in pregnant women. Non-A–E viral hepatitis has two distinct profiles: (1) a parenteral or community-acquired hepatitis with a benign course, and (2) a persistent viral infection that may have a fulminant course.

Alcohol-Induced Liver Injury. No particular quantity of alcohol is predictive of alcoholic liver disease. The incidence of serious liver disease begins to rise when the daily consumption of alcohol exceeds 60 g/d for men and 20 g/d for women. In addition to habitual alcohol consumption, other factors that predispose to alcohol-induced liver disease include: female gender, race, coexposure to other drugs, coinfection with the hepatotrophic viruses HBV and HCV, nutritional status, and immune dysfunction.

Drugs. Drugs causing liver injury can be "predictable," or "direct," hepatotoxins and "unpredictable," or "idiosyncratic," hepatotoxins. Direct hepatotoxins produce injury in a predictable, dose-dependent fashion. Characteristically, direct hepatotoxins produce liver cell necrosis in a predictable region of the hepatic lobule. Idiosyncractic hepatotoxins produce liver injury in an unpredictable manner. The pattern of injury is diffuse and consists of hepatocellular necrosis and/or cholestasis. Some idiosyncratic hepatotoxins are associated with fever, rash, eosinophilia, and autoantibody production. Examples of direct hepatotoxins include acetaminophen and carbon tetrachloride. Idiosyncratic hepatotoxins can be produced by isoniazid, and chloropromazine.

Autoimmune Hepatitis. A disease of unknown cause that occurs in individuals with a genetic predisoposition. Up to 5% of patients have a false-positive result for hepatitis C (anti-HCV). Most (2/3) patients have a positive antinuclear antibody and anti–smooth-muscle autoimmune markers. Others have autoantibodies against liver/kidney microsomes, type 1, liver cytosol antigen or asiloglycoprotein receptor. Supportive findings include: Concurrent immunologic disease (autoimmune thyroiditis, rheumatoid arthri-

tis, ulcerative colitis, Grave's disease), responsiveness to steroid therapy, hypergammaglobulinemia, and HLA-B8, Dr3, or Dr4.

Hereditary Disorders   AR

- *Hemochromatosis* (HCC), an HLA-linked autosomal recessive disorder of iron absorption, has a disease prevalence of 1/250. Symptomatic HCC presents with hepatomegaly, well-established hepatic fibrosis and cirrhosis, diabetes mellitus, and hyperpigmentation. AST and ALT may be slightly elevated.
- *Wilson's disease,* an HLA-linked autosomal recessive disorder of copper metabolism, has a disease prevelance of 1/30,000. Young patients (mean age 8–12 years) may present with hepatitis and fulminant hepatic failure.
- *Alpha$_1$-antitrypsin deficiency* is an important cause of neonatal hepatitis and cirrhosis in children and early emphysema in young adults. Fifteen percent to 30% of neonates with conjugated hyperbilirubinemia have alpha$_1$-antitrypsin deficiencies.

- **Management**

  Treatment. Treatment for acute hepatitis is primarily supportive care. Basic principles include:

- Avoidance of potentially liver-damaging circumstances, fluid and electrolyte replacement, ambulation within the bounds of fatigue, a regular or high-protein diet (in the absence of encephalopathy).
- Follow physical exam and biochemical tests: Prothrombin time is the best biochemical indicator of prognosis; also follow bilirubin, ALT, AST twice weekly while values are rising, weekly during the plateau, then at lesser intervals until normalized.
- Consideration for hospitalization is indicated for severe anorexia, vomiting, changes in mentation and biochemical changes, including a bilirubin value >15 or 20 mg/dL, persistence hyperbilirubinemia, rapidly falling aminotransferase activity with a rising bilirubin, increasing

protrombin time, and other evidence of hepatic failure.

Acute Viral Hepatitis. Most individuals with adequate family and medical support are treated in the outpatient setting. Hospitalization for isolation is not required (the period of infectivity precedes symptoms). Immunoprophylaxis (Tables 4–6 and 4–7).

Chronic Viral Hepatitis B. Preferred treatment is alpha-interferon, following quantitative serum HBV DNA.

Chronic Viral Hepatitis C. Treatment is also alpha-interferon, following quantitative serum HBV DNA.

Drug-Induced Liver Disease. Discontinue the implicated agent.

Alcoholic Liver Disease. Withdrawal of alcohol and substitution of a nutritious diet. Consider hospitalization for individuals with extrahepatic complications of alcohol ingestion (GI bleeding, coexistent infections, fluid and electrolyte abnormalities, pancreatitis, alcohol withdrawal syndromes).

Autoimmune Hepatitis. Responds to prednisone and/or azathioprine. Remission can be induced within 2 years of treatment in >70%. Relapse is common after withdrawal of drug therapy.

Hemachromatosis. Requires long-term phlebotomy and chelation therapy.

Wilson's Disease. Requires lifelong copper chelation therapy.

TABLE 4–6. INDICATIONS FOR HEPATITIS A VACCINATION

Travelers to endemic areas

Military personnel

Special populations where cyclic HAV epidemics occur

Homosexual males

Users of illicit intravenous drugs

Caretakers of the developmentally challenged

Employees of child day-care centers

Laboratory personnel handling live HAV

Handlers of primates that may be handling HAV

TABLE 4–7. PERSONS RECOMMENDED FOR HBV PROPHYLAXIS (VACCINE OR HBIG OR BOTH)

Preexposure prophylaxis

Persons with occupational risk, including clients and staff of institutions

Clients/staff of institutions for developmentally disabled

Patients on hemodialysis

Sexually active homosexual men

Sexually active heterosexual men and women

Users of illicit injectable drugs

Recipients of certain blood products, eg, clotting factors

Household and sexual contacts of HBV carriers

Adoptees from countries of high HBV endemicity

Populations with high endemicity

Inmates of long-term correctional facilities

Internaltional travelers to HBV endemic areas for >6 months

Postexposure immunoprophylaxis for hepatitis B

Type of Exposure	Immunoprophylaxis
Perinatal exposure	Vaccination + HBIG
Sexual, acute infection	HBIG ± vaccination
Sexual, carrier	Vaccination
Household contact, carrier	Vaccination
Household contact, known exposure	HBIG ± vaccination
Infant <12 months, acute case, primary caregiver	HBIG ± vaccination
Inadvertent percutaneous or permucosal	Vaccination + HBIG

Prevention. The health consequences of acute viral hepatitis are reduced by public health measures and immunization.

HAV. As the principle mode of transmission is person-to-person, prevention efforts are aimed at sanitation, chlorination, and proper handling of sewerage and identification of individuals at risk. The hepatitis A vaccine, used in Europe since 1991, is now approved by the FDA for use in the United States. It is indicated for persons traveling to or working in countries with intermediate or high HAV endemicity (countries other than Australia, Canada, Japan, New Zealand and in Western Europe and Scandinavia), military personnel, native peoples of Alaska and areas of the Americas where cyclic HAV epidemics occur, homosexual males, users of illicit intravenous drugs, employees of child day-care centers, laboratory workers who handle live HAV, and handlers of primates known to harbor the HAV virus (Table 4–6). Immune globulin (IG) is recommended for children under the age of 2 who are traveling to endemic areas (Havrix is not approved for children of less than 2 years of age) and postexposure, preferably within 2 weeks, for contacts of person with acute hepatitis A.

HBV. Despite the development and introduction of the hepatitis B vaccine in the 1980s, the incidence of hepatitis B has actually increased in the United States since 1980. One important reason for the failure of the vaccine has been an inability to reach an estimated 22 million people who are at highest risk. As a result, an expanded vaccination strategy focuses on the universal hepatitis B immunization for newborns, children, and adolescents, including infants born to HBeAg-positive mothers by vaccine plus HBIG within 12 hours of birth.

HCV. Development of specific serologic assays has dramatically decreased the dissemination of transfusion-related hepatitis. The residual risk is estimated to be 0.03%. The use of IG for percutaneous exposure to HCV-positive material is not recommended. No vaccine for hepatitis C is available.

HDV. No effective vaccine. However, transmission of HDV can be avoided with the hepatitis B vaccine. Carriers of HBsAg are at risk from continued IV drug abuse or sexual promiscuity.

B. Hepatocellular Carcinoma

H&P Keys

Hepatocellular carcinoma (HCC) has a specific geographic distribution. HCC is common in sub-Sahara Africa, China, Japan, and the Southeast, where it is strongly associated with chronic hepatitis HBV infection and repeated heavy exposure to the mycotoxin aflatoxin B. Intermediate risk for HCC in areas of southern Europe and Japan is associated with HCV infection. In other parts of the world, HCC occurs as a late complication of cirrhosis (particularly alcoholic liver disease and hemachromatosis).

Clinical Presentation. Amongst southern black Africans and Chinese patients, HCC occurs in relatively young (mean age 33 years) and apparently healthy individuals. Typically, the disease is silent in its early stages. Onset of symptoms: Abdominal pain, fullness, early satiety, anorexia, and weight loss corresponds to advanced disease. Physical findings include hepatomegaly, hepatic arterial bruit, ascites, splenomegaly, jaundice, fever. Among individuals with cirrhosis, an unexplained deterioration in liver function may be the only clue.

• Diagnosis

Tumor Markers. In high-incidence geographic regions, serum alpha-fetoprotein (AFP) is the most useful diagnostic test. Most symptomatic individuals (>75%) from these regions which will have a diagnostic level (>500 ng/mL) at presentation. In low-incidence regions, the AFP test is far less useful as a single tumor marker. A combination of tumor markers: tumor-associated isoenzymes of gamma-glutamyl transferase (elevated total GGT leads to isoenzyme fractionation) and the abnormal prothrombin, Desgamma-carboxy prothrombin may be abnormal when the AFP is nondiagnostic.

Newer molecular techniques amplify small amounts of tumor-specific gene-transcripts for albumin and alpha-fetoprotein mRNA promise to enhance detection of malignant hepatocytes in circulation.

Imaging. In patients with suspected HCC, the combination of arterial phase and portal venous phase CT imaging is superior to conventional dynamic incremental-bolus CT and will detect the majority of tumors. Magnetic resonance (MR) is useful for detecting small (<5 cm) HCC, differentiating HCC from hemangiomas and evaluating the proximity of HCC to adjacent blood vessels. Dynamic MR is now superior to hepatic arteriography. Ultrasound differentiates a cystic from solid mass but cannot distinguish HCC from other solid lesions. Hepatic sintography has surpassed other imaging modalities.

Pathology. A definitive diagnosis depends on histologic appearance. A percutaneous biopsy and/or aspiration cytology or biopsy carries the risk of systemic dissemination or seeding of the tumor and therefore is avoided when the tumor appears resectable.

- **Disease Severity**
Symptomatic HCC carries a poor prognosis. In Africa and China, average survival is less than 4 months from the onset of symptoms. In other geographic regions the course may be somewhat more indolent. Prognosis is more favorable when tumors are detected prior to the onset of symptoms. A high incidence of extrahepatic recurrance and reappearance of tumor in the donor liver after transplantation reflects early hematogenous spread of micrometastases. Recent advances in the use of reverse transcriptase polymerase chain reactions to amplify small amounts of tumor-specific gene-transcripts offer promising results to detect small numbers of malignant hepatocytes in peripheral blood.

- **Concept and Application**
HBV and HCV viruses promote mutagenesis indirectly by stimulating necroinflammatory activity in the liver. Emerging evidence indicates that both virus also have direct oncogenic potential. Geographic differences in the incidence of HCC among populations with comparable dietary aflotoxin B1 exposure may be due to individuals' capacity to detoxify mutagenic metabolites.

- **Management**
In areas where HBV-related HCC is common, there is some hope that early vaccination will decrease the incidence of HCC. For HCV-related HCC, vaccination remains a distant goal. Parenteral drug abuse and the high incidence of sporadic HCV infection in countries at intermediate risk for HCC offer little hope for reducing the incidence of HCV-related HCC.

    Dismal results are obtained with all forms of treatment for symptomatic tumors. Newer molecular markers and imaging modalities may increase the detection of small, asymptomatic and potentially resectable HCC in high-risk indivduals or populations. Small (<5 cm) lesions may be resectable when the tumor appears to be confined to one lobe and the remaining liver is noncirrhotic. Liver transplantation is considered for individuals with end-stage liver failure who coincidentally have a small single tumor without vascular invasion or extrahepatic spread. When operative treatment is not an option, dearterialization, embolization, and chemoembolization or injection of alcohol directly into the lesion may reduce the intrahepatic tumor burden.

C. Hepatic Fibrosis and Cirrhosis

- **H&P Keys**
In its early stages, the process may reverse on withdrawl of the injurious agent (early fibrosis). Persistent injury leads to irreversible scar tissue deposition, increased resistence to blood flow, impaired exchange of nutrients and metabolites, and failure of synthetic function. A gradual and tedious clinical course is typically interrupted by life-threatening complications: bleeding varices, decompensated ascites, peritonitis, or encephalopathy. Alcohol and chronic viral hepatitis B and C are the most common causes. Other etiologies include: drugs and toxins, autoimmune hepatitis, primary biliary cirrhosis, biliary obstruction, heart failure, metabolic and hereditary disorders (hemachromatosis, Wilson's disease, $alpha_1$-antitripson deficiency). Pertinent history includes alcohol use, risk factors for viral hepatitis, drug and toxin exposure, family history.

    Stigmata suggestive but not necessarily diagnostic of cirrhosis include: jaundice, spider angiomata, palmar erythema, Duputren's contracture, digital clubbing, easy bruising, loss of secondary sexual characteristics, skeletal muscle wasting, abdominal hernias, caput medusae.

- **Diagnosis**
Laboratory tests, imaging studies and liver biopsy screen for the presence, severity, potential causes, and prognosis of liver disease. No single battery of tests is applicable to all patients. The initial battery of biochemical tests, the so-called, liver function tests reflect:

- *Synthetic function:* Albumin, prothrombin time, coagulation factor levels, lipoproteins,
- *Hepatocellular injury:* Aminotransferases (ALT, AST)
- *Cholestatis:* Alkaline phosphatase
- *Excretory function and anion transport:* Bilirubin

Obtain additional tests when specific diagnoses are suspected:

- *Chronic viral hepatitis B and C:* HBsAg, anti-HCV
- *Autoimmune hepatitis:* ANA, SMA, serum globulins
- *Primary biliary cirrhosis:* Antimitochondrial antibody
- *Hemachromatosis:* Iron, transferrin, ferritin

Ultrasonography is the noninvasive imaging study of the liver for jaundice, suspected biliary obstruction, and mass lesion. The presence of cirrhosis is suggested by signs of portal hypertension: splenomegaly, ascites, decreased or reversed portal flow (via Doppler measurements). Supplemental diagnostic studies: ERCP, CT, and MR have value for specific situations:

- *Mass lesion:* MR, CT portography
- *Iron overlaod and fatty infiltration:* MR
- *Extrahepatic bile duct obstruction:* ERCP
- *Bleeding varices:* Upper endoscopy, ligation and/or sclerosis
- *New onset or decompensated ascites:* Diagnostic paracentesis

Liver biopsy plays a central role in the diagnosis of all stages of fibrosis and cirrhosis. Other indications for liver biopsy include otherwise unexplained hepatomegaly and/or liver biochemical abnormalities, documentation of neoplastic disease, assessment of chronic hepatitis, assessment of venoocclusive disease, and rejection after transplantation.

- **Disease Severity**
  Severity of cirrhosis is manifested by its clinical consequences: episodes of variceal bleeding, spontaneous bacterial peritonitis, intractable ascites, and poorly con-

TABLE 4–8. CHILD-TURCOTTE-PUGH SCORE

	Child-Turcotte-Pugh Score		
	1	2	3
Encephalopathy	None	1, 2	3, 4
Ascites	Absent	Slight	Moderate
Bilirubin (mg/dL)	1–2	2–3	>3
Albumin (g/dL)	>3.5	2.8–3.5	<2.8
Prothrombin time (s. prolonged)	1–4	4–6	>6
Total score			
1–6 = A			
7–9 = B			
10–15 = C			

trolled encephalopathy. The Child-Pugh scale (Table 4–8) provides a rough measure of prognosis by combining hepatic synthetic function (albumin, prothrombin time), excretory function (bilirubin), and portal hypertension (ascites, encephalopathy), potential candidates for liver transplantation need referral to the liver transplantation center well before they develop the following signs of decompensation: uncontrolled variceal bleeding, intractable ascites, poorly controlled encephalopathy, and fulminant hepatic failure.

- **Concept and Application**
  Fibrosis and cirrhosis are histologic terms that refer to the accumulation of excess extracellular matrix (ECM) within the liver with or without an accompanying inflammatory response. Recent evidence indicates that the ECM has important biologic effects of liver cell function in addition to its well-characterized effects on blood flow.

- **Management**

- *Cirrhotic ascites:* Dietary salt restriction, diuretic therapy. Consider large-volume paracentesis, peritoneovenous shunting, transjugular intrahepatic portovenous shunting (TIPS), and liver transplantation for refractory ascites.
- *Spontaneous bacterial peritonitis (SBP):* Cefotaxime is effective for initial therapy. Patients at risk (ascitic fluid protein <1 g/dL may benefit from Norfloxacin prophylaxis, particularly when hospitalized.

- *Encephalopathy:* Correction of any precipitant factors (GI bleeding, infection, electrolyte imbalance), reduction of dietary protein, and decrease in intestinal ammonia absorption of nonabsorbable carbohydrates, especially lactulose.
- *Acute Variceal Bleeding:* Variceal band ligation, sclerotherapy and/or pharmacologic therapy: somatostatin, octreotide, vasopressin, vasopressin/nitroglycerin. Consider TIPS for failure of urgent endoscopic and pharmacologic therapy.
- *Prevention of Rebleeding:* Variceal band ligation, sclerotherapy, nonselective β-blockade (nadalol, propranolol). Consider TIPS, shunt surgery, especially distal splenrenal shunt and small-diameter interposition portacaval graft, for endoscopic and pharmacologic failures.
- *Liver transplantation:* For all forms of cirrhosis, primary biliary cirrhosis, primary sclerosing cholangitis, biliary atresia, fulminant hepatic failure.

VIII. PANCREAS

A. Pancreatic Carcinoma

- **H&P Keys**

  Abdominal pain, weight loss, and jaundice are suggestive of pancreatic carcinoma. Other features include nausea, vomiting, anorexia, alteration in bowel function (typically constipation), steatorrhea, weakness.

  Physical findings include hepatomegaly, scleral icterus, progressive jaundice, pruritus, Courvoisier's sign (palpable gallbladder), ascites due to portal hypertension secondary to compression or occlusion of the splenic or portal vein by tumor, abdominal bruit, peripheral edema.

- **Diagnosis**

  Currently, there are no sensitive and specific methods for detection. Routine laboratory tests: Amylase, lipase, glucose, alkaline phosphatase, bilirubin, aspartate aminotransferase may be elevated in patients with pancreatic carcinoma. These values do not distinguish pancreatic carcinoma from pancreatitis. Although the tumor marker CA 19-9 (sensitivity 79%) is widely used, it is limited by the false-negative rate for localized tumors. CA 242 (a glycoconjugate expressed in mucin) is superior (equally sensitive yet more specific).

  Imaging: Spiral (helical) CT is superior to conventional dynamic CT scanning for suspected pancreatic masses. CT arterial portography (CTAP) is superior to arteriography for assessing vascular invasion and liver metastases. ERCP, transpapillary biopsy, and pancreatic duct cytology have an accuracy rate of 70%. Endoscopic ultrasound has emerged as the most accurate method available for diagnosis, N and M (including assessing vascular invasion). Ultrasonography-guided, real-time fine-needle-aspiration (FNA) carries the risk of tumor dissemination. It is applied to non-surgical candidates to confirm the diagnosis and guide treatment. Laparoscopy also is used for diagnosing and staging when the results of imaging studies are uncertain.

- **Disease Severity**

  Pancreatic carcinoma is the least likely malignancy to be confined to the organ of origin at the time of diagnosis. Most patients with pancreatic carcinoma present with advanced disease and generally have a poor prognosis. Only a fraction are candidates (<20%) for curative resection. Locoregional recurrence rates are high. Recent improvements in diagnostic imaging may improve the selection of candidates for resection.

- **Concept and Application**

  Epidemiology: The fifth leading cause of cancer-related mortality and the eleventh most common cancer in the United States. Risk factors include advanced age, smoking, urban location, high-fat diet, dichlorodiphenyltricholoroethane (DDT) exposure, and other chemical carcinogens, chronic pancreatitis, and hereditary pancreatitis. There appears to be little or no association between alcohol or caffeine consumption and pancreatic cancer.

  The molecular events leading to the development of pancreatic cancer are being

[handwritten: KRAS, P53]

intensely studied. K-ras mutations and abnormally high levels of p53 gene expression have been found in >60% of pancreatic tumors.

- **Management**
  Surgical resection for potentially curative tumors. Palliate all others for symptoms.
- Palliate obstructive jaundice with endoscopic stenting.
- Palliate duodenal obstruction with gastric bypass.
- Palliate abdominal pain with chemical splanchnicectomy or celic nerve block, which achieves pain control in 80% to 90% of patients. External beam radiation also controls pain in up to 50% of patients, but effective pain relief does not occur until several weeks after therapy.

B. Acute Pancreatitis

- **H&P Keys**
  Abdominal pain, nausea, vomiting. Patients appear ill, anxious, and restless. Hypotension, tachypnea, tachycardia, hyperthermia or hypothermia, jaundice, mild distention, involuntary guarding in upper abdomen, generalized abdominal tenderness, bowel sounds diminished, basilar atelectasis, pleural effusions, flank and periumbilical ecchymosis (Grey Turner's and Cullen's signs).

- **Diagnosis**
  Elevated serum amylase (within 2 to 12 hours, declining over next 3 to 5 days), elevated lipase (persists 5 to 7 days, can be detected after amylase normalizes), elevated hematocrit, leukocytosis with a leftward shift of the differential, hyperglycemia, hypoalbuminemia, hypocalcemia, prerenal azotemia with elevated blood urea nitrogen and serum creatinine, hyperbilirubinemia, hypertriglyceridemia. Routine roentgenography, ultrasonography, CT scanning.

- **Disease Severity**
  Ranson's criteria for prognosis on admission and during initial 48 hours don't predict course or outcome for individual patients.

- **Concept and Application**
  Biliary tract stone disease and alcohol abuse account for 60% to 80% of cases. Other causes: infections (*Mycoplasma pneumoniae,* mumps, coxsackie, *Ascaris, Opisthorchis*), drugs (azathioprine, thiazide diuretics, sulfonamides), lipid abnormalities, trauma, ERCP. Most attacks of acute pancreatitis result from injury to the pancreas by digestive enzymes.

- **Management**
  General supportive measures, with meticulous management of fluid, electrolyte, ventilatory, and hemodynamic alterations, parenteral alimentation. Early (within 72 hours) intervention (ERCP) to remove stones from the ductal system improves outcome. Anticipate possible local complications: pseudocyst infection, pancreatic ascites, abscess, blood vessel with or without rupture or thrombosis, bowel necrosis or stricture, esophageal varices, fistulas.

C. Chronic Pancreatitis

- **H&P Keys**
  Recurrent or persistent abdominal pain, weight loss, steatorrhea, glucose intolerance, epigastric tenderness.

- **Diagnosis**
  Plain roentgenogram of the abdomen may show pancreatic calcification; ultrasonography or CT scan may show enlarged gland, dilated pancreatic duct, or calculi; ERCP most sensitive and specific test for chronic pancreatitis. ERCP can differentiate chronic pancreatitis from pancreatic carcinoma. Tests of pancreatic exocrine function (secretin, cholecystokinin [CCK], or bentiromide test) for the rare patient with relatively minor ductal changes on ERCP in whom the diagnosis remains in doubt.

- **Disease Severity**
  Complications include pseudocyst, pancreatic ascites, fistula, splenic vein thrombosis. Suspect pseudocyst when a stable chronic pancreatitis patient experiences worsening of abdominal pain.

- **Concept and Application**
Alcohol in western societies (70% to 80%) and malnutrition worldwide represent major etiologies.

- **Management**
Avoidance of alcohol; analgesia; enzyme therapy for malabsorption and pain control, especially for patients with non–alcohol-induced chronic pancreatitis; celiac plexus block; surgery if all other measures have failed.

D. Cystic Fibrosis

- **H&P Keys**
Infants fail to gain weight despite vigorous appetite, watery stools; 80% have pancreatic exocrine insufficiency at diagnosis, hypoproteinemia with edema, "pot belly" on physical examination.

- **Diagnosis**
Sweat electrolytes: sodium and chloride are elevated in sweat in 99%; pancreatic stimulation test with CCK and secretin may confirm diagnosis when sweat test is equivocal; fetal screening and chromosomal analysis to diagnose cystic fibrosis by DNA analysis in the future.

- **Disease Severity**
Malnutrition and recurrent pulmonary infections are major concerns. Associated conditions include: Chronic meconium ileus in 15%, distal small-bowel obstruction ("meconium ileus equivalent") in older patients, rectal prolapse, intussusception, diabetes mellitus, chronic liver disease, abdominal pain, recurrent episodes of pancreatitis.

- **Concept and Application**
Increased viscosity of exocrine secretions leads to precipitation of exocrine secretions in all exocrine glands (pancreatic acini, intestinal glands, intrahepatic bile ducts, gallbladder, prostate, salivary glands) resulting in impaired pancreatic exocrine secretion, intestinal obstruction, focal biliary cirrhosis, obstructive pulmonary disease, and obstructive lesions of male genital tract.

- **Management**
Treatment of malnutrition with adequate caloric intake, balanced diet with vitamin supplementation (vitamins A, D, E, and K), pancreatic enzyme replacement, H_2-blockers to improve maldigestion.

IX. HERNIA

Indirect - Internal
Direct medial

A. External Hernias

Femoral inferior

- **H&P Keys**
Pain is derived from mechanical disruption of intestinal transit and tension exerted on the mesentery. Main symptom of groin hernia is an inguinal mass that may appear after activities that increase intra-abdominal pressure. Groin hernias are diagnosed by digital examination, with index finger introduced into inguinal canal through external inguinal ring by depressing the skin.

- **Diagnosis**
Examination is performed with the patient standing or in decubitus position. Palpate both sides of the groin and scrotum. Depress the skin of the area to introduce the finger into the inguinal canal through the external inguinal ring. Indirect hernias correspond to the internal inguinal ring; direct hernias lie more medially. Femoral hernias are palpated inferior to the inguinal ligament.

- **Disease Severity**
Hernia is reducible when herniation occurs intermittently and can be reversed spontaneously or by manipulation. An incarcerated hernia cannot be reversed. Sudden onset of pain in a previously asymptomatic hernia suggests compromise of the blood supply of the viscus or strangulation. Colicky abdominal pain, tenderness, nausea, vomiting, increased leukocytosis, fever indicates bowel obstruction.

- **Concept and Application**
Hernia, protrusion of any viscus from its proper cavity. Herniation occurs as a result

of increased intra-abdominal pressure, or decreased resistance of the abdominal wall. Most common hernias are umbilical, incisional, and groin. Groin hernias are classified by the anatomy of the area (indirect inguinal 60%, direct inguinal 30%, femoral 5%, combined 2%).

- **Management**
Surgical treatment is indicated for healthy patients. Symptomatic hernias in high-risk patients require further consideration. Strangulation and bowel obstruction are the acute complications that require surgical repair. Hernias with small hernial rings such as umbilical and femoral are at greater risk of strangulation. Manual reduction is effective in incarcerated or strangulated hernias of very short duration. Manual reduction is contraindicated when bowel necrosis is suspected or when symptoms have been present for more than 8 hours. A complication of manual reduction is reduction en masse. The hernia is returned to the abdominal cavity, but the bowel and blood supply remain constricted in the hernial sac. Colicky abdominal pain, tenderness, nausea, vomiting, increased leukocytosis, fever, signs of bowel obstruction demand laparotomy.

B. Traumatic Hernias of the Diaphragm

- **H&P Keys**
Penetrating or blunt trauma, left upper-quadrant pain that may be referred to the left shoulder, followed by nausea, vomiting, central abdominal pain, diaphoresis, respiratory distress.

- **Diagnosis**
Chest roentgenogram shows abdominal viscera in the thorax; fluoroscopy to evaluate diaphragmatic excursions, ultrasonography, and CT scan.

- **Disease Severity**
Principal complication is intestinal obstruction, often involving the intra-abdominal viscera more than the intrathoracic.

- **Concept and Application**
Most common injury is a large tear of the diaphragm from the esophageal hiatus to the left costal attachments. Herniated vis-

cera are stomach, spleen, colon, and left lobe of the liver.

- **Management**
Surgical repair.

X. ABDOMINAL AORTIC ANEURYSM

- **H&P Keys**
Usually asymptomatic until rupture. Physical examination may reveal tender, pulsatile mass. Abdominal discomfort, tenderness, ureteral obstruction suggest inflammatory aneurysms. Mycotic aneurysms present as tender enlarging masses.

- **Diagnosis**
Ultrasonography has a sensitivity approaching 100% and is cost-effective for aneurysm detection and sequential follow-up. CT scan is equally effective and should be used when ultrasonography is not possible and precise sizing is required. MRI may be better than either ultrasonography or CT, both for accurate aneurysm measurement and views of relevant vascular anatomy. Chest roentgenogram to exclude thoracic aortic aneurysm. Preoperative aortography if visceral, renal, or peripheral vascular disease is suspected. Selective screening of high-risk patients between the ages of 55 and 80: hypertension, aneurysms of femoral or popliteal artery, and family history of abdominal aortic aneurysm.

- **Disease Severity**
Most abdominal aneurysms remain asymptomatic until rupture. Symptoms and complications are related to aneurysm size and expansion rate. Aneurysms smaller than 4 cm have a risk of rupture of about 2%. From 25% to 41% of aneurysms larger than 5 cm rupture within 5 years. Risk factors for rupture include initial diameter of the aneurysm, elevated blood pressure, and presence of chronic obstructive pulmonary disease.

- **Concept and Application**
Pathogenesis is multifactorial: genetic predisposition, biochemical alterations of aor-

tic wall, and hemodynamic mechanical factors contributing. Inflammatory reaction can develop around the external calcified layer (inflammatory aneurysms). Mycotic aneurysms can be caused by bacterial or fungal infection and are rare.

- **Management**
Repair of symptomatic or ruptured abdominal aortic aneurysms and of all symptomatic aneurysms larger than 5 cm. Contraindications to elective aortic reconstruction: myocardial infarction (within 6 months), intractable angina pectoris, severe pulmonary insufficiency with dyspnea at rest, severe chronic renal insufficiency, incapacitating stroke, life expectancy of less than 2 years.

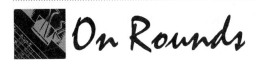
On Rounds

Inflammatory Bowel Disease

Ulcerative Colitis

- Bloody diarrhea, tenesmus, usually onset as child or young adult, pain relieved by bowel movement
- Affects colon only, mucosal disease
- Extraintestinal manifestations (arthritis, iritis, renal stones, etc.)
- Endoscopy for diagnosis
- Treatment: Sulfasalazine, corticosteroids, immunosuppressants

Crohn's Disease

- Bloating, weight loss, fever, fatigue, perianal disease, pain not relieved by bowel movement
- Affects small or large bowel, transmural disease
- Extraintestinal manifestations (same as above)
- Endoscopy for diagnosis
- Treatment: Similar to above

BIBLIOGRAPHY

Agrawal NM, Van Kerckhove HEJM, et al. Misoprostol coadministered with diclofenac for prevention of gastroduodenal ulcers: a one-year study. *Dig Dis Sci.* 1995;40:1125–31.

Alter HJ, Bradley DW. Non-A, non-B, hepatitis unrelated to the hepatitis C virus (non-ABC). *Sem Liver Dis.* 1995;15,1,110–20.

Baaer DM, Simons JL et al. Hemachromatosis screening asymptomatic ambulatory men 30 years of age and older. *Am J Med.* 1995;98:464–68.

Balthazar EJ, Freeny PC, VanSonnenberg E. Imaging and intervention in acute pancreatitis. *Radiology.* 1994; 193: 297–306.

Batey RG, Burns T, et al. Alcohol consumption and the risk of cirrhosis. *Med J Aust.* 1992;156:413–16.

Bazzoli F, Fossi S, et al. The risk of adenomatous polyps in asymptomatic first-degree relatives of persons with colon cancer. *Gastroenterology.* 1995;109:783–88.

Bond JH, for the Practice Parameters Committee of the ACG: Polyp guideline. Diagnosis, treatment, and surveillance for patients with nonfamilial colorectal polyps. *Ann Int Med.* 1993;199:836–43.

Cameron AJ, Lomboy CT, et al. Adenocarcinoma of the esophagogastric junction and Barrett's esophagus. *Gastroenterology.* 1995;109:1541–46.

Cutler AF, Prasad VM. Long-term follow-up of helicobacter pylori serology after successful eradication. *Am J Gastroenterol.* 1996;91:85–87.

deBoer W, Driessen W, et al. Effect of acid suppression on efficacy of treatment for helicobacter pylori infection. *Lancet* 1995;345:817–20.

Desmet VJ, Gerber M, et al. Classification of chronic hepatitis: diagnosis, grading and staging. *Hepatology.* 1994;19: 1513–16.

DeVault KR, Castell DO, et al. Guidelines for the diagnosis and treatment of gastroesophageal reflux disease. *Arch Int Med.* 1995;155:2165–73.

Elton E., Hanauer SB. Review article: the medical management of Crohn's disease. *Aliment Pharmacol Ther.* 1996:10:1–22.

Ernst CB. Abdominal aorta in aneurysm. *New Eng J Med.* 1993;328:1167–72.

Gallstones and laparoscopic cholecystectomy. *NIH Consensus Statement online* 1992;10(3):1–20.

Hanauer SB. Medical therapy for ulcerative colitis. *Ann Int Med.* 1993;118:540–49.

Isaacson PG. Gastrointestinal lymphoma. *Hum Pathol.* 1994;25:1020–29.

Lee WM. Drug-induced hepatotoxicity. *N Engl J Med.* 1995;333:1118–127.

Liskow B, Campbell J, Nickel EJ. Validity of the CAGE questionnaire in screening for alcohol dependence in a walk-in (triage) clinic. *J Stud Alcohol.* 1995;56:277–81.

Masuko K, Mitsui T, et al. Infection with hepatitis GB virus C in patients on maintenance hemodialysis. *N Engl J Med.* 1996;334;23:1485–89.

MMWR Morbid Mortal Wkly Rep. 1991.40:I.

Ottinger LW. Current concepts: mesenteric ischemia. *New Eng J Med.* 1982;307:535–37.

Owens DM, Nelson DK, Talley NJ. The irritable bowel syndrome: long-term prognosis and the physician–patient interaction. 1995;122:107–12.

Pasricha PJ, Ravich WJ, et al. Intrasphincteric botulinum toxin for the treatment of achalasia. *N Engl J Med.* 1995;322:774–78.

Rao SSC, Gregersen H, et al. Unexplained chest pain: the hypersensitive, hyperrreactive and poorly compliant esophagus. *Ann Intern Med.* 1996:124:950–58.

Rees JH, Soudain SE, et al. Camplobacter jejuni infection and Guillain-Barré syndrome. *N Engl J Med.* 1995;333:1374–79.

Rosch T, Braig C, et al. Staging of pancreatic and ampullary carcinoma by endoscopic ultrasonography: comparison with conventional sonography, computed tomography, and angiography. *Gastroenterology.* 1992;102:188.

Salam I, Katelaris P, et al. Randomised trial of single-dose ciprofloxacin for travellers' diarrhea. *Lancet* 1994;344: 1537–39.

Soll AH, for the Practice Parameters Committee of the ACG.

NIH consensus conference: medical treatment of peptic ulcer disease. *JAMA.* 1996;275:622–29.

Terrault N, Wright T. Interferon and hepatitis C. *N Engl J Med.* 1995;332:1509–11.

Toribara NW, Sleisenger MH. Screening for colorectal cancer. *N Engl J Med.* 1995;332:861–66.

Valdimarsson T, Franzen L, et al. Is small bowel biopsy necessary in adults with suspected celiac disease and IgA anti-endomysium antibodies? 100% positive predictive value for celiac disease in adults. *Dig Dis Sci.* 1996;41:83–7.

Warshaw AL, Gu Z, et al. Preoperative staging and assessment of resectability of pancreatic cancer. *Arch Surg.* 1990;125:230.

Winawer BJ, Zauber AG, et al. Risk of colorectal cancer in families of patients with adenomatous polyps. *N Engl J Med.* 1996;334:82–7.

Wright TL, Perreira B. Liver transplantation for chronic viral hepatitis. Liver Transplant Surg 1995;10:471–80.

5

Hematology and Oncology

Stephen D. Nimer, MD, and Anna Pavlick, MD

I. ANEMIA

[handwritten: Hypochromic microcytic ↓ mcv, mc H ↓ ferritin]

A. Iron-Deficiency Anemia *[handwritten: ↓ Fe ↑TIBC ↑RDW]*

- **H&P Keys**

Etiology. Menstruating women, iron-deficient diet, elderly with chronic gastrointestinal (GI) bleeding, chronic alcohol, aspirin, steroid, or nonsteroidal anti-inflammatory drug (NSAID) use.

Signs and Symptoms. Glossitis, spooning of nails, fatigue, weakness, dyspnea, pallor, pagophagia.

- **Diagnosis**
  Hypochromic, microcytic cells on peripheral smear. Mean corpuscular volume (MCV) and mean corpuscular hemoglobin (MCH) are low; low serum ferritin, low serum iron, increased total iron-binding capacity (TIBC), low percentage of saturation, increased red cell distribution width (RDW), thrombocytosis, and low reticulocyte count. Free erythrocytic porphyrin elevated.

- **Disease Severity**
  Absence of iron on bone marrow aspiration (Prussian blue staining).

- **Concept and Application**
  Underproduction anemia caused by inability to synthesize heme, which requires iron and porphyrin synthesis. Buildup of free porphyrin in red blood cells is present. May be the result of impaired iron absorption, deficient dietary intake, occult bleeding, chronic intravascular hemolysis.

- **Management**
  Determination of etiology. Supplemental iron. The hemoglobin deficit should be corrected by half within 3 weeks and fully corrected in 8 weeks, if iron loss terminates. Blood transfusion if patient has severe symptoms or if etiology is severe bleeding.

B. Blood-Loss Anemia

- **H&P Keys**

Etiology. GI bleeding (ulcer disease, gastritis, hemorrhoids, angiodysplasia, polyp, tumor, diverticulum); menstruation; massive hematuria.

Acute Symptoms. Fatigue, pallor, tachycardia, dyspnea, syncope.

- **Diagnosis**
  Complete blood count (CBC), reticulocyte count, stool guaiac.

Acute. Orthostatic changes; normochromic, normocytic anemia; elevated blood urea nitrogen (BUN) secondary to GI bleeding; reticulocytosis.

Chronic. Similar to iron deficiency. Microcytic anemia, low reticulocyte count, low serum iron and transferrin saturation.

- **Disease Severity**
  CBC, orthostatic hypotension, tachycardia, chest pain, and level of consciousness.

- **Concept and Application**
  Severe blood loss by any mechanism. Hematocrit (hct) may not fall if volume loss not repleted.

• **Management**
Determination of etiology. Check coagulation profile and platelet count.

Acute. Volume replacement, ie, blood products and IV fluids.

Chronic. Correction of etiology of bleeding, then supplemental iron replacement.

C. Folic Acid Deficiency

[handwritten: No neurologic Like B12 def.]

[handwritten margin: Macrocytic]

• **H&P Keys**
Symptoms of anemia. No neurologic sequelae as in B$_{12}$ deficiency. Nutritional deficiency (lack of green, leafy vegetables, fruit); patients with malabsorption syndromes. Increased losses or increased utilization (dialysis, pregnancy, hemolytic anemia).

• **Diagnosis**
Low serum and red blood cell (RBC) folate levels. Macrocytic anemia and hypersegmented neutrophils on peripheral smear. Megaloblastic bone marrow cells. Normal B$_{12}$ level. Increased lactase dehydrogenase (LDH). Increased bilirubin.

• **Disease Severity**
Observable pancytopenia; infertility, skin pigmentation abnormalities. Severe malabsorption syndromes diagnosed by jejunal biopsy. Neural tube defects if folate deficiency present during pregnancy.

• **Concept and Application**
Folic acid absorbed in the proximal jejunum. Folate deficiency leads to diminished thymidylate synthesis and abnormal DNA replication.

• **Management**
Determination of etiology, then replacement with oral folic acid 1 mg/d.

D. α-Thalassemia

• **H&P Keys**
An inherited disorder seen in American blacks and people of Mediterranean or Southeast Asian background. Carrier state (lack of one normal allele) is undetectable. Patients who lack two alleles (called α-thalassemia trait) are usually asymptomatic. Patients with deletion of three alleles (hemoglobin [HbH]) have moderately severe hemolytic anemia. Absence of α-chains is incompatible with life.

• **Diagnosis**
Microcytosis on peripheral smear in patients with α-thalassemia trait. Normal iron studies. Low RDW. Elevated RBC numbers. RBC inclusions in patients with HbH and evidence of hemolysis (elevated lactic dehydrogenese [LDH] and bilirubin). Coombs' test is negative. Molecular studies can identify precise abnormalities.

• **Disease Severity**
Hemolytic anemia and splenomegaly in patients with HbH. Hydrops fetalis occurs in homozygotes, in whom no α-globin is produced. Affected fetuses are either stillborn or die shortly after birth.

• **Concept and Application**
Caused by deletion of one or more α-globin genes. Presence or absence of symptoms depends on number of alleles deleted (or mutated). Inadequate production of α-globin leads to precipitation of β-globin (in HbH) or to β4 (beta chain tetramer) formation, which is incompatible with life.

• **Management**
Prenatal diagnosis can identify fetus at risk for fetal hydrops syndrome. Establishing diagnosis prevents confusion with iron deficiency. Patients with α-thalassemia trait may need transfusions. Splenectomy sometimes beneficial in patients with HbH.

E. β-Thalassemia

• **H&P Keys**
Most common in patients of Mediterranean background or from equatorial regions of Asia and Africa. Thalassemia minor patients (heterozygotes) usually have asymptomatic mild anemia. Thalassemia major (homozygotes) presents in childhood with symptoms of anemia. Splenomegaly occurs in thalassemia major. Frontal bossing from expansion of marrow cavity and bilirubin gallstones also seen.

• **Diagnosis**
Basophilic stippling and target cells on peripheral smear. Microcytic, hypochromic anemia, elevated RBC number. MCV usually <75. Hb electrophoresis.

• **Disease Severity**
Severity of disease depends on type of genetic abnormality and amount of HbF present. Some defects result in no β-chain production, others produce a decreased amount of β-chain. Thalassemia minor results in a mild hypochromic microcytic anemia. Elevated hemoglobin A_2 (HbA_2) on Hb electrophoresis is diagnostic. In thalassemia major, splenomegaly results in shortened RBC survival and at times thrombocytopenia or neutropenia. Serum ferritin to detect iron overload in transfused patients.

• **Concept and Application**
Hereditary anemia resulting from deletion or defective transcription of β-globin genes. Excess α-chains precipitate, causing rapid splenic clearing of RBCs. Frequent transfusions lead to iron overload.

• **Management**
Transfusions and iron chelation (desferoxamine should be initiated early). Genetic counseling. Bone marrow transplantation beneficial in thalassemia major.

F. Vitamin B$_{12}$ Deficiency

• **H&P Keys**
Symptoms of anemia (pallor, fatigue, weakness, dyspnea). Neurologic symptoms such as paresthesias, abnormal mental status, ataxia, and premature graying. History of autoimmune or intestinal diseases, such as atrophic gastritis, gastrectomy, sprue, and blind loop syndrome. Dietary deficiency rare.

• **Diagnosis**
Hypersegmented neutrophils, macrocytic, hyperchromic anemia (high MCV). Increased LDH, low serum B_{12} level. Document achlorhydria. Perform Schilling test to evaluate cause of pernicious anemia. Intrinsic factor antibody analysis. Bone marrow shows megaloblastic hematopoiesis with abnormally immature nucleus compared to cytoplasm (nuclear and cytoplasmic dissociation). Complete neurologic exam.

• **Disease Severity**
Serum B_{12} level <100 pg/mL. Neurologic symptoms consistent with long tract disease, then cerebral dysfunction. No correlation between anemia and neurologic symptoms.

• **Concept and Application**
Body stores of B_{12} last 3 to 4 years. B_{12} present in animal protein (meats, eggs, milk products). Impaired DNA synthesis, but normal RNA synthesis, induces ineffective erythropoiesis. Defective conversion of propionate to succinyl coenzyme A (CoA) may lead to defective myelin synthesis and patchy demyelination. Absorption of vitamin B_{12} requires secretion of intrinsic factor by the stomach and occurs in the terminal ileum.

• **Management**
B_{12} 100 µg given parenterally as a loading dose, then 100 µg per month for life.

G. Aplastic Anemia

• **H&P Keys**
Weakness, fatigue, pallor, petechiae, purpura, increased bruising and overt bleeding, fever or evidence of infection. Etiology may be idiopathic, familial (eg, Fanconi's syndrome) or acquired (eg, secondary to radiation, drugs, hepatitis, or autoimmune mechanisms).

• **Diagnosis**
Hypocellular bone marrow. Normal cytogenetics decreased reticulocyte count (<5%). Normochromic and normocytic RBCs. Rule out paroxysmal nocturnal hemoglobinuria with a Ham test.

• **Disease Severity**
Severe aplastic anemia defined as two or more of the following: absolute neutrophil count <500, reticulocyte count <1%, and platelets <20 000. Percentage of bone marrow cellularity.

- **Concept and Application**
  Immune suppression of hematopoiesis in most. Some patients have stem cell defect. No direct proof yet for an abnormal environment for hematopoietic development.

- **Management**
  HLA-matched sibling allogenic bone marrow transplant if patient has donor and is relatively young. Alternative treatment consists of antithymocyte globulin (ATG) or cyclosporin and corticosteroids. Avoid transfusions (if possible) if bone marrow transplant is planned.

H. Lead-Poisoning Anemia

- **H&P Keys**
  Autoimmune neuropathy (abdominal cramps, ileus). Renal dysfunction. Mental status changes. *Etiology:* Ingesting contaminated foods, inhaled particles, pica, lead cookware, frequent inhalation of gasoline.

- **Diagnosis**
  Mild anemia. Peripheral smear: RBCs hypochromic with basophilic stippling. Increased serum lead level.

- **Disease Severity**
  Measure erythrocyte aminolevulinic acid (ALA) dehydrogenase.

- **Concept and Application**
  Inhibition of ALA dehydrogenase leads to denaturing of proteins. Lead limits intestinal absorption of iron.

- **Management**
  Removal of lead source. Intravenous ethylenediaminetetraacetic acid (EDTA).

I. Anemia of Chronic Renal Disease

- **H&P Keys**
  Pallor and fatigue. Renal failure patients (not necessarily dialysis-dependent).

- **Diagnosis**
  Low Hb. Low reticulocyte count. Normochromic, normocytic RBCs, Burr cells, and schistocytes on peripheral smear. Increased serum creatinine, BUN. Serum erythropoietin level decreased. Iron deficiency, folate deficiency, and blood loss can complicate this disorder.

- **Disease Severity**
  Development of transfusion dependency.

- **Concept and Application**
  Decreased erythropoietin level. Iron and folate are lost during dialysis. Increased RBC loss and destruction; decreased RBC survival secondary to azotemia.

- **Management**
  Subcutaneous erythropoietin three times per week. Folate replacement.

J. Hemolytic Anemia

- **H&P Keys**
  Hereditary and acquired disorders. Intrinsic enzymatic defects, eg, pyruvate kinase and hexokinase deficiencies. Drug history: glucose-6-phosphate dehydrogenase (G6PD) deficiency leads to episodic hemolysis, after exposure to oxidative stress. Chronic hemolysis can result in splenomegaly. Some hemolytic conditions are secondary to lymphoid malignancies (chronic lymphocytic leukemia, lymphoma) or systemic lupus erythematosus (SLE) whereas others are associated with bacterial (mycoplasma) or viral (infectious mononucleosis) infections. Bilirubin gallstones.

- **Diagnosis**
  Elevated reticulocyte count. Coombs' test to determine autoimmune versus nonimmune (positive in autoimmune). Positive Coombs' test: detection of immunoglobulin and/or complement on RBC surface. Increased MCV. Elevated LDH, bilirubin (indirect).
  G6PD deficiency: can detect Heinz bodies on peripheral smear.
  Warm antibodies usually IgG: microspherocytes and reticulocytosis on peripheral smear.
  Cold antibodies usually IgM: Coombs' test: positive for complement.
  Microangiopathic hemolytic anemias (disseminated intravascular coagulation [DIC], thrombotic thrombocytopenic purpura [TTP], malfunctioning heart valve) show evidence of RBC fragmentation (schisto-

cytes, helmet cells). Intravascular hemolysis results in depletion of serum haptoglobin, formation of methemalbumin, urinary hemosiderin, and urinary free hemoglobin if severe.

- **Disease Severity**
Level of Hct, LDH, indirect bilirubin levels. Depletion of haptoglobin, free Hb in urine or serum.

- **Concept and Application**
May be autoimmune (antibody-mediated) or nonimmune (unstable hemoglobin, oxidative stress, as with deficiency of G6PD, an X-linked disorder). Intravascular versus extravascular hemolysis.

- **Management**
Avoidance of oxidative stress in patients with G6PD deficiency. Treatment of warm autoantibody by corticosteroids, splenectomy, or immunosuppression. Treatment of cold autoantibody by keeping the patient warm and using steroids and at times chlorambucil. Treatment of underlying disorder whenever possible.

K. Anemia of Chronic Disease

- **H&P Keys**
Symptoms of underlying disorder (weight loss, anorexias, myalgias, arthralgias).

- **Diagnosis**
  - Hb rarely count <9
  - Normochromic, normocytic anemia
  - Normal serum ferritin (or increased)
  - Decreased reticulocyte count
  - Decreased serum iron
  - Decreased TIBC
  - Decreased transferrin saturation
  - Bone marrow: adequate iron stores

- **Disease Severity**
Clinical signs of anemia.

- **Concept and Application**
Abnormal utilization of iron. Decreased RBC survival. Inadequate production of erythropoietin with respect to anemia.

- **Management**
Erythropoietin (EPO), treatment of underlying disease, transfusions.

L. Sickle Cell Anemia

- **H&P Keys**
Pallor; history of painful crises. Fatigue, tachycardia, leukocytosis, splenic infarctions, renal papillary necrosis, aseptic necrosis, cerebrovascular accident (CVA), priapism, hyposthenuria, bilirubin stones, infections such as pneumonias with encapsulated microorganisms, osteomyelitis with staphylococcus or salmonella.

- **Diagnosis**
Peripheral smear reveals sickle-shaped cells, Howell-Jolly bodies, nucleated RBCs, reticulocytosis, thrombocytosis. HbS on electrophoresis. Prenatal diagnosis by amniotic fluid DNA analysis.

- **Disease Severity**
Heterozygous state (sickle cell trait) asymptomatic. Homozygous state results in severe hemolytic anemia.

  Factors that induce sickling: infection, dehydration, low oxygen tension, low pH, increased serum osmolarity. Microvascular occlusion can lead to ischemia and tissue infarction. This is known as a sickle crisis. Aplastic crisis (abrupt halt in erythropoiesis) caused by parvovirus B19 infection.

- **Concept and Application**
Point mutation at position 6 of β-globin chains (glutamic acid to valine) allows for polymerization. Amount of Hb in cell important; thus sickle trait plus thalassemia less severe than homozygous sickle cell anemia.

- **Management**
Vigorous hydration, oxygen, transfusions if needed. Identification of initiating cause of crisis and treatment accordingly. Adequate analgesia. Pneumovax Folate. Genetic counseling.

  Drugs that can increase HbF levels under investigation.

II. MALIGNANT DISEASES

A. Acute Myelogenous Leukemia *Auer*
auer

- **H&P Keys**
Fatigue, bruising, petechiae, overt bleeding (eg, menorrhagia), fever or evidence of infection. In certain subtypes of acute myelogenous leukemia (AML), gingival hypertrophy, skin lesions or DIC; modest splenomegaly.

- **Diagnosis**
CBC reveals anemia and thrombocytopenia. White blood cells (WBC) can be elevated with increased blasts or depressed. Auer rods in some subtypes. Bone marrow is usually hypercellular, positive peroxidase or Sudan black staining, negative PAS staining. Flow cytometry to determine cell surface markers. Cytogenetic abnormalities include: t(8;21) (M2), t(15;17) (M3), inv16 (M4 with eosinophils). Central nervous system (CNS) involvement can be seen in M4 and M5 subtypes. Spuriously low Po_2 (oxygen tension) and serum glucose can be seen with high WBC.

- **Disease Severity**
Very high WBCs can cause leukostasis with CNS symptoms or pulmonary syndromes. AML in elderly patients and AML occurring after chemotherapy for other malignancies has a very poor prognosis.

French-American-British (FAB) Classification

- M1: undifferentiated cells
- M2: early differentiated cells, Auer rods
- M3: acute promyelocytic leukemia (APL), large granules, Auer rods
- M4: myelomonocytic leukemia
- M5: monocytic leukemia
- M6: erythrocytic leukemia
- M7: megakaryoblastic leukemia

- **Concept and Application**
Failure of myeloid stem cells to differentiate normally leads to progressive accumulation of leukemic blasts. Anemia and thrombocytopenia are due to lack of normal stem cells.

- **Management**
Pathologic diagnosis. Vigorous IV hydration, antibiotics if indicated for neutropenic fever, transfusions as needed, allopurinol to prevent uric acid nephropathy. Coagulation profile check and close monitoring for DIC. Monitoring for tumor lysis (serum K^+, creatinine, Po_4). Treatment consists of induction chemotherapy with cytarabine (Ara-C) and an anthracycline, followed by consolidation therapy. Bone marrow transplantation.

B. Acute Lymphocytic Leukemia

- **H&P Keys**
Fatigue, anorexia, easy bruising or overt bleeding (petechiae), fever or evidence of infection, lymphadenopathy, splenomegaly, or mediastinal mass. Headache, stiff neck suggest CNS disease. Testicular mass can be seen occasionally.

- **Diagnosis**
Hypercellular bone marrow with >30% blasts. Blasts are often positive for terminal deoxynucleotidyltransferase (TdT), common acute lymphoblastic leukemia antigen (CALLA) (CD10) and PAS; and negative for peroxidase and Sudan black. Elevated WBC. Anemia, thrombocytopenia. Lumbar puncture to rule out CNS leukemia. Elevated creatinine, LDH, Po_4, K^+ predict for tumor lysis syndrome. Philadelphia (Ph) chromosome t(9;22), seen in 10% of children and 30% of adults, confers a poor prognosis. Burkitt's type of acute lymphocytic leukemia (ALL) accompanied by t(8;14) or t(2;8) or t(8;22) involving c-myc oncogene.

- **Disease Severity**

Favorable Prognostic Factors. Young age, low WBC, Ph negative, no CNS disease, CALLA$^+$, rapid induction of remission.

Subclassifications

- L1: ALL
- L2: large cells with cleft nuclei

- L3: vacuolated, abundant cytoplasm, Burkitt's type

- **Concept and Application**
Block in differentiation results in the accumulation of immature cells with abnormal function.

- **Management**
IV hydration, transfusion of blood products and antibiotics for neutropenic fever. Induction chemotherapy, frequently with vincristine, prednisone, and either L-asparaginase or an anthracycline. Monitoring for tumor lysis. CNS prophylaxis with intrathecal chemotherapy. Long-term maintenance therapy.

C. Chronic Myelogenous Leukemia

- **H&P Keys**   BCR-abl
Nonspecific complaints most common; weakness, malaise, weight loss. Left upper quadrant fullness, early satiety and discomfort secondary to splenomegaly. In acute phase of disease, can present like acute leukemia.

- **Diagnosis**
Bone marrow is hypercellular with a marked proliferation of all granulocytic elements, increased eosinophils and basophils, and mild fibrosis. Ph chromosome t(9;22) positive, low leukocyte alkaline phosphatase (LAP) score. Increased WBC (50 000 to 300 000/μL), hyperuricemia, and increased serum B$_{12}$. Normal platelets and no or mild anemia in chronic phase.

- **Disease Severity**
Degree of splenomegaly, percentage of blasts, basophilia and eosinophilia can predict for survival. Presence of cytogenetic abnormalities in addition to Ph chromosome predicts for blastic transformation.

- **Concept and Application**
Myeloproliferative disorder characterized by an abnormal proliferation of myeloid cells without the loss of capacity to differentiate; bcr-abl rearrangement seen in nearly all patients.

- **Management**
HLA-identical sibling allogenic bone marrow transplant (BMT) if possible. Alpha interferon or hydroxyurea if no donor available or patient not a suitable BMT candidate. Allopurinol if high WBC.

D. Chronic Lymphocytic Leukemia

- **H&P Keys**
Usually a disease of elderly patients. Often asymptomatic leukocytosis. Some patients present with lymphadenopathy, hepatosplenomegaly, anemia, or thrombocytopenia.

- **Diagnosis**
Elevated WBC (>15 000 μL with lymphocytes greater than 60%). Look for kappa/lambda clonal excess or presence of CD5 + CD19+ cells to confirm diagnosis. Chromosomal abnormalities such as 14q+ and trisomy 12 can be seen. Bone marrow is hypercellular and monotonous with diffuse infiltration of small- and medium-size lymphocytes.

   Observable autoimmune phenomena (eg, Coombs' test positive, hemolytic anemia). Hypogammaglobulinemia.

- **Disease Severity**
Several staging systems. Rai staging best known:

  - Stage 0—lymphocytosis only
  - Stage 1—lymphocytosis with lymphadenopathy
  - Stage 2—lymphocytosis with splenomegaly
  - Stage 3—lymphocytosis with anemia
  - Stage 4—lymphocytosis with thrombocytopenia

Aggressive transformation into large-cell lymphoma, Richter's transformation.

- **Concept and Application**
Monoclonal proliferation of nonfunctioning mature β-lymphocytes. More frequent infections due to lack of opsonization.

- **Management**
Observation is appropriate for early stages. Treatment for later stages and for allevia-

tion of obstructive symptoms. Chemotherapy includes chlorambucil and prednisone or fludarabine.

E. Hodgkin's Disease

- **H&P Keys**
Frequently younger patients. Superficial, painless, enlarged "rubbery" lymph nodes (60% to 80% cervical or axillary, nontender), splenomegaly. "B" symptoms: fevers, night sweats, weight loss. Infections associated with depressed cell-mediated immunity. Bimodal peak incidence.

- **Diagnosis**
Lymph node biopsy reveals Reed-Sternberg cells with reactive lymphocytes. Disease spread by contiguous lymph node chains. Initial staging tests include computed tomography (CT) scans of the chest, abdomen, and pelvis, gallium scans, chest roentgenogram, bilateral bone marrow aspiration and biopsy. Laparotomy and lymphangiogram are rarely performed. Nodular sclerosing subtype most common. Lymphocyte-depleted histologic specimens associated with poor prognosis. Mixed cellularity and lymphocyte-predominant tissues offer better prognosis.

- **Disease Severity**

Ann Arbor Staging

- Stage I: single lymph node group
- Stage II: multiple lymph node groups on the same side of the diaphragm
- Stage III: involved lymph node groups on both sides of the diaphragm
- Stage IV: Extranodal disease (bone marrow involvement, liver involvement, lung or skin involvement)

"B" symptoms: fevers, night sweats, and 10% weight loss. Stage A: absence of "B" symptoms.

- **Concept and Application**
Cell of origin not clearly defined (possibly lymphoid or monocytoid). Defective T-cell function.

- **Management**
Early stages cured with a variety of approaches.

- Stage IA–IIA: extended field radiation
- Stage IB–IIB: Total nodal radiation or extended field and chemotherapy
- Stage IIIA/B and IVA/B: combination chemotherapy
- Bulky disease: radiation and chemotherapy

Chemotherapy consists of mechlorethamine, Oncovin (vincristine), procarbazine, and prednisone (MOPP) or Adriamycin (doxorubicin), bleomycin, vinblastine, and decarbazine (ABVD), MOPP alternating with ABVD, or Mopp/ABV hybrid.

F. Low-Grade Lymphoma

- **H&P Keys**
Lymphadenopathy usually diffuse and not necessarily contiguous. Splenomegaly can be seen. Extranodal disease (eg, bone marrow) common. Rarely fever, weight loss, night sweats.

- **Diagnosis**
Lymph node biopsy. Bone marrow aspiration and biopsy (bone marrow involvement common). Kappa/lambda clonal excess. Immunoglobulin gene rearrangement. Cytogenetic studies, eg, t(14;18), associated with follicular lymphoma.

- **Disease Severity**
Ann Arbor staging system (see Hodgkin's disease staging). Chest x-ray, CT scans of chest, abdomen, and pelvis. Often stage IV due to bone marrow infiltration. Presence of "B" symptoms, LDH, performance status.

- **Concept and Application**
Clonal proliferation of B-cell lymphocytes. Can transform into more aggressive lymphoma.

- **Management**
Conservative therapy if asymptomatic. Treatment to prevent obstruction of vital structures, autoimmune complications. Alkylating agents plus corticosteroids or ra-

diation if symptomatic. Fludarabine. Some patients will require aggressive chemotherapy.

G. Intermediate- or High-Grade Lymphoma

- **H&P Keys**
  Lymphadenopathy, splenomegaly. Extranodal disease can be seen. Fatigue, malaise. Rapidly enlarging lymphadenopathy can occur (especially Burkitt's lymphoma). Mediastinal mass can cause symptoms.

- **Diagnosis**
  Lymph node biopsy to make diagnosis. Needle biopsy not sufficient. Bone marrow aspiration and biopsy. Spinal tap to rule out meningeal spread. Burkitt's lymphoma associated with Epstein-Barr virus (EBV) and translocation t(8;14), t(2;8), or t(8;22). Increased LDH in aggressive disease. Chest roentgenogram to evaluate mediastinum. CT scans chest, abdomen, and pelvis. Testing for HIV. Tumor lysis can be seen with rapidly growing lymphomas (eg, Burkitt's). Monitor LDH, Po_4, creatinine, K^+, uric acid.

- **Disease Severity**
  Ann Arbor staging system. Bone marrow involvement or CNS involvement can have worse prognosis. Evidence of tumor lysis. HIV-associated lymphomas have poor prognosis. Poor prognosis, increased age, large tumor masses, "B" symptoms, bone marrow involvement, increased LDH, poor performance status.

- **Concept and Application**
  Most commonly clonal proliferation of B cells. Lymphoblastic lymphoma and cutaneous lymphomas frequently of T-cell origin. Different histologies represent block at different stages of B-cell development.

- **Management**
  Intensive combination chemotherapy with curative intent. If CNS positive, intrathecal therapy. Refractory or relapsed lymphomas: dose-intense chemotherapy with bone marrow transplant or peripheral stem cell transplant.

H. Multiple Myeloma

- **H&P Keys**
  Anemia, bone pain, increased susceptibility to infections, fatigue, weight loss, renal insufficiency, altered mental status.

- **Diagnosis**
  Anemia, hypercalcemia, presence of a paraprotein (or M-component) on serum protein electrophoresis (SPEP), Bence Jones proteins on urine protein electrophoresis (UPEP), lytic bone lesions on skeletal survey, bone marrow with greater than 30% plasma cells. Measure C-reactive protein and beta-2 microglobulin, serum creatinine. Quantitate amount of immunoglobulin present. Serum viscosity if altered mental status present.

- **Disease Severity**
- Stage I: Low tumor burden with Hb >10 g/dL, normal calcium, IgG <5 g/dL, IgA <3 g/dL, urine light chains <4 g/24 h and normal skeletal survey.
- Stage II: Intermediate tumor burden; patients who are neither stage I or stage III.
- Stage III: High tumor burden and any one of the following: Hb <8.5 g/dL, serum calcium >12 mg/dL, IgG >7 g/dL, IgA >5 g/dL, urine light chains >12 g/24 h, or extensive lytic bone lesions.

  Elevated beta-2 microglobulin at diagnosis reflects a poor prognosis.

- **Concept and Application**
  Monoclonal proliferation of plasma cells in the bone marrow. Osteoclastic activating factors (possibly interleukins [IL-1, IL-6], tumor necrosis factor [TNF]) responsible for bone lesions. Bone destruction leading to pathologic fractures, pain, hypercalcemia. Patients can develop amyloid over time.

- **Management**
  Low-stage disease can be conservatively treated. Chemotherapy used for symptomatic, more advanced disease. Radiation for palliation of localized lesions causing pain. Autologous or allogeneic BMT now used for eligible patients.

III. OTHER DISORDERS

A. Polycythemia Vera (Primary Erythrocytosis)

Associate ↑risk of non Hodgkins lymphoma, Multiple myeloma, leukemia

- **H&P Keys**
  Often asymptomatic, diagnosed on routine lab tests. Splenomegaly, early satiety, hypertension, facial plethora, venous thromboses, hemorrhages.

- **Diagnosis**
  Increased RBC mass with normal plasma volume key to diagnosis. Erythropoietin levels normal or low. Hypercellular bone marrow. WBC and platelet counts normal or elevated, increased LAP, increased B_{12}, low or absent iron stores.

- **Disease Severity**
  Degree of Hct elevation determines whole-blood viscosity. Decreased cerebral blood flow. Thromboembolism or life-threatening hemorrhage can occur. (Possibly iron deficiency exacerbates problem.) Can transform to myelofibrosis or acute leukemia.

- **Concept and Application**
  Autonomous proliferation of erythroid progenitors resulting from clonal proliferation of the pluripotent hematopoietic stem cell.

- **Management**
  Phlebotomy or therapy with hydroxyurea. Maintain Hct at approximately 45.

B. Secondary Erythrocytosis

- **H&P Keys**
  Spurious erythrocytosis may result from decreased plasma volume. If true erythrocytosis, consider if physiologically appropriate: chronic obstructive pulmonary disease (COPD), right-to-left cardiac shunt, high-affinity Hb, carboxyhemoglobinemia.

  Physiologically inappropriate: tumors producing erythropoietin (renal cell, hepatocellular carcinoma, cerebellar hemangioblastomas), renal disease, adrenal cortical hyperplasia, exogenous androgens.

- **Diagnosis**
  If true erythrocytosis (increased RBC mass with low plasma volume), look for no expansion of other cell lines, erythropoietin level normal or elevated (low in polycythemia vera). Arterial blood gas and determination of oxygen saturation.

- **Disease Severity**
  Level of Hct can predict. Hyperviscosity syndrome.

- **Concept and Application**
  Sometimes a result of reduced plasma volume (spurious erythrocytosis). It can be a physiologically appropriate response to decreased tissue oxygenation. It can also result from physiologically inappropriate production of erythropoietin or other factors that stimulate erythropoiesis. Higher Hct decreases cerebral blood flow.

- **Management**
  Determination of etiology. Correction of any factors that can exacerbate or cause erythrocytosis. Supplemental oxygen if needed. Phlebotomy if severe; maintenance of Hct ~45.

C. Transfusion Reactions

- **H&P Keys**
  Occur minutes to hours or even days after transfusion. Most severe is immune-mediated hemolytic reaction: fever, chest or back pain, hypotension, dyspnea, hemoglobinuria, shock. Most common are febrile reactions caused by contaminating WBCs, fever, chills. Rarely, febrile reactions are due to bacterial contamination.

  Patients with IgA deficiency can have anaphylactic reaction: sudden onset, no fever, may have cough, respiratory distress, hypotension, nausea, vomiting, abdominal pain, loss of consciousness, and shock. Delayed hemolytic transfusion reaction results from minor antigen mismatch (not detected by indirect Coombs' test).

- **Diagnosis**
  Stop transfusion and return unit to blood bank. Monitor Hg and Hct, hemoglobinuria, unconjugated bilirubin, serum hapto-

globin, LDH, coagulation profile, and renal profile. Repeat ABO, Rh, and compatibility screens. Direct antiglobulin test on post-transfusion blood sample from patient. Check IgA level if anaphylaxis. Culture remainder of blood product.

- **Disease Severity**
  Most severe reactions are major hemolytic transfusion reaction or anaphylaxis.

- **Concept and Application**
  Major hemolytic transfusion reaction caused by ABO incompatibility (immune-mediated destruction of RBCs after transfusion), often a result of clinical error.

- **Management**
  Stop transfusion! Maintenance of blood pressure and urinary output with IV fluids. If anaphylaxis: epinephrine, diphenhydramine hydrochloride (Benadryl), glucocorticoids, and aggressive hydration. Antibiotics if bacterial contamination suspected. Use of WBC filters to prevent febrile reactions.

D. Hemophilia A and B

- **H&P Keys**
  Hereditary bleeding disorders. Hemophilia A most common. A and B clinically indistinguishable. Frequent episodes of bleeding into joints, muscles, and skin with minimal or no trauma. Can result in chronic arthritis. Easy bruising. Prolonged postoperative hemorrhage. Intracranial hemorrhage can occur.

- **Diagnosis**
  Elevated partial prothrombin time (PTT) and low factor VIII (or IX) level. Normal bleeding time, normal prothrombin time (PT), normal thromboplastin time (TT). Specific assays for factor VIII or IX. 50:50 mixing study demonstrates factor deficiency. Polymerase chain reaction (PCR) analysis for prenatal detection.

- **Disease Severity**
  Patients with <1% factor VIII (or IX) level have severe disease; >5% factor VIII (or IX) results in mild disease. Clinical history very important in predicting bleeding tendency.

- **Concept and Application**
  X-linked recessive bleeding disorder resulting from deficiency of factor VIII (hemophilia A) or IX (hemophilia B).

- **Management**

  Mild Hemophilia A. First-line therapy is desmopressin (DDAVP) (stimulates immediate release of VIII:C and von Willebrand factor from endothelial cell stores). Second-line therapy is cryoprecipitate.

  Severe Hemophilia A. Factor VIII concentrate.

  Hemophilia B. Desmopressin not effective. Fresh-frozen plasma in mild cases; factor IX concentrates in more severe cases.

E. von Willebrand's Disease

- **H&P Keys**
  Mucocutaneous bleeding, epistaxis, GI bleeding, menorrhagia (can result in iron deficiency). Joint and intramuscular bleeding rare. Post-traumatic, postsurgical, and dental bleeding may be severe.

- **Diagnosis**
  (1) Prolonged bleeding time. PTT can be prolonged or normal. (2) Measure factor VIII:C activity. (3) Decreased ristocetin cofactor on platelet aggregation studies. (4) Measure von Willebrand factor (vWF) protein. (5) Measure activity levels.

  Type I. Generalized decrease in all multimeric forms of vWF.

  Type II. Selective deficiency of higher-molecular-weight forms. Perform crossed immunoelectrophoresis to make diagnosis.

- **Disease Severity**
  Repeat testing may be necessary to make diagnosis. Hemorrhagic tendency widely variable. Clinical history very important.

- **Concept and Application**
  Quantitative or qualitative abnormalities of the vWF protein, which is required for normal attachment of platelets to the endothelium. This interaction critical for normal platelet function. vWF also necessary for

normal factor VIII coagulant activity. Autosomal dominant trait with variable presentation.

- **Management**

  Assessment as to whether type I or type II disease.

  Mild Disease. Desmopressin (DDAVP) (contraindicated for some patients with type II), progesterone.

  Moderate to Severe Disease. Cryoprecipitate.

F. Vitamin K Deficiency

- **H&P Keys**

  Inadequate supply (dietary deficiency, antibiotic therapy). Surreptitious ingestion of warfarin anticoagulants. Purpura, ecchymoses, hematuria or gastrointestinal bleeding.

- **Diagnosis**

  Elevated PT, normal PTT, and normal bleeding time. A 50:50 mixing study corrects prolonged PT.

- **Disease Severity**

  Coagulopathy results in spontaneous overt bleeding.

- **Concept and Application**

  Vitamin K essential for final posttranslational carboxylation of factors II, VII, IX, and X synthesized by GI flora. No bile salt production impairs intestinal absorption and antibiotics destroy gut flora.

- **Management**

  Oral or subcutaneous vitamin K; IV vitamin K rarely indicated.

G. Lupus Anticoagulant

- **H&P Keys**

  Usually asymptomatic. Patients do not bleed spontaneously or postoperatively. Some patients have recurrent thromboembolisms or recurrent abortions. Seen in patients with autoimmune diseases, malignancies, and AIDS.

- **Diagnosis**

  Elevated PTT that does not correct with mixing studies. PT is normal or slightly elevated. Rat-brain clotting time, (TTI) test abnormal. Abnormal platelet aggregation studies. Thrombocytopenia. Positive anticardiolipin antibody or positive antiphospholipid antibody.

- **Disease Severity**

  Thromboses such as deep venous thrombosis, pulmonary embolism, or cerebrovascular accident (CVA).

- **Concept and Application**

  Immunoglobulin is directed against lipid components of the platelet membranes and prothrombin activator complex. It interferes with coagulation testing without inhibiting the activity of the coagulation factors; can be seen in SLE but usually occurs in patients with no obvious underlying disorder.

- **Management**

  Therapy not required for most patients. Rarely, patient may need lifelong anticoagulation.

H. Disseminated Intravascular Coagulation

- **H&P Keys**

  Activation of coagulation pathways resulting in both clotting and bleeding tendencies. Diffuse bleeding (IV sites, etc), petechiae, purpura, ecchymoses; may also see evidence of thrombosis. Caused by sepsis, cancers (particularly associated with acute promyelocytic leukemia), tissue damage, and amniotic fluid embolism. Bleeding and thrombotic events can lead to severe organ dysfunction.

- **Diagnosis**

  PT and PTT elevated. Low fibrinogen, increased fibrin split products (FSP), decreased factors V and VIII. Presence of D-dimers. Microangiopathic hemolytic anemia with schistocytes on peripheral smear; thrombocytopenia.

- **Disease Severity**

  Level of D-dimer formation. Fibrinogen level. PT prolongation. Uncontrolled bleeding leading to death.

- **Concept and Application**
Pathologic activation of coagulation with resultant intravascular generation of excess thrombin. Thrombin activates susceptible coagulation proteins and aggregates platelets, which become trapped in fibrin deposited in the microvasculature. Fibrin stimulates local fibrinolysis. Fibrin strands "clog" microvasculature and induce localized hemolysis.

- **Management**
Treatment of underlying disease. Replacement of clotting factors (especially fibrinogen) and platelets may be necessary. Use of heparin to stop ongoing consumption of clotting factors is controversial.

I. Antithrombin III Deficiency

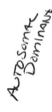

- **H&P Keys**
Family history of thromboembolic disease, recurrent venous thromboembolism (DVTs and pulmonary embolisms [PEs]). Unusual sites for clot formation, eg, mesenteric thrombosis. First episode in second or third decade. Family history of thromboembolic disease.

- **Diagnosis**
Low functional level of antithrombin III. Doppler studies or venograms revealing thromboembolism.

- **Disease Severity**
Arterial thrombosis or life-threatening PE.

- **Concept and Application**
Antithrombin III neutralizes the serine protease coagulation factors IXa, Xa, XIa, XIIa and inhibits thrombin by the formation of stable thrombin-antithrombin complexes. Inherited in an autosomal dominant fashion.

- **Management**
With active thrombosis, possible requirement of very high doses of heparin to achieve therapeutic anticoagulation. Switch to oral anticoagulation should be made as soon as possible. Patients require lifelong anticoagulation.

J. Protein-C Deficiency

- **H&P Keys**
Positive family history of thromboembolism. Recurrent venous thrombosis. Warfarin-induced skin necrosis. Purpura fulminans in newborns. Arterial thrombosis rare. Acquired protein-C deficiency has been reported (liver disease and DIC).

- **Diagnosis**
Normal PT and PTT, bleeding time, decreased protein-C level.

- **Disease Severity**
Massive pulmonary embolism, CVA.

- **Concept and Application**
Protein C requires vitamin K for its synthesis and is activated by thrombin on the surface of endothelial cells. Activated protein C acts as an anticoagulant by neutralizing factors Va and VIIIa and by stimulating fibrinolysis. Protein-C deficiency predisposes to thrombosis. Inherited as an autosomal dominant trait.

- **Management**
Long-term oral anticoagulation.

K. Activated Protein C (APC) Resistance

- **H&P Keys**
Positive family history of thromboembolism. Recurrent venous thrombosis.

- **Diagnosis**
Test for APC. PTT with and without addition of APC. Normal ratio >2. If <2, suggests APC resistence. Usually due to mutation of Factor V gene, leading to loss of cleavage site (Arg), that is, the site of APC action.

- **Disease Severity**
Life-threatening PE, CVA.

- **Concept and Application**
APC inactivates Factor Va and VIIIa, reducing clotting tendencies. APC resistance results in increased circulating Factor Va and risk for thrombosis.

- **Management**
Chronic anticoagulation in patients with repeated thrombosis. Aggressive prophylaxis in patients at risk for thrombosis.

L. Idiopathic Thrombocytopenia Purpura

- **H&P Keys**
Easy bruising, epistaxis, menorrhagia, gingival bleeding. Idiopathic thrombocytopenic purpura (ITP) in children has acute onset and is often a self-limited disease that develops after a viral infection, and lasts 5 to 6 months. Adults have a gradual onset with only 10% to 15% developing spontaneous remissions. Often ITP may be associated with SLE, Hodgkin's disease, chronic lymphocytic leukemia, pregnancy, ulcerative colitis, and infection.

- **Diagnosis**
Decreased platelet count. Normal number of megakaryocytes in bone marrow. Peripheral smear often reveals large platelets that are thought to represent young platelets.

- **Disease Severity**
Severity of thrombocytopenia (platelets <20 000 associated with significant risk of spontaneous bleeding).

- **Concepts and Application**
Usually autoimmune. Accelerated platelet destruction in spleen after coating of platelets by IgG autoantibody. Extravascular platelet destruction.

- **Management**
Treatment with corticosteroids as first-line therapy; splenectomy is often second-line therapy. IV IgG also effective.

M. Thrombotic Thrombocytopenic Purpura

- **H&P Keys**
Onset may be fulminant or subacute, single episode or recurring. Mental status changes result of intermittent ischemia. Classic pentad: fever, renal dysfunction, neurologic changes, thrombocytopenia, microangiopathic hemolytic anemia.

- **Diagnosis**
Low platelet count, normal or increased number of megakaryocytes in bone marrow, increased LDH, and increased RBC fragments on smear. Elevated BUN and creatinine or proteinuria reflect renal disease. DIC testing is negative. Usually a clinical diagnosis.

- **Disease Severity**
Severity of neurologic symptoms (patients can develop coma), and hemolysis (bilirubin, LDH, reticulocyte count).

- **Concept and Application**
Endothelial damage in microcirculation leads to platelet microthrombi, occlusion of small vessels, and ischemia in tissues. Abnormal vWf multimers.

- **Management**
Infusion of normal plasma and plasmapheresis acutely. Role of corticosteroids controversial.

N. Essential Thrombocythemia

- **H&P Keys**
Usually asymptomatic. Neurologic symptoms most common: recurrent or transient headache, visual changes. Episodes of thrombosis, embolism, or hemorrhage can occur.

- **Diagnosis**
Platelet count >800 000. Bone marrow: increased number of megakaryocytes. Normal Hb level. Mildly increased WBC (15 000 to 30 000). Platelet function testing usually abnormal. Rule out chronic inflammation, iron deficiency.

- **Disease Severity**
Complications infrequent in younger patients. In elderly patients, transient ischemic attack (TIA) most common complication. CNS hemorrhage or CVA secondary to emboli.

TTP   Fever
Renal dfcn.   thrombocytopene
neurologic Δ   microangiopathic hemolytic Aneme

- **Concept and Application**
Uncontrolled clonal proliferation of mega-karyocytic precursors.

- **Management**
Hydroxyurea, antiplatelet drugs for ischemia. Alpha-interferon, anagrelide (experimental). Splenectomy contraindicated.

O. Myelofibrosis

- **H&P Keys**
Often presents with symptoms of anemia or splenomegaly. Fever, weight loss, fatigue, early satiety, hepatomegaly, lymphadenopathy. Usually disease of elderly patients.

- **Diagnosis**
Anemia, nucleated RBCs, teardrop cells. Bone marrow biopsy shows increased fibrosis, increased megakaryocytes.

- **Disease Severity**
Extent of fibrosis on bone marrow and extramedullary hematopoiesis. Can evolve into acute leukemia.

- **Concept and Application**
Pathogenesis unclear. Replacement of normal bone marrow with fibrosis. Questionable whether fibrosis is due to megakaryocytic abnormalities.

- **Management**
Transfusions; splenectomy for painful splenomegaly or refractory cytopenia caused by splenic sequestration. Role of interferon not defined.

P. Platelet Dysfunction

- **H&P Keys**

Intrinsic. Congenital defect, easy bruising, epistaxis, menorrhagia with normal platelet count. Petechiae *not* common.

Extrinsic. Acquired defect secondary to myeloproliferative disease, uremia, malignancy, or drugs (aspirin).

- **Diagnosis**
Increased bleeding time. Abnormal aggregation studies.

- **Disease Severity**
Increased risk of postsurgical or post-traumatic bleeding.

- **Concept and Application**
Platelets fail to adhere to endothelium or to aggregate because of a deficiency of surface glycoproteins that bind fibrinogen or vWf. Failure to release platelet storage pool.

- **Management**

Intrinsic. In cases of severe bleeding, transfusion of platelets, administration of desmopressin (DDAVP).

Extrinsic. For myeloproliferative disease, platelet transfusions. For uremia, dialysis, cryoprecipitate, desmopressin (DDAVP). Discontinuation of offending drugs. Support with platelet transfusions if needed.

Q. Neutropenia

- **H&P Keys**
Acquired or congenital. Intrinsic or extrinsic abnormalities. Cyclic neutropenia: fatigue, decreased appetite, mouth sores that occur every 3 weeks and last 3 to 4 days. Hepatosplenomegaly. Evidence of infection: mouth sores, sore throat, skin infections, pneumonia, urinary tract infection.

- **Diagnosis**
CBC, follow sequential absolute neutrophil counts (ANCs). Perform bone marrow study to rule out malignancy. If febrile and ANC <500, obtain cultures and start broad-spectrum antibiotics.

- **Disease Severity**
Fungal infections or sepsis can develop. Agranulocytosis very serious (ANC <200).

- **Concept and Application**
Cyclic neutropenia results from stem cell defect. Infiltration of bone marrow by ma-

lignant neoplasm interferes with WBC maturation. Drug-induced marrow suppression often reversible if neutropenia; if agranulocytosis, often irreversible.

- **Management**
  If cyclic, and in other cases, administration of granulocyte-colony stimulating factor (G-CSF). Treatment of underlying disease. Administration of broad-spectrum antibiotics if febrile.

BIBLIOGRAPHY

Colman RW, ed. *Hemostasis and Thrombosis: Basic Principles and Clinical Practice.* Philadelphia: JB Lippincott Co; 1987.

Jandl JH, ed. *Blood Textbook of Hematology.* Boston: Little, Brown & Co; 1987.

Maxwell MW, ed. *Clinical Hematology.* Philadelphia: Lea & Febiger; 1981.

Williams J, Beutler E, Erslev A, et al, eds. *Hematology.* 4th ed. New York: McGraw-Hill Inc; 1990.

Zucker-Franklin D, ed. *Atlas of Blood Cells: Function and Pathology.* Philadelphia: Lea & Febiger; 1988.

6

Immunology and Allergy

Eliot Dunsky, MD

I. BRONCHIAL ASTHMA

- **H&P Keys**

Chronic or recurrent cough, dyspnea, or wheezing. Prolonged expiration and wheezing with or without use of accessory muscles. Allergic (extrinsic) asthma related to exposure to allergens (seasonal pollen, animals, dust, mold). Nonallergic asthma (intrinsic) asociated with infection, environmental pollution, exercise, cold air, and in a small percentage of patients, aspirin use.

- **Diagnosis**

Pulmonary function studies with a reversible obstructive pattern, positive methacholine challenge, sputum rich in eosinophils, and response to bronchodilator therapy. Chest roentgenogram, total eosinophil count, total IgE, and allergy skin tests. Arterial blood gases in acutely ill patients.

- **Disease Severity**
Disease-related lost days of school or work. Frequency of emergency room visits or hospitalizations. Frequency of nocturnal asthma or exertional asthma. Pulmonary function studies revealing severity of airway obstruction and desaturation of oxygen by oximetry or arterial blood gases.

- **Concept and Application**
Partial β-2 block leads to increased mast cell mediator release and airway hyperreactivity. Mast cell mediator release causes bronchospasm, production of tenacious mucus, and inflammation. Mediators include eosinophil chemotactic factor of anaphylaxis (ECF-A), neutrophil chemotactic factor of anaphylaxis (NCF-A), histamine, leukotrienes, prostaglandins, and platelet activating factor (PAF). Mast cell mediator release involves IgE trigger only in allergic type of asthma.

- **Management**

Early Disease. Environmental controls in allergic asthma, inhaled sympathomimetics (albuterol), inhaled cromolyn sodium, or oral theophylline.

Moderate Disease. Inhaled corticosteroids, hyposensitization in appropriate allergic asthma.

Severe Disease. Alternate or daily oral corticosteroids, immunosuppressive therapy.

Acute Episodes with Respiratory Distress. Nebulized sympathomimetic (albuterol), oxygen, IV corticosteroids, and in respiratory failure, intubation and mechanical ventilation.

II. ALLERGIC RHINITIS AND CONJUNCTIVITIS

- **H&P Keys**
Affects 20% of the population. Frequently affects other family members. Itchy eyes, nose, paroxysms of sneezing, pruritus of palate and throat. Postnasal drip, rhinorrhea, anosmia. Associated with serous otitis media or sinusitis. Seasonal symptoms caused by pollen or mold. Perennial symptoms result from exposure to animal dander, house dust mites, mold, and occupational allergens (eg, flour). More common in children than adults. Signs include: swollen bluish turbinates, nasal crease, injected conjunctivae, allergic shiners, allergic salute, and mouth breathing.

- **Diagnosis**
Positive allergy skin tests or radioallergosorbent test (RAST) assay to suspected allergens. Nasal or conjunctival smear filled with eosinophils. Elevated total IgE.

- **Concept and Application**
Patient develops specific IgE antibodies to offending allergens. IgE binds to mast cells of nasal and conjunctivae mucosa. Environmental allergens trigger mast cell mediator release including ECF-A, NCF-A, histamine, leukotrienes, prostaglandins, and PAF. Eosinophils and neutrophils are found at site of allergic reaction and participate in the inflammatory reaction.

- **Management**
Avoidance by removal of offending allergen from home (dog, cat), use of an air cleaner, or dustproofing home.

Mild Cases. Antihistamines and decongestants.

Moderate to Severe Cases. Nasal or ocular cromolyn sodium or topical corticosteroids (eg, beclomethasone). Nonresponding patients may also benefit from specific immunotherapy (hyposensitization).

III. ANAPHYLAXIS OR ANAPHYLACTOID REACTIONS

- **H&P Keys**
Sudden onset of urticaria, angioedema, wheezing, dyspnea, or hypotension. Patients may also have gastrointestinal or uterine cramps. Severe reaction may lead to hypovolemic shock and hypoxemia.

Symptoms occur soon after taking a medication (eg, penicillin, aspirin, IV contrast medium), exposure to allergen (food), or following an insect sting. Signs include pallor, cyanosis, diaphoresis, impaired or loss of consciousness, tachycardia, weak or irregular pulse, cold-clammy extremities, tachypnea, or stridor.

- **Diagnosis**
  Positive allergy skin tests or RAST assay to offending allergen. IgE-specific antibodies are not identified in anaphylactoid reactions. Other studies include: complete blood count (CBC), total IgE, total eosinophil count, elevated serum tryptase, and urine histamine.

- **Concept and Application**
  Mast cells and basophils rich in mediators (ECF-A, NCF-A, PAF, histamine, leukotriene, prostaglandins, etc) suddenly undergo degranulation following exposure to an allergen as a result of specific IgE directed against that allergen or, in the case of anaphylactic reactions, allergens cause mediator release through a non-IgE–mediated mechanism. Mast cell mediator release leads to shifting of intravascular fluid to interstitial tissues and hypotension, and may lead to hives and angioedema. Asthmatic patient will become dyspneic and wheeze.

- **Management**

  Mild Reaction. Oxygen, Trendelenburg position, subcutaneous epinephrine, and antihistamines.

  Moderate to Severe Reactions. IV fluids (often 4 to 5 L), corticosteroids, IV pressor agents (norepinephrine), shock trousers and intubation and ventilation. Prevention of future reaction by avoidance, hyposensitization in cases of insect venom hypersensitivity.

IV. URTICARIA

- **H&P Keys**
  Generalized pruritus; hives vary in size from 3 to 4 mm to giant lesion 10 to 15 cm in diameter. Usually have central clearing with peripheral erythema. Often associated with angioedema of soft tissues including eyes, lips, and tongue. Lesions leave no permanent changes in the skin. Acute urticaria: hives occur over a period of less than 6 weeks. Chronic urticaria: hives persist for period greater than 6 weeks. Hives may be induced by medications (eg, penicillin, aspirin), foods (eg, shrimp, peanut), physical exposure (cold, heat, dermatographism, pressure), and underlying systemic disease (eg, systemic lupus erythematosus [SLE], multiple myeloma).

- **Diagnosis**
  CBC, sedimentation rate, antinuclear antibodies (ANA), serum protein electrophoresis (SPEP), urine analysis (UA), and skin biopsy. Total IgE, allergy tests for suspected allergens.

- **Disease Severity**
  Mild disease includes intermittent hives responding to antihistamines. Moderate to severe disease includes persistent urticaria that requires corticosteroid treatment or is associated with angioedema of the respiratory or gastrointestinal tracts.

- **Management**
  Avoidance of known provocative factors. Antihistamines, classical or new nonsedating type, H_2 blockers, alternate corticosteroids, and epinephrine and daily steroid for angioedema.

V. IMMUNODEFICIENCY

A. Humoral Immunodeficiency

- **H&P Keys**
  Recurrent infections including pneumonia, sinusitis, otitis media, and skin infections. Frequent complaints of diarrhea and arthralgia or arthritis. Children may suffer from failure to thrive. Young males may have X-linked agammaglobulinemia. Older children and adults often suffer common variable hypogammaglobulinemia. Patients may have absent lymph nodes, and the

physical signs relate to the site of infection. Patients with recurrent bacterial infections usually lack immunoglobulins (humoral immunodeficiency); those with recurrent fungal or viral infection suffer from absent or defective T cells (cellular immunodeficiency).

- **Diagnosis**
  CBC, quantitative immunoglobulins (IgG, IgM, IgA), T- and B-cell enumeration, anergy panel, chest and sinus roentgenograms, sweat test, HIV testing.

- **Concept and Application**
  Failure of B cells to differentiate into immunoglobulin-producing cells or other defect in immunoglobulin production or secretion. Patients with IgA deficiency often have few symptoms.

- **Management**
  IV infusion of gamma globulin and early use of antibiotics in infections.

B. Cellular (T-Cell) Immunodeficiency

- **H&P Keys**
  Usually affects infants and young children. Patients often suffer from chronic diarrhea, failure to thrive, viral infections, or persistent fungal infections (*Candida*). Patients with combined immunodeficiency (loss of both T-cell and B-cell function) often fail to respond to therapy and die within the first year of life.

- **Diagnosis**
  Absence or diminution of T cells or their subsets. Decreased thymus on roentgenography. Diminished evidence of T-cell activity as assayed by the anergy panel or in vitro mitogen-induced lymphoblastic transformation.

- **Management**
  Supportive treatment. Infants with combined immunodeficiency may respond to transplant with fetal thymus tissues with total reconstitution of their immune system. Adults with chronic fungal infection may respond to ketoconazole treatment or treatment of lymphokines.

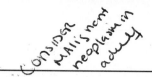
Consider malignant neoplasm in adults

VI. HEREDITARY ANGIOEDEMA

- **H&P Keys**
  This inherited disorder is seen in childhood, although an acquired form is seen mostly in adults. Patients develop nonpitting edema of the soft tissues including those of face, lips, tongue, and glottal structure. Upper airway obstruction may be fatal. Attacks may be precipitated by mild trauma (dental work). No pruritus is present. Patients do not respond to epinephrine. Gastrointestinal involvement may simulate an acute abdomen.

- **Diagnosis**
  C3, C4, CH$_{50}$, C1-esterase inhibitor (both functional and antigenic). Skin biopsy reveals no inflammatory changes and lacks eosinophilia.

- **Disease Severity**
  Severity can vary from episode to episode in an individual patient. Each episode involving the upper airway is potentially life-threatening. Severely affected patients have attacks of angioedema regularly every few weeks, and mildly affected patients may go many months between attacks.

- **Concept and Application**
  Most commonly is a congenital absence or decrease of the C1-esterase inhibitor levels. Adult with newly developed disease may have the acquired form, which may be associated with underlying malignant neoplasm.

- **Management**
  Treatment with attenuated androgens (stanozolol [Stanozol]) has been effective in long-term management. The infusion of C1-inhibitor quickly terminates an acute attack.

VII. ATOPIC DERMATITIS

- **H&P Keys**
  Atopic dermatitis is a very common chronic skin disorder seen mostly in in-

fants and children, although it occasionally occurs in adults. This highly pruritic rash often begins during the first few months of life and presents with a symmetrical eczemoid rash involving the extensor surfaces in infants. As the child grows, the rash becomes most prominent in the flexural areas (ie, popliteal fossae, antecubital fossae) and dry skin becomes a prominent feature. Over time the skin becomes lichenified and often hyperpigmented. Pruritus and scratching may lead to excoriation and infection of eczemoid lesions.

- **Diagnosis**

  Total IgE is often quite elevated, often beyond the levels seen in allergic rhinitis or allergic asthma. The total eosinophil count is frequently elevated during acute exacerbations of the rash. Allergy skin tests are usually positive to a wide variety of allergens, as is the RAST assay. However, it is often difficult to correlate these positive allergy tests with the clinical course of this disease.

- **Disease Severity**

  Although most infants presenting with atopic dermatitis have mild to moderate skin involvement, which can be managed on an outpatient basis, occasionally affected patients suffer from a generalized eczemoid rash involving much of the body surface. Severely affected patients may become acutely ill and develop generalized erythroderma and infection of their open skin lesions. This latter group require hospitalization, hydration, and intensive topical care as well as systemic antibiotics. On the other hand, mild to moderate cases of atopic dermatitis often respond to antihistamines and topical agents with gradual resolution of their skin rash over a period of years. Some adults diagnosed with atopic dermatitis during childhood continue to have dry skin and occasional hand eczema when they are exposed to irritants.

- **Concept and Application**

  The mechanism for atopic dermatitis is not well understood. However, most patients are clearly atopic, having high levels of IgE, positive allergy skin tests, and high incidence of allergic rhinitis and conjunctivitis. Paradoxically, these patients may reveal minor defects in their cellular immunity with suppressed delayed hypersensitivity tests, and decreased T-suppressor cell counts. Patients also demonstrate abnormal cutaneous vascular responses. Defects in cellular immunity are demonstrated clinically by patients with atopic dermatitis who contract herpes, which may lead to life-threatening infection.

- **Management**

  Patients with mild to moderate disease suffer from severe pruritus, which often responds in part to antihistamines. Hydroxyzine has been particularly effective in controlling pruritus. Dry skin is treated with frequent application of moisturizers. Direct irritation of sensitive skin is managed by educating patients to wear light cotton clothes and avoid irritating soaps. Topical corticosteroids are used on recalcitrant lesions and are the only effective treatment for lichenified lesions.

VIII. CONTACT DERMATITIS

- **H&P Keys**

  Contact dermatitis is a common occupational skin disease. Most of the skin is simply inflamed as a result of exposure to a nonspecific irritating substance (eg, detergents, solvents, water), which is referred to as irritant dermatitis. Allergic contact dermatitis is related to a delayed hypersensitivity reaction and may be due to a natural exposure to antigens, such as those in poison ivy plants, or may result from exposure to nickel in tools, watches, or jewelry, or allergens in hair dye, rubber products, makeup, or preservatives (parabens) in creams and lotions. Allergic contact dermatitis can occur at any age but is most often seen in adults. The lesions are initially pruritic but with time become lichenified. The location of the rash usually indicates the site of exposure. For example, allergy to a leather dye may cause shoe dermatitis.

- **Diagnosis**
Allergy patch testing to common contact allergens will usually be positive within 72 hours of application. A skin biopsy of the affected skin reveals an intense inflammatory infiltrate characterized by a marked infiltration of lymphocytes and macrophages, which typify a delayed hypersensitivity reaction.

- **Disease Severity**
Acute contact dermatitis such as widespread poison ivy may incapacitate the patient. The lesions are highly pruritic and often blisters, erythema, and edema are noted in acute reactor. Moderate reaction: often limited areas of eczema, which ultimately become lichenified. Dark-skinned patients develop hyperpigmentation at the site of the rash. Once the allergen is identified and eliminated, the rash will gradually resolve. Patients with unavoidable chronic exposure will continue to have a rash even if they receive medication.

- **Concept and Application**
Allergic contact dermatitis is a type IV delayed or cellular allergic reaction. The hapten of the allergen passes into the skin, combining with Langerhans' cells, lymphocytes, and other carrier molecules to form a complete allergen. With repeated allergen exposure, hypersensitivity increases. Lymphocytes release mediators (macrophage inhibiting factor) that recruit macrophages, which attack the allergen and surrounding tissues.

- **Management**
For acute vesiculating allergic contact dermatitis, wet dressings are best. Wetting with saline or aluminum sulfate and slow drying over 1 to 2 days will dry wet, oozing lesions. If secondary infection has occurred, antibiotics are appropriate. The mainstay of treatment is topical corticosteroids. However, oral corticosteroids may be used for extensive allergic contact reactions. Although antihistamines may help control pruritus, they do not affect the rash.

IX. ALLERGIC BRONCHOPULMONARY ASPERGILLOSIS

- **H&P Keys**
Allergic bronchopulmonary aspergillosis (ABPA) results from a manipulation reaction resulting from the presence of the fungus *Aspergillus fumigatus* present in the bronchial tree of asthmatic patients. Patients typically present with difficult-to-manage bronchial asthma associated with peripheral eosinophilia and high total IgE. Of asthmatic patients 1% to 2% are affected by ABPA. Affected patients often have a history of frequent use of or dependence on corticosteroids. At times, patients may complain of fever, general malaise, productive cough, and wheezing. Mucoid impaction may lead to atelectasis. Severely affected patients with pulmonary fibrosis may exhibit signs of chronic hypoxemia, including digital clubbing.

- **Diagnosis**
Total IgE is significantly elevated (>1000 ng/mL); elevated total eosinophil count (>1000/mm^3); positive immediate type hypersensitivity reaction to *A. fumigatus*. Roentgenograms often reveal transient infiltrates. The presence of central or proximal bronchiectasis and absence of distal bronchiectasis is highly suggestive of ABPA. Patients often have significant titers of precipitating antibodies to *Aspergillus*, and *A. fumigatus* may be cultured from sputum of some patients. Examination of sputum may identify *A. fumigatus* hyphae and intense eosinophilia.

- **Disease Severity**
ABPA may vary from mild to moderate disease, with intermittent flares of asth-

matic symptoms that quickly respond to corticosteroids, to severe progressive asthma associated with pulmonary fibrosis, progressive hypoxemia, digital clubbing, and end-stage pulmonary disease. ABPA can be staged as follows: acute, remission, exacerbation, corticosteroid-dependent asthma, and fibrotic.

- **Concept and Application**

  The mechanism for ABPA is not entirely understood. However, it appears that certain asthmatic patients have a propensity to colonize *A. fumigatus* along their bronchial tree. The fungus does not infiltrate but remains in close proximity to the respiratory mucosa. *Aspergillus* antigens apparently diffuse to the mucosa and elicit a variety of reactions including a type I–IgE reaction as well as an Arthus phenomenon. Specific IgE and IgG antibodies are produced against *Aspergillus*. Eventually an acute inflammatory reaction ensues, leading to clinical symptoms.

- **Management**

  Corticosteroids are the only known effective treatment for ABPA. Oral prednisone can reduce clinical symptoms, with attendant changes including decreased total IgE and clearing of chest roentgenogram. Initially symptomatic patients may be given 0.5 mg/kg/d until symptoms improve and chest roentgenogram clears. They are then changed over to a lower-dose maintenance program, which may consist of alternate day treatment or daily treatment. The total IgE will gradually decrease in successfully treated cases.

X. HYPERSENSITIVITY PNEUMONITIS

- **H&P Keys**

  Hypersensitivity pneumonitis or allergic alveolitis is caused by an immunopathologic reaction involving the alveoli, bronchioles, and surrounding pulmonary tissues resulting from exposure to fungi (eg, *Microsporum faeni*). Most commonly result of an occupational or hobby exposure, as with farmer's lung, bird-fancier's disease, or mushroom-pickers lung. Allergens are usually inhaled as part of an organic dust and, depending on their concentration and other factors, cause either an acute reaction or an insidious chronic disease. Acute disease is associated with fever, chills, sweats, myalgia, dyspnea, and coughing; symptoms last for hours to days following exposure. Chronic disease usually lacks systemic symptoms, with patients complaining of dyspnea and perhaps cough. Physical examination may reveal bilateral fine rales and signs of hypoxemia. Patients with chronic disease may lack clinical symptoms initially but over time develop symptoms of dyspnea resulting from chronic pulmonary fibrosis and other signs of hypoxemia.

- **Diagnosis**

  In part the diagnosis is based on evidence of the immunologic reaction to the inhaled antigen. Affected patients reveal evidence of the presence of precipitating (IgG) antibody directed against the offending antigen. Pulmonary function tests identify the presence of a restrictive lung disease, decreased diffusing capacity for carbon monoxide (DLCO), and arterial blood gases identify hypoxemia. Chest roentgenogram may be normal initially. However, eventually repeated or prolonged exposure to the antigen will be associated with roentgenologic evidence of interstitial fibrosis. Inhalation challenge is rarely used today because of the potential for serious damage.

- **Disease Severity**

  Hypersensitivity pneumonitis may present as an acute disease associated with fever and elevated white count and sedimentation rates. Within a short time signs, symptoms, and findings resolve. Repeated allergen exposure may lead to subacute episode in which pulmonary functions do not return to normal, and patients with chronic exposure to the allergen will develop irreversible restrictive lung disease and eventually end-stage lung disease.

- **Concept and Application**
  Cell-mediated and antigen-antibody hypersensitivity reactions to inhaled organic matter.

- **Management**
  Avoid offending agent; corticosteroids may be of value.

XI. HYPEREOSINOPHILIC SYNDROME

- **H&P Keys**
  Hypereosinophilic syndrome is characterized by high levels of peripheral eosinophilia and pulmonary infiltrates associated with eosinophilic infiltration into tissues and organs. Patients may initially be asymptomatic but over time show symptoms of organ pathology. Organs frequently infiltrated with eosinophils include the lung, heart, neurologic tissue, skin, bone marrow, and gastrointestinal tract. Symptoms may include coughing, dyspnea, symptoms of congestive heart failure, abdominal pain, and intravascular clotting abnormalities. Hypereosinophilic syndrome often affects young and middle-aged adult men.

- **Diagnosis**
  Eosinophilia often exceeds 50% of the peripheral white count. The total IgE is not particularly elevated. Bone marrow biopsy reveals an intense myeloid hyperplasia of eosinophils. Biopsy of affected organs (eg, lungs, heart, gastrointestinal tract) reveals an eosinophil infiltrate. The criteria for diagnosis include: eosinophilia of 1500/mm^3 for at least 6 months, tissue eosinophilia as exhibited on biopsy of specific organs, and no other known etiology for eosinophilia.

- **Disease Severity**
  Hypereosinophilic syndrome can remain a limited disease with few clinical symptoms and marked primarily by very high eosinophil counts. Or vital organs can sustain irreversible damage that ultimately results in the demise of the patient. Cardiac

infiltration may lead to a restrictive carditis and congestive heart failure.

- **Concept and Application**
  The mechanism for hypereosinophilic syndrome is unknown. It is thought to be related to overactive T-cell secretion of lymphokines, which stimulate the eosinophil line.

- **Management**
  Corticosteroids and at times cytotoxic agents are used to manage patients with significant organ involvement. With the use of corticosteroids in patients with congestive heart failure secondary to cardiac involvement, the 3-year survival has increased to 96%.

XII. DRUG ALLERGY

- **H&P Keys**
  Drug allergy is an adverse immunologic reaction to an administered medication. The development of drug allergy is influenced by the type of medication, route of administration, frequency of administration, and underlying reactivity of the patient. Patients may suffer adverse drug reactions that are not immunologic in nature and are therefore nonallergic reactions. Drug allergies can present as anaphylaxis, urticaria, or angioedema, serum-sickness—like disease, vasculitis, ptomaine disease, drug fever, nephritis, or patholic cutaneous conditions. Penicillin allergy is quite common and is often IgE-mediated, presenting as urticaria or anaphylaxis. Nonimmunologic reactions simulating drug allergy often occur with aspirin, IV contrast medium, and mast cell degranulators, such as meperidine hydrochloride (Demerol) and codeine.

- **Diagnosis**
  A good temporal correlation between the use of a medication and the onset of typical allergic symptoms (eg, anaphylaxis, urticaria) sets the stage for a diagnosis of drug allergy. However, some supporting

evidence of an immunologic reaction is needed to indicate that the origin of the reaction is immunologic. An elevated total or specific IgE, as well as eosinophilia, is supportive of the diagnosis of drug allergy. One of the most commonly diagnosed drug allergies is that of penicillin, confirmed by positive allergy skin test reactions to penicillin major or minor determinants.

- **Disease Severity**

Mild reversible or transient symptoms of drug allergy include cutaneous reactions, including urticaria, angioedema, and various exanthems. With cessation of the medications, symptoms subside without sequelae. On the other hand, drug reactions causing exfoliative dermatitis (eg, sulfa drugs), severe anaphylaxis (eg, penicillin), hepatitis (eg, phenytoin [Dilantin]), pulmonary interstitial fibrosis (eg, nitrofurantoin), interstitial nephritis (eg, methicillin), Stevens-Johnson syndrome (eg, sulfa) in some cases has led to permanent impairment and even death.

- **Concept and Application**

The drug itself or its metabolite is often a low-molecular-weight hapten, which joins with body proteins to become an allergen. IgE-mediated drug reactions usually result in urticaria, angioedema, or anaphylaxis. Autoimmune disease or vasculitis may be a result of a reaction involving immune complexes containing antigen, antibody, and complement, whereas fixed drug eruptions and contact dermatitis appear to be caused by cellular or delayed-hypersensitivity reactions.

- **Management**

Discontinuing the offending medications is often enough treatment to resolve the reaction. Antihistamines may be helpful with urticaria. Patients with angioedema and severe cutaneous exanthems benefit from corticosteroids. IgE-mediated life-threatening penicillin anaphylaxis can be effectively treated when no alternative is available with a desensitization protocol. Contact dermatitis is treated with corticosteroids. In fact, most severe drug reactions respond to corticosteroid when treated with adequate doses (eg, 2 mg/kg/d). Management of anaphylaxis may require IV medications and fluids. Adrenalin is often helpful in acute and severe IgE-mediated reactions.

BIBLIOGRAPHY

Ball GV. *Clinical Rheumatology*. Philadelphia: WB Saunders Co; 1986.

Behrman RE. *Nelson Textbook of Pediatrics*. 13th ed. Philadelphia: WB Saunders Co; 1987.

Bierman CW. *Allergic Diseases from Infancy to Adulthood*. 2nd ed. Philadelphia: WB Saunders Co; 1988.

Callen JP. *The Medical Clinics of North America, Collagen Vascular Diseases*. Philadelphia: WB Saunders Co; 1989; vol. 73.

Cohen PT. *The AIDS Knowledge Base*. Waltham, MA: The Medical Publishing Group; 1990.

Corless IB. *AIDS, Principles, Practices and Politics*. New York: Hemisphere Publishing Corp; 1989.

Dieppe PA. *Atlas of Clinical Rheumatology*. Philadelphia: Lea & Febiger; 1986.

Lawlor GJ. *Manual of Allergy and Immunology, Diagnosis and Therapy*. 2nd ed. Boston, MA: Little, Brown & Co; 1988.

Mindel A. *AIDS, A Pocketbook of Diagnosis and Management*. Baltimore: Urban & Schwarzenberg, Inc; 1990.

Moskowitz RW. *Clinical Rheumatology*. 2nd ed. Philadelphia: Lea & Febiger; 1982.

Roitt IM. *Essential Immunology*. 7th ed. London: Blackwell Scientific Publications; 1991.

Stites DP. *Basic and Clinical Immunology*. 7th ed. Norwalk, CT: Appleton & Lange; 1991.

7

Injuries, Wounds, Toxicology, and Burns

Joel S. Goldberg, DO

I. EPISTAXIS

- **H&P Keys**
  Remove blood, proceed with a careful exam to pinpoint the source of bleeding. Evaluate history for bleeding disorders and medication.

- **Diagnosis**
  If indicated, rule out bleeding disorders (prothrombin time [PT], partial prothrombin time [PTT], platelets), leukemia, and severe liver disease.

- **Disease Severity**
  Severe bleeding, most often posterior. Monitor vital signs including pulse oximetry (hypoxemia may occur from nasopulmonary reflex). Evaluate underlying conditions that exacerbate the bleeding (hypertension, liver disease).

- **Concept and Application**
  Anterior bleeding arises from Kiesselbach's plexus; posterior, from external or internal carotids. Most often trauma-induced.

- **Management**

  Anterior. Pressure or packing, topical vasoconstrictors, cauterization (silver nitrate).

  Posterior. Posterior packing, antibiotics, volume resuscitation if indicated, surgery.

II. CRANIAL INJURY

A. Facial Fracture (Frontal Bone, Mandible, Maxilla, Orbits, or Nose)

- **H&P Keys**
  History and physical exam, roentgenographic studies, information from witness.

- **Diagnosis**
  Primarily include physical exam and roentgenographic studies. Pain, cerebrospinal fluid (CSF) rhinorrhea, diplopia, deformity, and tenderness suggest fracture.

Orbital Fracture. Swelling, difficulty with eye movement, vertical diplopia, and facial emphysema.

Frontal or Ethmoid. May have CSF rhinorrhea.

Nasal Bones. Deformity, epistaxis.

Mandible or Maxilla. Swelling, pain, airway compromise, jaw pain or deformity upon opening or closing the mouth (abnormal occlusion).

- **Disease Severity**
  Neurologic deficits indicate poorer prognosis. Assess degree of trauma, neurologic status, and associated injuries via physical exam and roentgenograms.

- **Concepd Application**
  Trauma. Evaluate neurologic status at intervals.

- **Management**
  Control of airway and hemorrhage, antibiotics, fracture reduction.

Nasal. Closed reduction for simple fracture, open reduction in severe fracture cases.

Maxillary. Reduction, interdental wiring (simple fractures), orbital or zygoma wiring and traction (complex fractures).

Mandibular. Internal fixation.

Orbital. Surgery to resupport orbit.

B. Skull Trauma or Fracture

- **H&P Keys**
  May be asymptomatic, or pain or swelling, central nervous system (CNS) signs, CSF leak (nose or ears). If CSF in nose or ears or blood in the middle ear, think basilar skull fracture. If ecchymosis behind ear (Battle's sign), think mastoid fracture. With raccoon eyes, think orbital roof or basilar fracture.

- **Diagnosis**
  History and physical exam, roentgenographic exam (remember, basilar fractures may not be evident on roentgenograms).

- **Disease Severity**
  Frequent neurologic exams. Observe for epidural hematoma with linear fracture across middle meningeal artery.

- **Concept and Application**
  Skull trauma may result in hemorrhage, CSF leak, cranial nerve damage, or meningitis.

- **Management**
  Cardiopulmonary resuscitation (CPR) and ABCs (airway, breathing, circulation) then:

  Simple Linear (Closed). Observation.

  Compound Linear (Open) . Antibiotics.

  Simple Depressed. Surgical treatment (fragment elevation).

  Compound Depressed. Urgent surgical treatment.

C. Concussion

- **H&P Keys**
  Neurologic exam may be normal. History reveals a brief loss of consciousness, headache, amnesia, nausea, and vomiting.

- **Diagnosis**
  History and physical exam (roentgenogram, computed tomography [CT] scan and magnetic resonance imaging [MRI] are all normal in concussions).

- **Disease Severity**
  Determine neurologic status, degree of injury.

- **Concept and Application**
  Head trauma, resulting in head injury and brief unconsciousness, without physical brain damage, secondary to disruption of the reticular activating system. Condition is the result of brain acceleration or deceleration.

- **Management**
  Careful observation (neurologic watch).

D. Subdural Hematoma

- **H&P Keys**
  After brief or prolonged time from injury: lethargy, headache, seizures, and coma. May have dilated ipsilateral pupil.

- **Diagnosis**
  History and physical exam, radiography (CT) or MRI.

- **Disease Severity**
  Severity determined by neurologic exam and rate of deterioration.

- **Concept and Application**
  Trauma resulting in vein or brain tear and hemorrhage under the dura.

- **Management**
  Surgical (especially in acute subdural), observation in some cases (small amount of bleeding, high-risk patient).

E. Epidural Hematoma

- **H&P Keys**
  Very shortly after injury: lethargy, headache, seizures, and hemiplegia. May have brief loss of consciousness (lucid interval).

- **Diagnosis**
  History and physical exam, radiography (CT) or MRI.

- **Disease Severity**
  Evaluate neurologic status.

- **Concept and Application**
  Trauma-induced artery or vein tear (middle meningeal artery or vein common). Associated temporal bone fractures are common.

- **Management**
  Urgent surgery to avoid brain herniation.

F. Ocular Injury

- **H&P Keys**
  May have pain, vision loss, subconjunctival hemorrhage. If light flashes noted, rule out retinal detachment.

- **Diagnosis**
  History and physical exam, ophthalmoscopic and slit-lamp exam.

- **Disease Severity**
  Evaluate vision. In chemical exposure, prognosis varies with type of agent, duration of exposure, and emergency care provided.

- **Concept and Application**

Chemicals. Chemical conjunctivitis, blindness.

Trauma. Hyphema, laceration, abrasion.

- **Management**

Hyphema. (Anterior chamber hemorrhage) ophthalmologist's evaluation needed as soon as possible.

Chemicals. Irrigation with normal saline.

Corneal Abrasion. Antibiotic ointment, patch.

Corneal Laceration. Patch, refer to ophthalmologist.

G. Auditory Injury

- **H&P Keys**
  Swelling, pain, hearing loss, vertigo, and hemorrhage.

- **Diagnosis**
  History, physical exam, and audiometric exam, roentgenogram of skull and temporal bone (rule out associated fracture).

- **Disease Severity**
  Evaluate trauma to the pinna, external ear canal, and tympanic membrane.

- **Concept and Application**
  Trauma.

- **Management**

Tympanic Membrane Perforation. If small, supportive treatment (cotton earplug, systemic antibiotic for infection); if large, surgical treatment.

Noise-induced Hearing Loss. No treatment (except hearing aid).

Additional Information

Trauma may cause subperichondral hematoma. Calcified hematoma results in cauliflower ear. Prevent with early drainage.

H. Epidemiology and Prevention of Ocular and Auditory Injury

Epidemiology. Includes blunt ocular trauma (occupational, recreational, environmental), and ophthalmic foreign bodies and lacerations. Auditory injury may affect children (fireworks), teens (high-decibel music), and adults (occupational).

Prevention. Involves eye and ear protection along with education.

III. CHEST AND ABDOMINAL INJURY

A. Rib Cage

Rib fracture.

- **H&P Keys**
  Pain following trauma, increased with inspiration and palpation, ecchymosis. Rib roentgenograms may be negative shortly after injury, yet show a "healing fracture" several weeks later.

- **Diagnosis**
  History and physical exam, roentgenographic exam.

- **Disease Severity**
  Assess cardiopulmonary status and consider possible trauma in adjacent areas. Rule out pneumothorax if patient remains dyspneic.

- **Concept and Application**
  Fracture secondary to trauma. Without trauma, consider pathologic fracture causes.

- **Management**
  Simple rib fracture: Analgesics, ice initially, injection of local anesthetic (into intercostal nerve) as an option.

B. Pneumothorax

- **H&P Keys**
  Dyspnea, chest pain, absent breath sounds, decreased tactile fremitus, hyperresonance. Tachycardia and hypotension may present in tension pneumothorax.

- **Diagnosis**
  History and physical exam, chest roentgenogram.

- **Disease Severity**
  Evaluate cardiovascular status, mentation, coexisting problems, oxygenation. Reduced venous return resulting from tension pneumothorax requires urgent treatment.

- **Concept and Application**
  Air in pleural space, as a result of blunt or penetrating trauma (including iatrogenic trauma). May also be spontaneous, in patients with pulmonary disease, or menses-associated (catamenial).

- **Management**

  Tube Thoracostomy. Best treatment if over 50% or recurrent. Use fifth intercostal space, anterior axillary line.

  Small (Under 15%) or Stable Pneumothorax. Observe.

  Urgent Tension Pneumothorax. Insert large-bore needle into second intercostal space, mid-clavicular line (MCL).

  Catamenial. Medication to suppress ovulation.

C. Hemothorax

- **H&P Keys**
  Dyspnea, chest pain.

- **Diagnosis**
  History and physical exam (absent breath sounds), chest roentgenogram.

- **Disease Severity**
  Evaluate and monitor cardiac and pulmonary status. Prognosis worse in patients with significant preexisting condition.

- **Concept and Application**
  Trauma or spontaneous. May be iatrogenic (cultural venous pressure [CVP] monitor insertion).

- **Management**
  Chest tube (32 to 40 French, with 20-cm water suction).

  Open Thoracotomy. For persisting hemorrhage or massive initial blood loss. Inadequate hemothorax drainage results in fibrothorax.

D. Flail Chest

- **H&P Keys**
  Paradoxic chest wall motion, respiratory distress.

- **Diagnosis**
  History and physical exam (chest palpation), roentgenographic exam.

- **Disease Severity**
  Monitor for reduced vital capacity and respiratory distress secondary to multiple fractures.

- **Concept and Application**
  Respiratory paradox with inspiration, secondary to multiple rib fractures.

- **Management**
  Intubation and positive pressure ventilation with positive end-expiratory pressure (PEEP).

E. Additional Information

Pericardial Tamponade Symptoms

Diminished heart tones, narrow pulse pressure, electrocardiogram (ECG) with low voltage. Also Beck's triad (hypotension, reduced cardiac tones, high central venous pressure [CVP].

F. Perforation of Viscus

- **H&P Keys**
  Abdominal rigidity, pain, peritoneal irritation, reduced or absent bowel sounds, shoulder pain.

- **Diagnosis**
  History and physical exam, roentgenography, CT scan, diagnostic peritoneal lavage, exploratory laparotomy.

- **Disease Severity**
  Determined by initial presentation, presence of coexisting medical problems, and baseline condition.

- **Concept and Application**
  Trauma.

- **Management**
  Laparotomy and surgical repair.

Spleen. Repair or splenectomy.

Colon. Repair (resection if severe injury).

Stomach. Repair.

Additional Information

Blunt Abdominal Trauma. Spleen most often injured.

Penetrating Abdominal Trauma. Small bowel most often injured.

Positive Peritoneal Lavage Criteria. Red blood cells (RBC) over 20 000 (in penetrating injury) or RBC over 100 000 (in blunt injury).

G. Pelvic Fractures

- **H&P Keys**
  Pain, with history of significant injury.

- **Diagnosis**
  History and physical exam, roentgenographic studies, CT exam.

- **Disease Severity**
  Review roentgenogram. Prognosis worse in elderly and with coexisting medical problems.

- **Concept and Application**
  Trauma via falls, motor vehicle accidents, sports injuries, etc, resulting in fracture of innominate bone (ilium, ischium, or pubis), sacrum.

- **Management**
  Depends on multiple factors, with open reduction and internal fixation, traction, and external fixation as choices. Evaluation for coexisting injuries or trauma and treatment accordingly.

Fracture of Ilium. Rest.

Fracture of Anterior Superior Spine. Surgery.

Fracture of Sacrum. Rest and support.

Additional Information
Hemorrhage is the most important complication of pelvic fracture. Angiography or embolization may be required for severe, persisting hemorrhage.

H. Epidemiology and Prevention of Chest and Abdominal Injury

Epidemiology. Etiology most often cites motor vehicle accidents. Blunt injury, occupational injury, falls, and trauma play a role. Increased incidence of trauma-related abdominal and chest injury in low-socioeconomic (SES) areas. Pneumothorax and hemothorax, perforation of viscera, and vascular tears are common.

Prevention. Involves driver education and vehicle safety modifications for automobiles. Community programs, education, job opportunity, and effective law enforcement reduce the incidence of street crime trauma.

IV. Lacerations

- **H&P Keys**
  Observation; consider both history and source of injury; ascertain tetanus immunization status.

- **Diagnosis**
  History and physical exam.

- **Disease Severity**
  Evaluate neurovascular status and check for associated injuries, fractures, and hypotension.

- **Concept and Application**
  Soft-tissue injury secondary to trauma.

- **Management**
Irrigation and debridement, antibiotics if indicated, tetanus toxoid, and primary closure (maintaining minimal wound tension and everting wound edges). Use 1% to 2% lidocaine for anesthesia (with epinephrine, except for digits and end organs). Remove facial sutures in 3 to 5 days. All other areas 7 to 14 days.

Additional Information
Increased infection is noted with primary closure of human bites.

V. FOREIGN BODIES

A. Eye, Ear, and Nose

- **H&P Keys**

Ear and Nose. Asymptomatic or odor, unilateral purulent drainage.

Eye. Pain, decreased visual acuity.

- **Diagnosis**
Physical exam.

- **Disease Severity**

Ear and Nose. Check tympanic membrane, test hearing.

Eye. Full ophthalmoscopic exam.

- **Concept and Application**

Ear and Nose. Commonly children.

Eye. Often work-related, trauma.

- **Management**

Ear and Nose. Gentle removal (forceps, irrigation).

Eye. Removal of foreign body under local anesthesia. Avoid additional trauma during object removal. Ensure anesthesia is adequate and, in pediatric patient, control movement.

B. Aspiration

- **H&P Keys**
Wheezing and dyspnea may be present. History of child with object in mouth, reduced cough reflex secondary to anesthesia, disease, etc. Often an abrupt onset of cough or wheezing, dyspnea, and voice change. Most common in children under age 4.

- **Diagnosis**
Chest roentgenogram (opaque foreign body, atelectasis, mediastinal shift).

- **Disease Severity**
Evaluate degree of respiratory distress.

- **Concept and Application**
Obstruction of trachea or bronchi by a foreign body.

- **Management**
Removal via bronchoscopy

Additional Information

Epidemiology. Children are a high-risk group.

Prevention. Includes identification and management of high-risk patients (postop, sedated, or overdosed, with nasogastric [NG] tube, with neuromuscular disorders), reduction of gastric acidity (ranitidine [Zantac], etc). In children: avoidance of grapes, hot dogs; checking toys and objects for small parts, and maintaining alertness. Peanuts are the most frequently aspirated object in children. Instruction in the Heimlich maneuver.

C. Swallowed

- **H&P Keys**
Sudden onset of gagging, pain, and choking.

- **Diagnosis**
Indirect laryngoscopy, roentgenography, including barium swallow.

- **Disease Severity**
Observation and evaluation for esophageal perforation.

- **Concept and Application**
Increased frequency with motility disorders, stricture, and children results in lodged foreign body. Most common location is at the cricopharyngeus muscle.

- **Management**
Endoscopic removal. If perforation, antibiotics are given to avoid mediastinitis. Do not give meat tenderizer for obstruction by meat.

VI. BURNS

A. Eye Burns

See Ocular Injury section on page 132.

B. Thermal Burns

- **H&P Keys**
Assess degree of burn depth, determine etiology (thermal, chemical, etc), duration of exposure, and emergency or home treatment rendered.

- **Diagnosis**
History and physical exam.

- **Disease Severity**
Erythema minor (first degree). Blisters (split thickness; second degree). Pain (first and second degree). No pain (third degree).

- **Concept and Application**
Burns result in thermal skin and tissue injury. Total epidermis destruction with partial dermis destruction is typical of second-degree burns. Total epidermis and dermis destruction is noted in third-degree burns.

- **Management**
Removal of patient from source of burn, CPR, cooling burn, cleaning and debridement of burn, fluids (Ringer's initially), determination of area of burn, full history and physical exam, antibiotics, tetanus toxoid, grafting. For minor burn: loose gauze wrap on nonadhering dressing. For severe burns: CPR and airway control, fluid replacement (monitoring CVP and output), NG tube,

pain and sepsis control (morphine), surgical treatment (grafting, etc).

Additional Information
Rule of nines to estimate burn extent: Each leg is 18%, each arm is 9%, body front is 18%, back is 18%, head is 9%, groin 1%.

C. Electrical Burns

- **H&P Keys**
Look for an entry or exit wound (high-voltage, lightning). Massive tissue and bone destruction may be noted. Patients may be comatose and in cardiac arrest.

- **Diagnosis**
History and physical exam, serial arterial blood gases (ABGs), and hematocrit.

- **Disease Severity**
Prognostic factors include duration of electrical contact, amount of grounding present, path of the current, and amount of moisture present (moisture lowers skin resistance).
    Massive tissue necrosis may precede infection, rhabdomyolysis. Assess and monitor cardiac and pulmonary status. Persisting myoglobinuria indicates significant muscle injury.

- **Concept and Application**
Direct electrical tissue trauma.

- **Management**
Removal of patient from source safely, CPR, fluids and electrolyte treatment, cleaning and debridement of burns, surgical evaluation (fasciotomy, amputation), tetanus toxoid. Significant fluid replacement may be required. Monitoring for arrhythmias. Silver sulfadiazine cream may be employed topically.

VII. POISONING

A. Acetaminophen

- **H&P Keys**
Nausea and vomiting and diaphoresis.

- **Diagnosis**
  Serum acetaminophen level.

- **Disease Severity**
  Plot acetaminophen level on Rumack-Matthew normogram to define risk. Monitor vital signs; may have hepatic failure or hepatic necrosis (jaundice, abnormal liver functions, right upper abdominal pain).

- **Management**
  Activated charcoal, then ipecac or gastric lavage; antidote is acetylcysteine (Mucomyst).

B. Tricyclic Antidepressants

- **H&P Keys**
  Transient hypertension, then hypotension, tachycardia, arrhythmias, conduction blocks, seizures, anticholinergic symptoms (dry mucosa or skin, urinary retention).

- **Diagnosis**
  History and physical exam, blood level, ECG (wide QRS).

- **Disease Severity**
  Increasing serum levels correlated with increasing risk (seizures, arrhythmias). Monitor mentation, cardiac status, respiratory rate and exchange.

- **Management**
  Gastric lavage, activated charcoal, NG tube suction, sodium bicarbonate to correct acidosis, physostigmine, phenytoin (Dilantin) for seizures.

C. Sedatives

- **H&P Keys**
  Lethargy, confusion, coma, hypotension, respiratory depression, disconjugate eye motion.

- **Diagnosis**
  History and physical exam, blood drug level.

- **Disease Severity**
  Coma scale, respiration depression. Length of time since ingestion and history of amount ingested may assist in severity determination.

- **Management**
  Control of airway, activated charcoal (if patient awake), cautious gastric lavage, supportive care.

D. Stimulants

- **H&P Keys**
  Euphoria, dilated pupils, hypertension, tremors, tachycardia, hyperactivity, psychosis, hyperthermia, seizures, anxiety, nausea and vomiting.

- **Diagnosis**
  History and physical exam (tremor, increased bowel sounds, etc), blood drug level.

- **Disease Severity**
  Determined by amount ingested (peak effects 1 to 2 hours after ingestion), coexisting medical problems, cardiac status.

- **Management**
  Supportive (treatment of hypertension, seizures, arrhythmias), gastric lavage, charcoal. Emesis may cause seizures.

E. Cocaine

- **H&P Keys**
  Agitation, hyperthermia, hypertension, cardiac arrhythmia, tachycardia, seizures, pulmonary edema.

- **Diagnosis**
  History and physical exam, blood drug level.

- **Disease Severity**
  Assess by history, cardiac status.

- **Management**
  Supportive treatment, control of airway.

F. PCP (Phenylcyclidine)

- **H&P Keys**
  Nystagmus, blank stare, psychosis, lethargy, incoordination, violent behavior, self-destructive behavior.

- **Diagnosis**
  History and physical exam, blood drug level. May have elevated creatine phosphokinase and myoglobinuria.

- **Disease Severity**
  Physical exam.

- **Management**
  Control of airway, activated charcoal, supportive therapy.

G. Alcohol

- **H&P Keys**

Methanol. Blurry vision, headache, vomiting.

Ethanol. Incoordination, diplopia, drunkenness.

- **Diagnosis**
  History and physical exam, blood alcohol level. May have elevated triglycerides, uric acid, and γ-glutamyl transferase (GGT).

- **Disease Severity**
  Assess history, impact on the individual and the family, and clinical picture (withdrawal, abnormal lab tests, hepatic function).

- **Management**

Methanol. Ipecac, antidote (ethanol), sodium bicarbonate, detoxification, and rehabilitation.

Ethanol. Ipecac, sodium bicarbonate. Prevention includes continued support (AA meetings) and medication (disulfiram).

H. Solvent Sniffing

- **H&P Keys**
  Gastrointestinal (GI) irritation, CNS symptoms. Skin injury.

- **Diagnosis**
  History and physical exam.

- **Disease Severity**
  Assess duration and frequency of abuse; neurologic exam.

- **Management**
  Supportive treatment, control of airway, oxygen. Ipecac for massive ingestion only.

I. Heavy Metals and Arsenic

- **H&P Keys**
  GI symptoms, arrhythmia, CNS symptoms, skin bronzing, cyanosis, delirium, Mees' lines, renal failure, vomiting, garlic odor.

- **Diagnosis**
  History and physical exam, roentgenogram of abdomen (arsenic, lead, and iodides may be radiopaque), anemia, hematuria.

- **Disease Severity**
  Assess by clinical exam (neurologic, cardiac, and pulmonary status).

- **Management**
  Emesis, gastric lavage, dimercaprol (BAL), 3 to 5 mg/kg IM q 4 to 6 h.

Additional Information

Lead. Vomiting, lethargy, blue gum line; lavage, then use edetate calcium disodium (EDTA calcium).

Mercury. Give milk, gastric lavage, then dimercaprol. Chelators such as edetate calcium disodium (EDTA calcium), penicillamine, and dimercaprol (BAL) may be used for treatment of heavy metal toxicity.

J. Carbon Monoxide

- **H&P Keys**
  Headache, confusion, nausea, dyspnea, clumsiness, cyanosis, or cherry-red skin.

- **Diagnosis**
  History and physical exam (cyanosis), elevated blood carboxyhemoglobin.

- **Disease Severity**
  Chronic exposure associated with parkinsonism.

- **Management**
  Removal from source, 100% oxygen. Hyperbaric oxygen (if available) for comatose patients.

K. Deet

- **H&P Keys**
  CNS symptoms, seizures, coma, hypotension, GI irritation.

- **Diagnosis**
  History and physical exam.

- **Disease Severity**
  By clinical exam (neurologic status, time since exposure, degree of exposure).

- **Management**
  Emesis, gastric lavage.

L. Additional Information

1. Other Poisonings

Iron. Symptoms include diarrhea, abdominal pain, and bloody stools. Gastric lavage with Fleet's Phospho-Soda, parenteral deferoxamine.

Aspirin. Causes respiratory alkalosis and metabolic acidosis. Patient may be hyperventilating, diaphoretic, and report tinnitus.

Theophylline. Look for tremor, nausea and vomiting, and metabolic acidosis.

Narcotics. Pinpoint pupils, hypotension; administration of naloxone hydrochloride (Narcan).

Barbiturates. Respiratory depression, hypotension; supportive care, charcoal, and alkalinization of urine.

2. Selected Antidotes

Folic acid for methyl alcohol poisoning. D-Penicillamine for copper poisoning. Protamine sulfate for heparin overdose. Latrodectus antivenin for black widow spider bites.

3. Drugs Visible on Roentgenogram

Heavy metals, phenothiazines, iodides, and chloral hydrate.

4. Poisoning Management Overview

CPR, maintain airway, history and physical exam, lab studies, gastric lavage and emesis, antidote after lavage, supportive care, laboratory workup. Avoid ipecac with caustic ingestion and in somnolent patient. If antidote available, don't give charcoal in addition.

VIII. FRACTURES

A. Vertebral Column

- **H&P Keys**
  Pain, neurologic abnormalities.

- **Diagnosis**
  History and physical exam, roentgenographic exam, CT exam.

- **Disease Severity**
  Neurologic status, serial evaluations.

- **Concept and Application**
  Vertebral body fracture (wedging, body fracture), articular process fracture, transverse process fracture.

- **Management**

Simple Compression Fracture. Brace (some advocate surgical intervention, especially in young individual).

Initial Cervical Spine Treatment. Ensure airway, control shock and hemorrhage. For unstable fracture or progressing neurologic deficit, cranial traction followed by surgical internal fixation. Most other simple spinal fractures are treated with bracing or casting, with surgical intervention reserved for progressive neurologic symptoms.

B. Extremities

1. Tibia

- **H&P Keys**
  Pain when pressure applied to the tibia.

- **Diagnosis**
  History and physical exam, roentgenogram.

- **Disease Severity**
  Determine severity via roentgenogram, co-existing medical problems.

- **Concept and Application**
  Trauma.

- **Management**

Tibia Shaft. Closed reduction and cast.

Medial Tibial Condyle. Open reduction and internal fixation (ORIF).

Lateral Tibial Condyle. External reduction.

2. Fibula

- **H&P Keys**
  Pain and swelling, with retained ability to walk.

- **Diagnosis**
  History and physical exam, roentgenographic exam.

- **Disease Severity**
  Rule out coexisting ankle injury.

- **Concept and Application**
  Trauma.

- **Management**
  Walking cast or boot, followed by therapy.

3. Femur

- **H&P Keys**
  Pain, swelling, deformity.

- **Diagnosis**
  History and physical exam, roentgenographic studies.

- **Disease Severity**
  Evaluate for coexisting medical problems, hypotension.

- **Concept and Application**
  Usually significant trauma. With children, rule out child abuse.

- **Management**

Femoral Neck. Long-term traction (usually in immobile patients) versus ORIF. *Complications* of femoral neck fractures include avascular necrosis and nonunion of fracture.

4. Radius

- **H&P Keys**
  Pain, reduced elbow-joint motion.

- **Diagnosis**
  History and physical exam, roentgenographic studies.

- **Disease Severity**
  Check neurovascular status.

- **Concept and Application**
  Fall on hand common.

Colles' Fracture. Fall on extended wrist, fracture of distal radius and ulnar styloid (volar angulation and dorsal displacement).

Smith's Fracture. Fall on flexed wrist (dorsal angulation and volar displacement).

- **Management**

Radial Head. Hemarthrosis aspiration and mobilization if simple, surgical (ORIF) if complete or displaced fracture.

Distal Radius Undisplaced. Cast 4 to 6 weeks, therapy.

5. Ulna

- **H&P Keys**
  Pain, swelling, deformity.

- **Diagnosis**
  History and physical exam, roentgenogram.

- **Disease Severity**
  Check neurovascular status.

- **Concept and Application**
  Trauma.

- **Management**

Undisplaced. Closed or open reduction.

Displaced. ORIF.

Greenstick Radius or Ulna Fractures in Children. Complete the break, then cast.

6. Humerus

- **H&P Keys**
  Pain, swelling.

- **Diagnosis**
  History and physical exam, roentgenographic studies.

- **Disease Severity**
  Evaluate neurovascular status.

- **Concept and Application**
  Trauma.

- Management

Humeral Shaft or Distal Humerus. Reduction (traction), then splint and sling.

Surgical Neck of Humerus. Avoid immobilization, instead gentle range of motion. ORIF for displaced tuberosity fracture.

Additional Information

Childhood Medial or Lateral Epicondyle Fractures. If without displacement, splint elbow at 90°. With any displacement, ORIF.

IX. SPRAINS AND DISLOCATIONS

Sprains involve ligament injury; strains affect muscle; dislocations affect joints.

A. Hands

1. Distal Interphalangeal (DIP) Sprain

- **H&P Keys**
  Pain, difficulty with joint flexion or extension.

- **Diagnosis**
  History and physical exam, roentgenographic exam.

- **Disease Severity**
  Evaluate strength and range of motion.

- **Concept and Application**
  DIP joint injury or sprain, resulting in possible flexor-extensor tendon disruption.

- **Management**
  Symptomatic (if able to bend or extend joint).

Additional Information

Mallet Finger. Tendon disruption, with loss of joint extension. Treat with splinting in hyperextension or surgery.

2. Proximal Interphalangeal (PIP) Dislocation

- **H&P Keys**
  Pain. Displaced digit and motion loss.

- **Diagnosis**
  History and physical exam. Roentgenogram to rule out fracture.

- **Disease Severity**
  Examine for neurovascular status.

- **Concept and Application**
  Injury secondary to hyperextension, trauma.

- **Management**
  Flexion splint 2 weeks.

Additional Information

PIP Sprain. Splint if a hyperextension injury or collateral ligament sprain (flexion splint). Extensor slip tear-splint in hyperextension.

3. Metacarpal Phalangeal (MCP) Sprain

- **H&P Keys**
  Sprained finger or thumb MCP joint resulting in pain and motion loss.

- **Diagnosis**
  History and physical exam, roentgenographic exam.

- **Disease Severity**
  Evaluate for pinch, laxity of thumb ligaments. Use of hand contingent on adequate thumb strength.

- **Concept and Application**
  Trauma, often hyperextension.

- **Management**
  Splint.

Additional Information

Gamekeeper's Thumb. MCP joint of thumb sprained, affecting the ulnar collateral ligament. May need cast or surgical treatment.

B. Ankle

1. Lateral Ankle Pain
Injury to anterior talofibular ligament. May also include injury to fibulocalcaneal and posterior talofibular ligaments.

2. Medial Pain
Deltoid ligament injury.

- **Management**
RICE (rest, ice, compression, elevation), nonsteroidal anti-inflammatory drugs (NSAIDs), ankle splint for second-degree sprain; cast for third-degree sprain.

C. Elbow Dislocation

Check vascular and neurologic status; if urgent reduction indicated, splint.

D. Shoulder Dislocation or Injury

Anterior-inferior dislocation most common (in young patients).

- **Management**

Dislocation. Urgent reduction (slow traction, Kocher maneuver, or reduction under anesthesia). Other dislocations include posterior and inferior.

Mild Sprain. Prevent external rotation for 6 weeks; sling.

X. DROWNING

- **H&P Keys**
Wheezing, tachypnea, vomiting, pulmonary edema, unconsciousness, shock, and cardiac arrest.

- **Diagnosis**
History and physical exam, chest roentgenogram, ABGs, ECG.

- **Disease Severity**
Consider duration of immersion, patient's baseline medical status, water temperature, timing of rescue measures, cardiac and pulmonary status, electroencephalogram (EEG).

- **Concept and Application**
Dry (laryngospasm) or water-induced asphyxia results in hypoxia and brain damage.

- **Management**
Urgent CPR and 100% oxygen. Remember to continue CPR in hypothermic or prolonged cold-water submersion victims.

XI. INSECT AND SNAKE BITES

- **H&P Keys**

Insect Bite. Mild erythema to anaphylaxis and hypotension.

Snake Bite. Pain, swelling, hemorrhage, weakness, disseminated intravascular coagulation (DIC), possible systemic signs (lethargy, vomiting, shock).

- **Diagnosis**
History and physical exam. Leukocytosis and coagulation disorders.

- **Disease Severity**
Assess cardiac and pulmonary status. Consider patient's age and preexisting medical problems, time since envenomation, location of bite (trunk has worse outcome than extremity), snake size (larger worse), and emergency treatment received.

- **Concept and Application**

Insects. Hymenoptera species commonly.

Snakes. In United States, pit vipers (copperhead, rattlesnake, water moccasin) are responsible for poisonous bites and are toxic to cardiac, vascular, and hematologic systems.

- **Management**

Insect Bite. Remove stinger, ice, diphenhydramine hydrochloride (Benadryl).

Anaphylaxis. Epinephrine (1:1000 0.4 mL SQ), CPR, antihistamines, prednisone.

Snake Bite. Tourniquet, antivenin.

Additional Information

Black Widow Spider (Latrodectus mactans). Red hourglass pattern on abdomen, bite results in muscle spasm and cramping. First, clean wound, give tetanus toxoid, muscle relaxant, antivenin.

Brown Recluse Spider (Loxosceles reclusa). Violin design on back; possible skin necrosis; treat by cleaning wound and tetanus toxoid.

XII. ANAPHYLACTIC SHOCK

Systemic severe IgE-induced allergic reaction.

- **H&P Keys**
  Hypotension, urticaria, dyspnea, tachycardia, vascular collapse and pruritus.

- **Diagnosis**
  History (onset of symptoms in seconds to minutes) and physical exam.

- **Disease Severity**
  Assess cardiac and pulmonary systems. Prognosis worse without early intervention.

- **Concept and Application**
  Mast cell and basophils release histamine, platelet-activating factor (PAF), and arachidonic acid.

- **Management**
  CPR and control airway, epinephrine (1 : 1000 0.3 to 0.5 mL SQ), diphenhydramine hydrochloride (Benadryl), fluids, dopamine, beta-agonists, corticosteroids, oxygen, aminophylline.

XIII. ADDITIONAL MANAGEMENT INFORMATION

A. Traumatic Injury

Administer CPR, control airway, treat urgent problems (large pneumothorax, hemorrhage, etc), administer oxygen, insert IV line, give fluids and medications, obtain history and physical exam, roentgenographic and lab studies.

B. Shock

Administer CPR, control airway, obtain history and physical exam, administer fluids (caution with cardiogenic shock, check CPV and output), administer vasopressors (dopamine), get lab studies, administer: corticosteroids, diuretic (protects kidneys), buffers, antibiotics (septic shock).

C. Child Abuse, Sexual Abuse, Rape

History and physical exam, medical treatment, documentation of evidence and appropriate reporting, psychologic evaluation and support, separation from danger (child abuse), and long-term care plan.

D. Thermal Injuries

1. Frostbite

- **H&P Keys**
  Tissue cold and hard without feeling.

- **Diagnosis**
  History and physical exam; affected area may be white (superficial injury) or firm and frozen (deep injury).

- **Disease Severity**
  Duration of exposure, prior presence of peripheral vascular disease or other medical problems.

- **Concept and Application**
  Tissue damage as a direct result of thermal trauma. Skin and tissue damage from ice crystal formation. May be superficial or deep. Line of demarcation may develop.

- **Management**
  Rapid rewarming after body-core temperature warming, tetanus toxoid, possibly antibiotics, surgical evaluation, amputation.

2. Hypothermia

- **H&P Keys**
  Reduced core temperature (under 35°C), lethargy, coma, hypotension, confusion, miotic pupils.

- **Diagnosis**
  History and physical exam, core temperature at or below 95°F (35°C), ECG (Osborne wave, elevated J-point; bradycardia; arrhythmias), flat EEG, metabolic acidosis.

- **Disease Severity**
  Assess duration of exposure, age (mortality much worse in the elderly), emergency treatment rendered, and preexisting med-

ical problems. Worse prognosis with lower temperatures.

- **Concept and Application**
Reduced core temperature from cold exposure resulting in decreased cardiac output, hypotension.

- **Management**
CPR, core rewarming (heated oxygen), warming blankets, volume expansion. Monitor ABGs, electrolytes, and rule out sepsis.

Additional Information

Hypothermia Complications. DIC, pneumonia.

Hypothermic Death. Never declare dead unless patient rewarmed to 98.6°F.

3. Heatstroke

- **H&P Keys**
Confusion, elevated core temperature with or without diaphoresis, tachycardia, hypotension, hot skin, and headache.

- **Diagnosis**
History and physical exam, core temperature high, combined with CNS signs.

- **Disease Severity**
Assess cardiovascular status. Worse prognosis with significant preexisting disease.

- **Concept and Application**
Tissue injury from elevated temperature, with children and elderly at most risk.

- **Management**
Urgent cooling (water spray, fans, ice packs), skin massage to reduce peripheral vasoconstriction.

Additional Information

Heat Cramps. Cramps from salt depletion; skin cool; give fluids and salt, keep cool.

Heat Exhaustion. Salt and water loss; nausea, weakness, headache, thirst; give fluids and salt, keep cool.

Complications of Heat Stroke. DIC, rhabdomyolysis, acidosis.

XIV. EPIDEMIOLOGY AND PREVENTION OF SELECTED ACCIDENTS

A. Home Accidents

Epidemiology. Involves all age groups and consists of a wide variety of hazards (electrical, thermal, poisoning, and trauma).

Prevention. Includes education, preventive planning (bicycle helmets, toy and playground equipment checks, removal of dangerous objects, obstacles, etc).

B. Workplace Accidents

Epidemiology. Includes increased risk groups (meatcutters and -packers, steelworkers, etc), along with all employees.

Prevention. Includes both education and exercise of precautions (eye shield, hearing protection, hard hats, steel-tip shoes, etc) and elimination of dangerous materials, practices, and procedures.

C. Athletic Accidents

Epidemiology. Includes home, school, recreational, and professional accidents. Impact and type of injuries are multiple, including falls, trauma, thermal injury, sprains and strains, fractures, concussions, contusions, and death.

Prevention. Includes education, correction of both training and performance errors (spearing in football), providing protective equipment of correct fit.

D. Automobile Accidents and Drunk Driving

Epidemiology. Includes all ages of society, with increased risk for both teenagers (drunk and reckless driving) and the elderly (visual impairment, cognitive functioning, and reaction time). Increased risk is associated with motorcycle and three-wheel all-terrain vehicle use.

Prevention. Includes education (driving, using seat belts, avoidance of drugs and alcohol), reduced speed limits, better roads, improved roadway markings and median barriers, and abutment protection. Numerous other factors play a role, such as larger-size vehicles, air bags, collapsible steering wheel, and padded dash regulations. Drunk driving prevention includes both education and modification of drinking age, along with effective legal deterrents (fines and jail terms).

E. Head and Spinal Cord Injury and Whiplash

Epidemiology. Includes motor vehicle accidents (the major cause of these injuries), falls, child abuse, occupational and trauma-induced accidents.

Prevention. Includes education, safety devices (automotive: air bags, seat and shoulder belts, padded dashboards, headrests; work: hard hats, etc), and behavior modification (avoidance of high-risk activities or behavior). Appropriate emergency care may prevent permanent neurologic sequelae (sandbag, head stabilization).

F. Drowning

Epidemiology. Involves children most often.

Prevention. Centers on education (parents and children), swimming instruction, water and boating safety, dangers of hyperventilation, dangers of drug and alcohol use, and CPR training. Recognition of high-risk patients (epilepsy, syncope, divers, children, etc).

G. Ingestion of Poisonous and Toxic Agents

Epidemiology. Includes accidental overdose in both children and adults and work and environmental toxicology and suicide in adolescents and adults.

Prevention. Includes education, awareness and labeling of dangerous substances, prevention of child access (keeping medication and toxins locked and in unaccessible locations, "child-proof" containers), and easy access to emergency advice and treatment. Importance of home supply of ipecac.

H. Gunshot and Stab Wounds

Epidemiology. Demonstrates an increasing rate of violent crime and increasing use of handguns and automatic weapons. Elevated level of crime in poor SES areas. Impact includes an ever-increasing utilization of medical emergency facilities, financial burden on the medical insurance system, and morbidity and mortality, including innocent bystanders.

Prevention. Includes education, gun control, control of alcohol and drug use and abuse, law enforcement, and society efforts to diffuse inner-city neglect.

I. Thermal Injury

Prevention. Key points include education (increased heat disorders with alcohol; cystic fibrosis patients; dehydration; dark, nonbreathable clothing; use of antipsychotics and diuretic; high-humidity days) and need for increased fluid intake and gradual heat acclimatization. Skin protection and early recognition of symptoms in frostbite and hypothermia patients is critical. Increased awareness for high-risk patients (elderly and children, alcohol and drug abusers, CNS disease, and sepsis) is important.

J. Child, Spouse, and Elderly Abuse

Epidemiology. Suggests that susceptible abuse victims include children, spouses, and the elderly. Impact is significant as a frequent society malady with great morbidity, mortality, and possible permanent psychologic impact. Difficulty in obtaining accurate numbers of cases involved because of sensitivity of the subject and reluctance of many abused individuals to tell their stories.

Prevention. Physician and family education to obtain early diagnosis and screen for potentially abusive parents (observe and evaluate mother for postpartum depression). High index of suspicion may be required. Past medical history (abusers may have been abused themselves as children).

K. Sexual Abuse and Rape

Epidemiology. Suggests that adolescents and young children are at risk for sexual abuse (usually by family member).

Prevention. Includes early recognition by health care workers, and education. Rape prevention includes patient education (how to avoid being a target) and self-defense.

L. Fire Prevention

Prevention. Includes education (not smoking in bed, proper storage of flammables, etc), home precautions (smoke detector and fire extinguisher, fireplace glass screen, fire safety plan, escape route, upkeep of electrical systems, etc).

M. Falls

Epidemiology. Affect children, elderly, and adults (workplace injury, seizure-disorder patients, alcoholics) and are a frequent cause of accidental death. Significant morbidity and mortality associated with hip fractures.

Prevention. For children includes child-proofing the house, covering sharp corners, window locks, stair gates, and control of obstacles. For the elderly, medical and family assessment for need of cane, walker, or wheelchair; medical treatment or control of contributing illness (Parkinson's disease, visual impairment, anemia, stroke, etc).

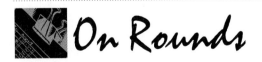

Poisoning Symptoms at a Glance

• Carbon Monoxide:	Headache, confusion, cyanosis, cherry-red skin
• DEET:	CNS symptoms
• Iron:	Diarrhea, abdominal pain, bloody stools
• Theophylline:	Tremor, nausea, vomiting
• Aspirin:	Respiratory alkalosis, metabolic acidosis, hyperventilation, tinnitus
• Stimulants:	Dilated pupils, euphoria, hypertension, tremor
• Cocaine:	Agitation, hyperthermia, hypertension, arrhythmia
• PCP:	Nystagmus, blank stare, violent behavior, incoordination
• Acetaminophen:	Nausea and vomiting
• Sedatives:	Lethargy, confusion, coma, hypotension
• Heavy metal and Arsenic:	GI symptoms, CNS symptoms, skin bronzing

BIBLIOGRAPHY

Ballenger JJ. *Diseases of the Nose, Throat, Ear, Head, and Neck.* 14th ed. Philadelphia: Lea & Febiger; 1991.

Behrman RE. *Nelson Textbook of Pediatrics.* 13th ed. Philadelphia: WB Saunders Co; 1987.

Birnbaum JS. *The Musculoskeletal Manual.* Orlando, FL: Academic Press Inc; 1982.

Bryson PD. *Comprehensive Review in Toxicology.* 2nd ed. Rockville, MD: Aspen Publishers Inc; 1989.

Cailliet R. *Neck and Arm Pain.* 3rd ed. Philadelphia: FA Davis Co; 1991.

D'Ambrosia RD. *Musculoskeletal Disorders, Regional Examination and Differential Diagnosis.* 2nd ed. Philadelphia: JB Lippincott Co; 1986.

Dreisbach RH. *Handbook of Poisoning: Prevention, Diagnosis and Treatment.* 12th ed. Norwalk, CT: Appleton & Lange; 1987.

Goldfrank LR. *Toxicologic Emergencies.* 4th ed. Norwalk, CT: Appleton & Lange; 1990.

Hardy JD. *Textbook of Surgery.* 2nd ed. Philadelphia: JB Lippincott Co; 1988.

Rockwood CA. *Fractures in Adults.* 3rd ed. Philadelphia: JB Lippincott Co; 1991; 1, 2.

Schroeder SA. *Current Medical Diagnosis and Treatment.* 30th ed. Norwalk, CT: Appleton & Lange; 1991.

Turek SL. *Orthopaedic Principles and Their Application.* 4th ed. Philadelphia: JB Lippincott Co; 1984; 1, 2.

Upton AC. Environmental medicine. *Med Clin North Am.* Philadelphia: WB Saunders Co; 1990.

8

Infectious Disease

Craig A. Wood, MD

I. HUMAN IMMUNODEFICIENCY VIRUS INFECTION AND THE ACQUIRED IMMUNE DEFICIENCY SYNDROME

A. Human Immunodeficiency Virus Infection

- **H&P Keys**

  Human immunodeficiency virus (HIV) infection is acquired by sexual transmission (heterosexual, homosexual), parenteral transmission (transfusion, intravenous drug use), and perinatal transmission. Primary HIV infection may be followed 4 to 6 weeks later by an acute mononucleosis-like illness lasting for 1 to 2 weeks consisting of fever, malaise, lymphadenopathy, rash, headache, arthralgias, or myalgias. Following primary infection, there is an asymptomatic period of variable duration. Ultimately, the patient may present with systemic complaints (fever, sweats, weight loss, diarrhea), opportunistic infection (see individual descriptions of common opportunistic infections [OI] for clinical clues), or malignant disease associated with the HIV-related immunosuppression. Rate of progression of disease is highly variable, with an average period of 10 years from HIV infection to acquired immune deficiency syndrome (AIDS).

- **Diagnosis**

  HIV serologic testing (enzyme-linked immunosorbent assay [ELISA] screen, Western blot test) indicated for workup of unexplained symptoms or risk group. Further workup in the HIV-positive patient for baseline and follow-up: CD4-positive T-lymphocyte count (CD4), complete blood count (CBC), chemistry (including liver tests), VDRL or rapid plasma reagin (RPR), purified protein derivative (PPD), hepatitis B serology, cytomegalovirus (CMV) serology, toxoplasmosis serology, Pap smear. HIV viral load (or burden) now may be measured by quantifying plasma HIV RNA. The two most frequently used assays are polymerase chain reaction (PCR) and branched DNA (bDNA). Viral load measurements appear to help to predict the initial rate of progression to AIDS and to select, maintain, and modify effective antiretroviral therapy.

- **Disease Severity**

  Association between development of OIs and absolute or percentage CD4. As CD4 declines, risk of OI increases substantially. With CD4 >800, risk of OI very small; CD4 200 to 500, increasing risk for *Mycobacterium tuberculosis, Histoplasma, Cryptococcus;* CD4 <200, risk for *Pneumocystis carinii* pneumonia (PCP); CD4 <100, increasing risk for *Toxoplasma,* CMV, *Mycobacterium avium* complex (MAC). OIs associated with the majority of AIDS deaths. Classification of HIV infection modified to include CD4 as marker for HIV-related immunodeficiency (Table 8–1). Categorization is based on clinical conditions associated with HIV infection and CD4 count. Clinical category A includes acute primary infection, asymptomatic HIV infection, and persistent generalized lymphadenopathy (PGL). Conditions in category B include bacillary angiomatosis, oropharyngeal candidiasis, persistent vulvovaginal candidiasis, cervical dysplasia or carcinoma in situ, constitutional symptoms (fever or diarrhea for more than 1 month), hairy leukoplakia, herpes zoster (more than two episodes or more than one dermatome), idiopathic thrombocytopenic purpura (ITP), listeriosis, pelvic inflammatory disease (PID), or peripheral neuropathy. Category C includes the clinical conditions listed in the AIDS surveillance case definition (Table 8–2). All patients in clinical category C as well as all with a CD4 <200 meet the case definition of AIDS. People with a high HIV viral load are at increased risk for disease progression. Initiation or modification of antiretroviral therapy may be dictated based on these results.

- **Concept and Application**

  The etiologic agent of AIDS is the human retrovirus, HIV. The CD4-positive T lymphocyte is the primary target of infection because of the CD4 surface marker. Loss of

TABLE 8-1. 1993 REVISED CLASSIFICATION SYSTEM FOR HIV INFECTION AND EXPANDED AIDS SURVEILLANCE CASE DEFINITION FOR ADOLESCENTS AND ADULTS*

CD4 + T-Cell Categories	Clinical Categories		
	(A) Asymptomatic, Acute (Primary) HIV or PGL	(B) Symptomatic, not (A) or (C) Conditions	(C) AIDS-Indicator Conditions[†]
1. ≥500/μL	A1	B1	C1
2. 200–499/μL	A2	B2	C2
3. <200/μL AIDS-indicator T-cell count	A3	B3	C3

* Persons with the AIDS-indicator conditions (category C) as well as those with CD4-positive T-lymphocyte counts <200/μL are reportable as AIDS cases.

† See text AIDS case definition.

PGL, persistent generalized lymphadenopathy.

TABLE 8-2. CONDITIONS INCLUDED IN THE 1993 AIDS SURVEILLANCE CASE DEFINITION

- Candidiasis of bronchi, trachea, or lungs
- Candidiasis, esophageal
- Cervical cancer, invasive
- Coccidioidomycosis, disseminated or extrapulmonary
- Cryptococcosis, extrapulmonary
- Cryptosporidiosis, chronic intestinal (>1 mo duration)
- Cytomegalovirus disease (other than liver, spleen, or nodes)
- Cytomegalovirus retinitis (with loss of vision)
- Encephalopathy (HIV-related)
- Herpes simplex: chronic ulcer(s) (>1 mo duration), or bronchitis, pneumonitis, or esophagitis
- Histoplasmosis, disseminated or extrapulmonary
- Isosporiasis, chronic intestinal (>1 mo duration)
- Kaposi's sarcoma
- Lymphoma, Burkitt's (or equivalent term)
- Lymphoma, immunoblastic (or equivalent term)
- Lymphoma, primary, of brain
- *Mycobacterium avium-intracellulare* complex of *M. kansasii,* disseminated or extrapulmonary
- *M. Tuberculosis,* any site (pulmonary or extrapulmonary)
- *Pneumocystis carinii* pneumonia
- Penumonia, recurrent
- Progressive multifocal leukoencephalopathy
- *Salmonella,* septicemia, recurrent
- Toxoplasmosis of brain
- Wasting syndrome caused by HIV

CD4 T lymphocytes results in progressive impairment of the immune response. There is a wide spectrum of disease, from asymptomatic infection to life-threatening illness caused by OI or cancer. HIV binds CD4-positive cells and then fuses with the membrane to enter the cell. The virus uncoats, and reverse transcriptase transcribes viral RNA into DNA, which is integrated into the host chromosome. The latent virus reactivates, DNA is transcribed into RNA, viral proteins are synthesized, and new virus is assembled (mediated by HIV protease) budding from the cell membrane. Antiviral chemotherapy may be aimed at any point in the viral life cycle. Reverse transcriptase (nucleoside and nonnucleoside reverse transcriptase inhibitors) and protease (protease inhibitors) are the only viral targets thus far utilized in antiretroviral therapy. Our knowledge concerning HIV viral dynamics and host CD4 dynamics has recently expanded markedly. The HIV viral load is quite high during initial infection and then, after approximately 3 months, falls to a steady-state level. These steady-state levels vary considerably from person to person (approximately 10^2 to 10^6 HIV RNA copies/mL). The CD4 count also falls during acute HIV infection and then rebounds to a steady-state level. We now appreciate that even during the so-called latent phase of infection when the HIV viral load and CD4 count appear stable, there is tremendous daily turnover of both HIV and CD4. Understanding these dynamics has important treatment implications. The high mutational rate of HIV, occurring constantly, has greatly influenced the rapid acceptance of combination therapy in an effort to escape or delay antiretroviral resistance. The initial steady-state HIV load has great predictive value for the rapidity of disease progression. People with very high viral load are at risk for rapid progression, whereas those with very low viral burden may be long-term nonprogressors. The HIV viral load has also important implications for monitoring and modifying antiretroviral therapy (see Management). Some AIDS-indicator conditions are caused directly by HIV infection (AIDS encephalopathy, wasting syndrome [cytokine dysregulation], enteropathy, nephropathy).

- **Management**

Our antiretroviral armamentarium has expanded markedly. There are now nine antiretroviral agents approved for use in the United States. There are five nucleoside reverse transcriptase inhibitors, including zidovudine (AZT, ZDV, Retrovir), didanosine (ddI, Videx), zalcitabine (ddC, Hivid), stavudine (d4T, Zerit), and lamivudine (3TC, Epivir). There are three HIV protease inhibitors approved, including saquinavir (Invirase), ritonavir (Norvir), and indinavir (Crixivan). There is a single nonnucleoside reverse transcriptase inhibitor currently available, nevirapine (Viramune), but others are being developed and will likely follow. Therapy of HIV infection is based on CD4 count, HIV RNA level, and clinical status. The optimal time to initiate antiretroviral is unknown and remains an area of controversy. Most would initiate antiretroviral therapy in symptomatic HIV disease, in asymptomatic individuals with a CD4 of <500, and in asymptomatic persons with a CD4 of >500 but with a high viral load and/or a rapidly declining CD4 count. Preferred initial antiretroviral regimens include nucleoside combinations such as AZT + 3TC, ddI, ddC, or d4T, or ddI + d4T. The protease inhibitors should probably be reserved for patients at higher risk for progression. The role of the nonnucleoside reverse transcriptase inhibitors has not yet been determined. The minimal decrease in HIV RNA indicative of effective therapy is >0.5 log decrease. The goal level of HIV RNA after initiation of treatment is undetectable or at least <5000 copies/mL. A return of the HIV RNA level to within 0.3–0.5 log of the pretreatment value suggests drug treatment failure and the need to modify therapy. HIV RNA measurements should be obtained at baseline, 3 to 4 weeks after initiating or changing therapy, and every 3 to 4 months along with CD4 counts.

Health Maintenance. Annual influenza vaccine, pneumococcal vaccine, hepatitis B vaccine (if seronegative). (See comments in the specific OI section for prophylaxis recommendations for PCP, MAC, etc.) Counseling and HIV testing should be offered to all pregnant women. AZT administration has been shown to reduce significantly perinatal transmission of HIV. Postexposure prophylaxis for health care workers reduces the frequency of HIV transmission. The Centers for Disease Control and Prevention has recently published recommendations for this indication depending on the type and source of the exposure. Combination prophylaxis with ZDV + 3TC +/− indinavir has been recommended.

B. *Pneumocystis carinii* Pneumonia

silver stain

- **H&P Keys**

Most common AIDS-defining OI in the United States. Symptoms include fever, nonproductive cough, tachypnea, and shortness of breath.

- **Diagnosis**

Usually develops when CD4 <200. Arterial blood gas: hypoxemia, increased alveolar–arterial (A–a) gradient. Chest roentgenogram usually shows bilateral infiltrates. Definitive diagnosis by demonstrating organism in pulmonary specimen (induced sputum, bronchoalveolar lavage [BAL], biopsy). Cysts commonly visualized with silver stain, trophozoites with Giemsa stain.

- **Disease Severity**

Mild disease (patient may be candidate for oral, outpatient therapy): Po_2 >70 mm Hg, able to take oral medication, reliable follow-up. More severe hypoxemia and tachypnea are poor prognostic features.

- **Concept and Application**

Controversy as to whether *P. carinii* is a protozoan or a fungus. Infection with *P. carinii* common early in life but rarely causes disease in the normal host. HIV-related immunosuppression allows *P. carinii* to cause disease.

- **Management**

Mild disease may be treated orally; severe disease is treated parenterally. Drug of choice is considered to be trimethoprim and sulfamethoxazole (TMP-SMX). Alternative agents include pentamidine, dapsone and trimethoprim, clindamycin and primaquine, atovaquone, or trimetrexate and leucovorin. Duration of therapy is usually 21 days. For nonventilated patients with more severe disease (room air Po_2 <70, A–a gradient >35 mm Hg), adjunctive corticosteroids are recommended.

BACTRIM (handwritten annotation in left margin)

Health Maintenance. Primary PCP prophylaxis is recommended for all HIV-infected individuals with a CD4 <200. Secondary prophylaxis is indicated for all with a previous episode of PCP. Drug of choice is trimethoprim-sulfamethoxazole with alternatives, including dapsone with or without trimethoprim or pyrimethamine, aerosolized or IV pentamidine, or clindamycin and primaquine.

C. Cytomegalovirus Infection

- **H&P Keys**

CMV infection is the most common viral OI in advanced AIDS. The most common infections are retinitis, gastrointestinal (GI) tract (colitis, esophagitis), and systemic (viremia associated with wasting syndrome). Ocular complaints include "floaters," decreased vision, or blindness. Ophthalmoscopic exam is diagnostic. Colitis is associated with persistent diarrhea and crampy abdominal pain. Esophagitis presents with dysphagia. Wasting syndrome consists of significant weight loss with fever or diarrhea.

- **Diagnosis**

CMV retinitis diagnosed by ophthalmoscopic exam revealing exudates and inflammatory changes following a vascular distribution. Isolation of CMV from other body sites confirms the ophthalmoscopic impression. CMV colitis or esophagitis is diagnosed by endoscopy revealing edema, erythema, erosions, and hemorrhage. Cyto-

megalic inclusions seen on histopathologic exam are diagnostic. CMV may be recovered from buffy coat blood culture in the wasting syndrome.

- **Disease Severity**

The severity of CMV retinitis often is dictated by the anatomic location of lesions. Macular involvement severely affects vision; optic nerve involvement may cause blindness.

- **Concept and Application**

CMV infection is extremely common in the general population, but disease is rare in the normal host. HIV-related immunosuppression allows for reactivation of latent viral infection. Shedding of virus in urine, saliva, or blood documents active infection but does not prove disease.

- **Management**

Induction antiviral therapy is given with either ganciclovir or foscarnet for an average of 14 to 21 days. Both drugs effectively suppress retinitis but cannot cure infection. Maintenance therapy must be given lifelong to prevent recurrence. Efficacy of either agent for disease other than retinitis is less well documented. Neutropenia or thrombocytopenia with ganciclovir and renal insufficiency with foscarnet are frequently dose-limiting. Long-term maintenance therapy with ganciclovir is associated with a risk of emergence of ganciclovir resistance, dictating treatment with foscarnet. Cidofovir recently approved for the treatment and maintenance therapy of CMV retinitis in patients with AIDS. Because of its long half-life, cidofovir is given once weekly for therapy and every other week for maintenance. Pharmacokinetics may allow for outpatient induction and maintenance without long-term IV access. Nephrotoxicity and neutropenia have limited the initial enthusiasm for this therapy, and the role of cidofovir is still being clarified. Oral ganciclovir also approved for maintenance therapy of CMV retinitis, but high cost and inferior efficacy have limited its application. Ganciclovir intraocular implants are available therapy but, without systemic therapy, there is a risk of disease in the contralateral eye or of systemic disease.

Health Maintenance. Oral granciclovir recently approved as prophylaxis for CMV disease in AIDS. Current use is unclear as toxicity, cost, and resistance issues are resolved.

D. Tuberculosis

- **H&P Keys**

  Since the mid-1980s, there has been a resurgence of tuberculosis (TB) in the United States with many of the cases present in HIV-infected individuals. Symptoms may be predominantly pulmonary in nature or may reflect extrapulmonary disease. The most common extrapulmonary sites are peripheral lymph nodes and bone marrow. Other extrapulmonary sites include bone and joint, urine, liver, spleen, GI mucosa, and cerebrospinal fluid (CSF). TB may present as wasting syndrome. TB in early HIV infection tends to be similar to disease in non–HIV-infected patients. TB in later-stage HIV disease is more commonly atypical.

- **Diagnosis**

  Pulmonary TB often occurs at a CD4 of 250 to 500; extrapulmonary TB more commonly occurs at a lower CD4, often <200. Skin testing with PPD may be unreliable because of skin test anergy. Chest roentgenography may show typical nodular infiltrates, with or without cavitation (apical lung fields most common), or more atypical lesions. Isolation of *M. tuberculosis* from pulmonary or other sites is diagnostic.

- **Disease Severity**

  Though response to therapy is often good, the prognosis for AIDS patients with tuberculosis is worse than in HIV-seronegative individuals and worsens with progressive immunosuppression. Mortality rates are higher and median survival time shorter in the AIDS patient. Disseminated or extrapulmonary disease is more common with advanced immunodeficiency.

- **Concept and Application**

  HIV-related immunosuppression increases the frequency and severity of TB disease. The HIV-infected person is at risk for developing active disease from an exposure as well as from reactivation of previously acquired, inactive disease.

- **Management**

  A minimum treatment course of 9 months is recommended in AIDS patients. In patients without previous treatment for TB and living in an area where drug resistance is low, a four-drug regimen (isoniazid [INH], rifampin, pyrazinamide, and ethambutol) is recommended for initial treatment. In patients with a history of previous TB treatment, contact with multidrug-resistant TB, or living in an area with frequent drug resistance, five or more initial anti-TB drugs are indicated. These regimens consist of the standard four drugs with ofloxacin, ciprofloxacin, or streptomycin. Direct observed therapy (DOT) should be used whenever possible.

Health Maintenance. Twelve months of isoniazid is indicated for all HIV-infected people with a positive PPD.

E. Disseminated *Mycobacterium avium-intracellulare* Complex

< 100 CD4

- **H&P Keys**

  Disseminated MAC is the most common systemic opportunistic bacterial infection in patients with AIDS. MAC most commonly causes lymphadenitis and disseminated infection. Persistent fever and significant weight loss are common. Other frequent symptoms include chronic diarrhea or malabsorption and abdominal pain. Lymphadenopathy, organomegaly, or an abdominal mass may be present.

- **Diagnosis**

  Abnormal liver tests, anemia, and leukopenia are common. Diagnosis requires isolation of the organism from blood or tissue (bone marrow, lymph node, or liver are commonly positive).

- **Disease Severity**
  There are a tremendous number of organisms present in the blood and tissues of AIDS patients with disseminated MAC. Despite the number of organisms, most patients remain asymptomatic until late-stage disease. Survival without therapy is only about 4 months.

- **Concept and Application**
  MAC are ubiquitous in the environment and acquisition in AIDS is thought to result from ingestion or inhalation of organisms. MAC are minimally virulent and rarely cause disease in the immunocompetent host. The immune dysfunction in AIDS allows for disseminated infection. Disseminated MAC almost always occurs when the CD4 is <100, often when the CD4 is <50.

- **Management**
  MAC are generally resistant to usual antimycobacterial agents. Effective therapy has been shown to sterilize blood cultures and reduce the symptoms associated with infection, such as fever and night sweats. Current recommendations for therapy include either clarithromycin or azithromycin with ethambutol. Sicker patients should receive one or more additional drugs from among rifabutin, clofazimine, ciprofloxacin, and amikacin. Therapy is continued for life.

Health Maintenance. Prophylaxis is indicated for HIV-positive patients with a CD4 of <100, as it appears to reduce disseminated MAC by approximately 55% to 85%. In order of decreasing efficacy, azithromycin + rifabutin, clarithromycin, azithromycin, and rifabutin, are all approved for MAC prophylaxis. The combination regimen is the least tolerated and most expensive. There is a risk of emergence of resistance with a macrolide regimen, potentially risking a loss of efficacy if a therapeutic regimen is needed.

F. Toxoplasma Encephalitis

- **H&P Keys**   *CD4 <100*
  Toxoplasma gondii is the most common cause of latent central nervous system (CNS) infection in AIDS patients. Toxoplasma encephalitis is a multifocal process often involving the brainstem or basal ganglia with associated neurologic abnormalities that may include focal deficit, change in reflexes or sensation, ataxia, or decreased cognition.

- **Diagnosis**
  Patients with toxoplasma encephalitis are almost always seropositive. Computerized tomographic (CT) scan or magnetic resonance imaging (MRI) will typically reveal multifocal disease. Serologic and radiographic studies lead to a presumptive diagnosis for which empiric therapy is often prescribed. Definitive diagnosis requires isolation of the organism from brain tissue.

- **Disease Severity**
  Brain biopsy for definitive diagnosis usually is reserved for patients who are seronegative, have atypical radiologic imaging (single lesions), or do not improve on empiric therapy.

- **Concept and Application**
  Serologic evidence suggests that up to one third of the U.S. population has been infected with toxoplasma. Reactivation of a latent infection generally occurs when the CD4 is <100. Up to one third of seropositive AIDS patients may ultimately develop toxoplasma encephalitis. The immunosuppression associated with AIDS allows for the release of tachyzoites from tissue cysts, resulting in necrotic foci of infection.

- **Management**   *Pyrimethamine   Folinic Acid   Sulfadiazine*
  The initial 6 weeks of therapy commonly consists of pyrimethamine, sulfadiazine, and folinic acid. Response rates are quite high, approximately 85%. Clindamycin may replace sulfadiazine in the sulfa-allergic patient. Chronic maintenance, often at reduced dose, is required lifelong to prevent relapse.

Health Maintenance. There is evidence that trimethoprim-sulfamethoxazole used for PCP prophylaxis may also be effective prophylaxis for toxoplasma encephalitis.

G. Cryptococcal Infection

[handwritten: India ink]

[handwritten margin: Fluconazole maintenance]

- **H&P Keys**
Cryptococcal infections are the most common disseminated fungal infections in patients with AIDS. *Cryptococcus* may involve the lungs, skin, blood, bone marrow, prostate, and genitourinary tract, but more than one half of the time it causes meningitis. The symptoms of cryptococcal meningitis are often subacute and nonspecific. The most common symptoms are fever and headache, with nausea, vomiting, and mental status changes occurring less frequently. Classic symptoms of meningismus, neck stiffness, and photophobia are uncommon.

- **Diagnosis**
Serum cryptococcal antigen may be used to screen patients with nonspecific symptoms. CSF cryptococcal antigen allows for the most rapid diagnosis of cryptococcal meningitis, though culture is the standard diagnostic test. The India ink exam is usually positive in patients with AIDS.

- **Disease Severity**
Mental status changes and very high serum or CSF cryptococcal antigen titers are associated with poor prognosis.

- **Concept and Application**
Cryptococcus neoformans is an encapsulated yeast commonly found in soil and associated with pigeon feces. Disease is acquired by inhalation and primarily infects the lungs. The humoral and cell-mediated immune defects in AIDS predispose to dissemination.

- **Management**
Standard acute therapy includes an approximate 2-week course of amphotericin B with or without flucytosine. All patients receive lifelong maintenance therapy to prevent relapse. Fluconazole is most frequently prescribed for maintenance therapy.

H. Herpes Simplex Virus

- **H&P Keys**
Herpes simplex virus (HSV)-1 and HSV-2 may cause ulcerative lesions at a variety of sites including orolabial, genital, anorectal, and esophageal ones. Lesions are characterized by pain and vesicle formation, followed by ulceration. Crusting and epithelialization may be quite delayed or may not occur without specific therapy. Regional lymphadenopathy may be present. Esophagitis is associated with retrosternal pain and dysphagia.

- **Diagnosis**
The diagnosis of mucocutaneous HSV should be confirmed with HSV culture. Esophagitis requires endoscopy, with histopathologic and culture confirmation.

- **Disease Severity**
Severity depends on the site of infection and degree of immunosuppression.

- **Concept and Application**
Most AIDS patients have previously been infected with HSV and have latent infection in nerve root ganglia. Latent HSV more often reactivates in the immunocompromised patient and can cause severe, prolonged disease.

- **Management**
Usual therapy consists of oral or parenteral acyclovir until the lesions are healed. Many patients will relapse after initial therapy and will require reinduction therapy, followed by long-term maintenance. Long-term maintenance therapy with acyclovir is associated with a risk of development of acyclovir resistance, dictating therapy with foscarnet.

II. SEXUALLY TRANSMITTED DISEASES

A. Gonorrhea

- **H&P Keys**
Uncomplicated gonococcal infections include urethritis, cervicitis, anoproctitis, and pharyngitis (pelvic inflammatory disease [PID] is discussed separately). Urethritis in men causes discharge and dysuria, whereas women report only dysuria. Cervicitis is

generally asymptomatic. Pharyngitis generally causes no symptoms, but erythema and exudate may be present on exam. Anoproctitis often is associated with pain, and discharge may be present. Disseminated gonococcal infection resulting from bacteremia may cause petechial or pustular skin lesions, tenosynovitis, septic arthritis, and occasionally hepatitis, endocarditis, or meningitis.

- **Diagnosis**
  Specific diagnosis is made by recovery of *Neisseria gonorrhoeae* from discharge, blood, or other body fluid. Therapy for uncomplicated disease is often empiric, without benefit of culture.

- **Disease Severity**
  Of the uncomplicated gonococcal infections, pharyngitis is the most difficult to cure and dictates more specific therapy than does anal or genital infection (see Management, below). Hospitalization is generally recommended for initial therapy of disseminated infection.

- **Concept and Application**
  It is estimated that 1 million new infections with *N. gonorrhoeae* occur each year in the United States. Most infections in men produce symptoms for which they seek medical care, though often not before transmitting the disease. Many infections in women produce minimal or no symptoms and medical care is delayed until serious complications such as PID occur. PID may cause tubal scarring, resulting in infertility or ectopic pregnancy.

- **Management**
  Coinfection with *Chlamydia* is common in people treated for gonococcal infections. Treatment for gonorrhea should include therapy that is effective against *C. trachomatis* (see *Chlamydia* management recommendations). Resistance to penicillin and tetracycline largely dictates current treatment regimens. Recommended regimens for uncomplicated gonorrhea include ceftriaxone, cefixime, ciprofloxacin, or ofloxacin, all as a single dose, plus a regimen effective against *Chlamydia*. Ceftriaxone or ciprofloxacin

should be used for pharyngeal disease. Many additional antibiotics are effective for uncomplicated gonorrhea, including spectinomycin, ceftizoxime, cefotaxime, cefotetan, cefoxitin, cefuroxime axetil, cefpodoxime proxetil, enoxacin, lomefloxacin, and norfloxacin. The initial treatment of disseminated gonococcal infection consists of a parenteral cephalosporin (ceftriaxone, cefotaxime, ceftizoxime) or spectinomycin. After clinical improvement, oral therapy with cefixime or ciprofloxacin is given to complete a week of treatment.

Health Maintenance. Persons treated for gonorrhea should be screened for syphilis by serologic testing. Sex partners should be referred for treatment. Safer sex is encouraged.

B. *Chlamydia*

- **H&P Keys**
  C. trachomatis causes urethritis and cervicitis (PID is discussed separately). Urethritis is characterized by mucoid or purulent discharge and dysuria. Cervicitis is characterized by yellow endocervical exudate.

- **Diagnosis**
  A number of nonculture chlamydial tests may aid in the rapid, presumptive diagnosis of *Chlamydia* infection; however, these tests are less specific than standard culture and may yield false-positive results. Chlamydial infection may be confirmed by standard cell culture methods or by an additional nonculture test.

- **Disease Severity**
  As with gonococcal disease, chlamydial infection may go untreated in the female patient and result in tubal scarring, infertility, or ectopic pregnancy.

- **Concept and Application**
  C. trachomatis is an obligate intracellular parasite of columnar or pseudostratified cells. It is estimated that the incidence of chlamydial infection is greater than that of gonorrhea.

- **Management**
  Coinfection with the gonococcus is common in patients treated for chlamydial in-

fection. Treatment for *Chlamydia* should include therapy effective for gonococcal infection (see gonorrhea management recommendations). Recommended regimens for chlamydial urethritis or cervicitis include doxycycline or azithromycin. Alternatives include ofloxacin or erythromycin. These antibiotic therapies (with the exception of ofloxacin, which is active against gonorrhea) should include an antigonococcal regimen.

Health Maintenance. Sex partners should be referred for evaluation and treatment. Safer sex is encouraged.

C. Syphilis

- **H&P Keys**
  Patients may seek treatment for signs or symptoms of primary infection (ulcer at the site of infection), secondary infection (rash, mucocutaneous lesions, adenopathy), or tertiary disease (cardiac, neurologic, ophthalmic, auditory, or gummatous lesions). Patients with latent infection may be identified by serologic testing.

- **Diagnosis**
  Darkfield exam and direct fluorescent antibody tests of exudates or tissue allow the diagnosis of early syphilis. Presumptive diagnosis may be made serologically (a nontreponemal test: Venereal Disease Research Laboratory (VDRL) or RPR, confirmed with a treponemal test: fluorescent treponemal antibody absorption [FTA-ABS] or *Treponemal pallidum* hemagglutination assay [MHA-TP]). Neurosyphilis is diagnosed by CSF examination (cell count, protein, VDRL). Patients with primary, secondary, or latent syphilis need not undergo CSF exam unless there are: neurologic or ophthalmic signs or symptoms, other evidence of active disease (aortitis, gumma, iritis), treatment failure, HIV infection, nontreponemal titer $\geq 1:32$ (unless duration less than 1 year), or therapy not involving penicillin is planned.

- **Disease Severity**
  Patients are staged and treated according to clinical signs and symptoms (see above) or

the duration of latency. Patients with latent disease for less than 1 year are considered to have early latent disease, whereas others have late latent syphilis or syphilis of unknown duration. The duration or intensity of therapy is largely dictated by stage. The titer of the nontreponemal test correlates with disease activity.

- **Concept and Application**
  Syphilis is a systemic disease caused by *T. pallidum*. Though CSF invasion in primary or secondary syphilis is common, few patients develop neurologic disease when treated appropriately.

- **Management**
  Patients with primary, secondary, and early latent syphilis are treated with one 2.4 mouse units IM injection of benzathine penicillin. Nonpregnant penicillin-allergic patients can be treated with a tetracycline for 2 weeks. Patients with late latent and tertiary syphilis are treated with three weekly 2.4-MU IM injections of benzathine penicillin G. Four weeks of a tetracycline offers alternative therapy. Neurosyphilis is treated for 10 to 14 days with high-dose penicillin. All patients require follow-up serologic testing (CSF if appropriate) to monitor response. Though data are incomplete, HIV-infected patients are generally treated as above (though some recommend more intense treatment than is dictated by stage).

Health Maintenance. Sex partners should be referred for evaluation, though transmission occurs only when mucocutaneous lesions are present (uncommon after the first year). Patients should be considered for HIV testing.

D. Chancroid

- **H&P Keys**
  One or more painful genital ulcers, often in association with tender inguinal lymphadenopathy. Inguinal adenopathy may be suppurative.

- **Diagnosis**
  Special cultures not readily available. Diagnosis probable with clinical signs and no evidence of syphilis or HSV.

- **Disease Severity**
  In extensive cases, scarring may occur despite successful therapy.

- **Concept and Application**
  Chancroid is caused by *Haemophilus ducreyi* and is endemic in many areas of the United States. It is a well-established cofactor for HIV transmission.

- **Management**
  Azithromycin or ceftriaxone single-dose therapy and 7 days of erythromycin are all successful. Alternatives include 7 days of amoxicillin and clavulanate potassium or 3 days of ciprofloxacin.

Health Maintenance. Patients should be tested for HIV infection. ✳

E. Pelvic Inflammatory Disease

- **H&P Keys**
  PID represents a spectrum of upper genital tract inflammatory disorders, including endometritis, salpingitis, tubo-ovarian abscess, and pelvic peritonitis. Minimal clinical criteria for diagnosis of PID include lower abdominal tenderness, adnexal tenderness, and cervical motion tenderness. Fever and cervical discharge may be present.

- **Diagnosis**
  Evidence for cervical infection with *N. gonorrhoeae* or *C. trachomatis* may be present. Endometritis on endometrial biopsy, tubo-ovarian abscess on ultrasound exam, or laparoscopic evidence is more definitive.

- **Disease Severity**
  Patients with mild disease may be considered for outpatient therapy. Initial hospitalization is recommended if: diagnosis is uncertain, abscess is suspected, pregnancy or HIV infection is present, patient is unable to tolerate oral medication, or compliance or follow-up are in question.

- **Concept and Application**
  PID is caused by sexually transmitted organisms such as *N. gonorrhoeae* or *C. trachomatis,* as well as genital tract flora such as anaerobes *Enterobacteriaceae* and group B streptococcus.

- **Management**
  Outpatient regimens include cefoxitin plus probenecid or a third-generation cephalosporin plus 14 days of doxycycline or ofloxacin plus either clindamycin or metronidazole for 14 days. Common parenteral regimens include cefoxitin or cefotetan plus doxycycline or clindamycin plus gentamicin.

Health Maintenance. Sex partners should be referred for evaluation and treatment.

F. Epididymo-Orchitis

- **H&P Keys**
  Unilateral testicular pain and tenderness and palpable swelling of the epididymis are common.

- **Diagnosis**
  Culture for *N. gonorrhoeae* and *C. trachomatis* and urine culture.

- **Disease Severity**
  Failure to improve within 3 days requires reevaluation and consideration of hospitalization.

- **Concept and Application**
  In men under 35 years of age, epididymo-orchitis is caused by gonococcal or chlamydial infection. Nonsexually transmitted disease associated with urinary tract infection caused by enteric bacilli is more common in men over 35 years of age.

- **Management**
  Treatment of sexually transmitted epididymo-orchitis includes therapy for both *Chlamydia* and gonorrhea. Single-dose ceftriaxone and 10 days of doxycycline or of ofloxacin are recommended.

Health Maintenance. Sex partners should be referred for evaluation and treatment.

G. Genital Herpes

- **H&P Keys**
  Groups of painful vesicles that progress to shallow ulcerative lesions prior to crusting and healing. Commonly seen on external genitalia and on the cervix. Systemic symptoms such as fever, headache, and myalgias are not uncommon with initial episodes.

- **Diagnosis**
  Viral culture for HSV.

- **Disease Severity**
  Most infected persons never recognize signs of genital herpes; some have symptoms during the initial episode and then never again. A minority of infected persons have recurrent genital lesions.

- **Concept and Application**
  Genital herpes, usually caused by HSV-2, is a recurrent disease without cure. Serologic evidence suggests that 30 million people in the United States have been infected.

- **Management**
  Acyclovir therapy speeds recovery from initial episodes or recurrences and can be used to suppress recurrent disease. Therapy cannot eradicate latent virus.

III. OTHER INFECTIOUS DISEASES

A. Infectious Mononucleosis

- **H&P Keys**
  Fever, sore throat, lymphadenopathy, splenomegaly. Headache, myalgias, sweats, anorexia, and abdominal pain may also be present.

- **Diagnosis**
  Atypical lymphocytosis, positive test for heterophile antibody (positive Monospot or Mono-Diff test), positive serology for Epstein-Barr virus (especially IgM antibody to viral capsid antigen [VCA-IgM]).

- **Disease Severity**
  Complications of infectious mononucleosis include hemolytic anemia (positive Coombs' test), thrombocytopenia, granulocytopenia, splenic rupture rarely, neurologic syndromes (including Landry-Guillain-Barré syndrome), myocarditis, or pericarditis.

- **Concept and Application**
  Infectious mononucleosis is an acute, self-limited infection predominantly occurring in children and young adults and caused by

the herpesvirus, Epstein-Barr virus (EBV). Usual course of illness is 2 to 4 weeks.

- **Management**
  There is no specific therapy for EBV infection. Corticosteroids are occasionally prescribed for severe tonsillitis with airway compromise, severe hemolytic anemia or thrombocytopenia, neurologic complications, myocarditis, or pericarditis.

B. Varicella (Chickenpox)

- **H&P Keys**
  Erythematous, maculopapular lesions that rapidly become vesicular and then pustular. The lesions then crust and heal. Spread of the rash is centripetal.

- **Diagnosis**
  Positive Tzanck preparation for multinucleate giant cells and isolation of varicella-zoster virus (VZV).

- **Disease Severity**
  Varicella is occasionally complicated by pneumonia, encephalitis, or Reye's syndrome. Infection in the compromised host often includes severe skin disease and dissemination to visceral organs.

- **Concept and Application**
  Varicella, or chickenpox, is caused by the herpesvirus VZV. Varicella is the primary infection in the nonimmune host, whereas zoster (shingles) is a reactivation of latent virus. Transmission of infection is very efficient from 1 day before skin lesions appear to approximately 5 days after onset.

- **Management**
  The use of acyclovir in a usual episode of varicella, though approved, is controversial. Acyclovir therapy is routinely used for disseminated disease, CNS involvement, and pneumonia (zoster is discussed in Chapter 2).

Health Maintenance. Vaccine for VZV has recently been approved and is indicated for everyone older than 1 year without a history of clinical varicella. The duration of protection and the need for a booster remain to be determined. Zoster-immune globulin is given

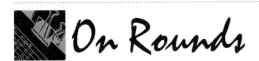

AIDS at a Glance

- **Cause:** Human retrovirus, HIV
- **Primary Target:** CD4-positive T lymphocyte
- **Transmission:** Sexual, parenteral and perinatal
- **Early Symptoms:** Primary HIV infection may be followed in 4–6 weeks by a mono-like illness
- **HIV to AIDS:** 10 years
- **Diagnosis:** HIV serologic testing (ELISA screen, Western Blot)
- **Disease Severity:** As CD4 declines, risk of opportunistic infection increases

BIBLIOGRAPHY

ACP Task Force on Adult Immunization and Infectious Diseases Society of America. *Guide for Adult Immunization.* 3rd ed. Philadelphia: American College of Physicians; 1994.

Carpenter CCJ, Fischel MA, Hammer SM, et al. Antiretroviral therapy for HIV infection in 1996. *JAMA.* 1996;276:146–54.

Centers for Disease Control and Prevention. General recommendations on immunization. Recommendations of the Advisory Committee on Immunization Practices (ACIP). *MMWR.* 1994;43 (No. RR-1).

Centers for Disease Control. 1993 revised classification system for HIV infection and expanded surveillance case definition for AIDS among adolescents and adults. *MMWR.* 1992;41 (No. RR-17).

Centers for Disease Control. Pelvic inflammatory disease: guidelines for prevention and management. *MMWR.* 1991;40 (No. RR-5).

Centers for Disease Control and Prevention. Prevention of varicella. Recommendations of the Advisory Committee on Immunization Practices (ACIP). *MMWR.* 1996;45 (No. RR-11).

Centers for Disease Control. Recommendations of the Advisory Committee on Immunization Practices (ACIP): use of vaccines and immune globulins in persons with altered immunocompetence. *MMWR.* 1993;42 (No. RR-4).

Centers for Disease Control. Recommendations for the prevention and management of *Chlamydia trachomatis* infections, 1993. *MMWR.* 1993;42 (No. RR-12).

Centers for Disease Control and Prevention. Recommendations of the U.S. Public Health Service task force on the use of zidovudine to reduce perinatal transmission of the human immunodeficiency virus. *MMWR.* 1994;43 (No. RR-11).

Centers for Disease Control. Sexually transmitted diseases treatment guidelines, 1993. *MMWR.* 1993;42 (No. RR-14).

Centers for Disease Control and Prevention. Update: Provisional Public Health Service recommendations for chemoprophylaxis after occupational exposure to HIV. *MMWR.* 1996;45:468–72.

Centers for Disease Control and Prevention. USPHS/IDSA guidelines for the prevention of opportunistic infections in persons infected with human immunodeficiency virus: a summary. *MMWR.* 1995;44 (No. RR-8).

Fauci, AS. Immunopathogenic mechanisms of HIV infection. *Ann Intern Med.* 1996;124:654–63.

Gorbach SL. *Infectious Diseases.* Philadelphia: WB Saunders Co; 1992.

Havlir DV, Richman DD. Viral dynamics of HIV: implications for drug development and therapeutic strategies. *Ann Intern Med.* 1996;124:984–94.

Mandell GL. *Principles and Practice of Infectious Diseases.* 4th ed. New York: Churchill Livingstone Inc; 1995.

Medical Letter. The choice of antibacterial drugs. *Med Lett Drugs Ther.* 1996;38:25–34.

Medical Letter. The treatment of Lyme disease. *Med Lett Drugs Ther.* 1992;34:95–97.

Medical Letter. Drugs for AIDS and associated infections. *Med Lett Drugs Ther.* 1995;37:87–94.

Medical Letter. Drugs for non-HIV viral infections. *Med Lett Drugs Ther.* 1994;36:27–32.

Medical Letter. Drugs for sexually transmitted diseases. *Med Lett Drugs Ther.* 1995;37:117–122.

Medical Letter. Drugs for tuberculosis. *Med Lett Drugs Ther.* 1995;37:67–70.

Medical Letter. New drugs for HIV infection. *Med Lett Drugs Ther.* 1996;38:35–37.

Sande MA. *The Medical Management of AIDS.* 4th ed. Philadelphia: WB Saunders Co; 1995.

Schacker T. Collier AC, Hughes J, et al. Clinical and epidemiologic features of primary HIV infection. *Ann Intern Med.* 1996;125:257–264.

9

Musculoskeletal and Connective Tissue Disease

Pekka Mooar, MD

I. INFECTIONS

A. Osteomyelitis

[handwritten: • STAPH AUREUS • neonates - STREP B 6mo 5yr ↑ H.inf]

- **H&P Keys**
  More common in children, may be triggered by trauma, usual seeding is hematogenous. Presents with refusal to bear weight or move extremity. Fever usually present.

- **Diagnosis**
  White blood cell count (WBC), erythrocyte sedimentation rate (ESR), blood cultures. Radiographs may show soft-tissue swelling, early followed by periosteal elevation and finally bone infarct and involucrum. Bone scan shows focal increased activity.

- **Disease Severity**
  Clinical evaluation following a change in ESR may be useful.

- **Concept and Application**
  In children, osteomyelitis is usually hematogenous. Seeding occurs in the small arterioles of the metaphysis where there is sluggish blood flow. Infection elevates pressure, creating pain. Pus lifts the periosteum and may cause cortical necrosis, resulting in a sequestrum. The most common organism is *Staphylococcus aureus,* except in neonates, where *Streptococcus* B is most common. From 6 months to 5 years *Haemophilus influenzae* is the most common.

- **Management**
  Aspiration is useful to recover organisms for antibiotic selection. Blood cultures may substitute if positive. IV antibiotics, followed by oral medication after temperature normalized for 6 weeks or until ESR normal. Immobilization for symptomatic relief. Surgical debridement for refractory cases with involucrum and sequestra.

B. Septic Arthritis *[handwritten: >100,000 Diagnostic]*

- **H&P Keys**
  Pain, erythema, joint effusion, and soft-tissue swelling. Refusal to bend joint or bear weight in children.

- **Diagnosis**
  Joint aspirate, high white count >50 000 suspicious, >100 000 diagnostic of infection. Polymorphonuclear leukocytes predominate. High peripheral WBC, elevated ESR.

[handwritten notes at top left: Septic Arthritis / H Infl < 5yr / Saureus > 5yr / Gcaureus]

- **Disease Severity**
Coexisting morbidity predisposes to infection (chronic disease, cancer, drug abuse, immune deficiency).

- **Concept and Application**
H. influenzae most common in children under 5 years old, *S. aureus* in children over 5 years old, gonococci in adults and adolescents. In children, joint may be seeded from area of contiguous osteomyelitis.

- **Management**
In children, hip joint requires early surgical drainage to prevent joint destruction. Adults may be treated with serial aspiration, following the WBC in the fluid. If no response, surgical debridement, often arthroscopically. IV antibiotics, followed by oral antibiotics.

C. Lyme Disease   *[handwritten: Erythema chronicum MIGRANS]*

- **H&P Keys**   *[handwritten: Bell's palsy]*
Variable presentation: joint effusions, arthralgia, myalgia, fatigue, occasional cardiac arrhythmia, central nervous system (CNS) involvement (Bell's palsy, headaches). May have characteristic rash, erythema chronicum migrans ("bull's-eye" rash).

- **Diagnosis**
Joint aspirates negative by culture, radiographs normal, serologic testing: enzyme-linked immunosorbent assay (ELISA) screen confirmatory Western blot.

- **Disease Severity**
Cardiac and CNS symptoms.

- **Concept and Application**
Disease caused by *Borrelia burgdorferi*, a spirochete borne by the deer tick (*Ixodes dammini*). The disease occurs in three stages: rash, neurologic symptoms (neuritis, neuropathy, encephalopathy), arthritis. Immune complexes and cryoglobulin accumulate in the synovial fluid and tissues of the host.   *[handwritten: ① RASH / ② Neurological / ③ ARTHRITIS]*

- **Management**
Treatment with oral doxycycline 100 mg b.i.d. or amoxicillin 2 g/d for 3 weeks.

[handwritten: Doxycline / Amoxicillin]

Recalcitrant cases: IV ceftriaxone (Rocephin) 2 g/d for 6 weeks.

D. Gonococcal Tenosynovitis

- **H&P Keys**
Acute loss of joint motion with fusiform swelling of digit. Erythema, redness, fever, migratory polyarthritis, multiple arthralgia.

- **Diagnosis**
History and physical diagnosis confirmed by aspiration and culture. Radiographs normal.

- **Disease Severity**
Multiple-location presentation.

- **Concept and Application**
Presentation of systemic gonococcal infection.

- **Management**
Penicillin G or ceftriaxone.

II. DEGENERATIVE DISORDERS

A. Degenerative Joint Disease; Arthralgia   *[handwritten: OSTEOARTHRIS = DJD / ARTICULAR CART.]*

- **H&P Keys**
Eighty percent of adults 65 years and older demonstrate radiographic signs of osteoarthritis (OA). Signs and symptoms are usually localized. If diffuse symptoms exist, collagen vascular disease should be considered. Pain occurs after use and is relieved with rest; in later stages rest pain and night pain may be present. Crepitation occurs with passive motion and may be associated with pain. Joint enlargement from osteophyte and synovial hypertrophy is present late.

- **Diagnosis**
Characteristic radiographic findings are joint-space narrowing, subchondral bony sclerosis, marginal osteophyte formation, subchondral cyst formation. Laboratory findings are normal.

Qs 1) Pain - worsen C ACTIVITY
relieve by rest
2) morning STIFFness
3) gelling phenomenon - sensation
renew stiffness after
prolong inactivity

Heberden's nodes - enlg DIP
BOUCHARDS   PIP

Differential Diagnosis. Roentgenographic findings of OA of the hands are also seen with seronegative arthritis. OA of the hip may be avascular necrosis or pigmented villonodular synovitis. OA of the knee may be meniscus pathology, osteochondritis dessicans, or a sequela of septic arthritis.

• **Disease Severity**
Disease severity is a clinical diagnosis with severe restriction of activities of daily living. Radiographs may be normal early, weight-bearing films demonstrate joint-space narrowing. Osteophyte formation with sclerosis and cyst formation occur late.

• **Concept and Application**
Disease is characterized by progressive loss of articular cartilage, followed by formation of new bone and cartilage at the joint margins (osteophyte). Incidence increases with age, obesity, repetitive occupational activities (coal miners, jackhammer operators, etc). The pathology of OA reflects the damage to the joint and reaction of the surrounding tissues. There is an increase in water content of the cartilage, with increased proteoglycan synthesis. As the disease progresses, the joint surface thins and becomes fibrillated. Appositional bone growth in the subchondral region leads to the sclerosis seen on radiographs. With further decrease, progression clefts and fractures of the subchondral plate occur, with the formation of subchondral cysts. Growth of bone and cartilage at the joint margins form osteophytes. Synovitis and joint effusions may be present.

• **Management**
Protection of the joints from excessive force and chronic overuse. Supportive splints and the use of ambulatory aides (cane, crutches, walker) are protective. Avoidance of repetitive impact loading (jumping, running) in lower-extremity OA. Weight loss is beneficial. Physical therapy to increase joint motion and strength is beneficial. Drug therapy consists of analgesics (acetaminophen), aspirin, and nonsteroidal anti-inflammatory drugs (NSAIDs). Narcotics should be used only as short-term mea-

Capsaicin (substance P inhibitor)

sures. Intra-articular corticosteroid may be helpful in the management of acute flares. Surgery is reserved for cases in which conservative therapy fails. Options include arthroscopic lavage and debridement, osteotomy, arthroplasty, fusion.

B. Low-Back Pain

• **H&P Keys**
Predisposing factors include age 30 to 50, repetitive movements such as lifting, pulling, bending, and twisting. Exposure to chronic vibration and prolonged sitting. Personal behavior (sedentary life-style, cigarette smoking, poor posture, emotional stress, obesity).

Etiologic Factors. Acute or chronic muscle, tendon, or ligamentous strain, lumbar disk herniation, degenerative changes of the spine, facet joint dysfunction, metabolic conditions that result in mechanical failure (osteoporosis).

• **Diagnosis**
Radiographs show age-related changes. Magnetic resonance imaging (MRI), computerized tomographic (CT) scan not necessary for initial evaluation; indicated when symptoms persist with radicular neurologic symptoms.

• **Disease Severity**
Physical evaluation, with loss of spine motion in all planes. Perivertebral muscle spasm. The presence of radicular pain below the knee suggests neurologic involvement (eg, disk disease).
Below knee

• **Concept and Application**
Back pain is usually a self-limiting condition resulting from an acute strain or repetitive overload. The resulting inflammation and pain of ligaments, muscles, and tendons creates the short-term disability. Treatment addresses the cause of the overload and the underlying inflammation.

• **Management**
Short period of rest (3 to 5 days). Treatment of muscle spasm with ice massage and lumbar support. Acetaminophen or NSAIDs for anti-inflammatory effect. Major treatment is education to prevent recurrence and in

proper body mechanics. Muscle strengthening for the back and abdomen, combined with a flexibility program, complete the treatment.

C. Lumbar Disk Disease

- **H&P Keys**
Low-back pain with radiation below the knee; leg pain is usually greater than back pain. Ten percent of backaches are related to some sort of nerve root irritation. Altered sensation, pins and needles, numbness may be present in the lower extremity. Pain increases with coughing, sneezing. Weakness may be present. Central disk may cause bilateral symptoms. Signs of limited spine motion, antalgic gait, sciatic list. Hip and knee flexed with standing, extended with sitting, absent or diminished reflexes, diminished sensation in a dermatome pattern. Positive tension signs with straight leg raising or sitting root tests.

- **Diagnosis**
Radiographic evaluation may demonstrate disk space narrowing or may be normal. CT scan and MRI allow visualization of the disk and neural elements. Electromyogram (EMG) will show changes only after several weeks of symptoms.

- **Disease Severity**
Dense parasthesias with complete motor loss are signs of severe nerve root impingement. Progressive loss of motor function and sensation an indication for early surgical intervention. Loss of bowel and bladder function (cauda equina syndrome) requires emergency treatment with surgical decompression of the neural elements to prevent permanent dysfunction.

- **Concept and Application**
Nuclear material bulges, protrudes, or extrudes from the disk space to put pressure on the ligaments and nerve roots. Molecular changes in the disk with aging alter the structural properties of the disk and the annulus fibrosis that contains the disk. The disk loses water and becomes dry and friable, decreasing its ability to withstand axial loads. With sudden loading or repetitive loading in flexion and rotation, disk material is extruded beyond the confines of the annulus, resulting in the neurologic symptoms.

- **Management**
Early intervention with a short period of bed rest 3 to 5 days, in conjunction with anti-inflammatory medication and ice. This is followed by mobilization with back rehabilitation exercises. Zero percent of patients obtain relief in 4 weeks, 90% in 3 months, 96% in 6 months. Surgical intervention is required for progression of symptoms and for those who are unresponsive to conservative management.

D. Disorders Secondary to Neurologic Disease

- **H&P Keys**
Stroke, diabetes, muscular dystrophy, cerebral palsy, neuropathies all have musculoskeletal consequences.

- **Diagnosis**
Physical examination of joint motion and muscle balance. Examination for altered sensation. Painless swelling and joint deformity may be present with Charcot's joint arthropathy.

- **Disease Severity**
Clinical evaluation. Radiographs show progressive joint destruction and loss of position.

- **Concept and Application**
Neurologic conditions that alter muscle strength, balance, and protective sensation have musculoskeletal manifestations. Increased spasticity after stroke creates flexion deformities of the affected joints because of the increased strength of flexor over extensor musculature. This may result in functional problems, such as thumb-in-palm deformity, equinus deformity, gait abnormality. The loss of protective sensation and proprioceptive sensation as a result of neuropathy from diabetes leads to Charcot's arthropathy (painless destruction of a joint) as well as problems of skin ulceration from excess pressure (dropped metatarsal heads).

• **Management**
Protective splinting to prevent contractures and physical therapy to preserve joint motion may prevent surgical intervention. For severe muscle imbalance, corrective surgery with release and weakening of the flexors or augmentation of the extensors with muscle transfers may be required. Protection of insensate joints with bracing and full-contact orthotics may delay or prevent joint destruction.

III. INHERITED, CONGENITAL, OR DEVELOPMENTAL DISORDERS

A. Congenital Hip Disorders U/S

• **H&P Keys**
Congenital hip dislocation (CDH) is a serious condition if not diagnosed and treated in the first weeks of life. Girls are affected eight times more often than boys. Diagnosis is made by clinical exam at the time of birth. Backward and forward pressure on the femur in full flexion and abduction can demonstrate the femoral head moving in and out of the acetabulum.

Femoral head not calcified until 10wk Xrays not Helpful

• **Diagnosis**
Radiographs are not helpful because the femoral head is not calcified until at least 10 weeks of age. Ultrasonography of the hip is the diagnostic procedure of choice in the first weeks of life.

• **Disease Severity**
Delay in diagnosis gravely affects prognosis and treatment. If diagnosis delayed until 12 to 18 months as walking begins demonstrating a limp and rolling gait, surgery will only achieve a useful hip but one that will not be normal.

• **Concept and Application**
Risk factors include family history of dislocations, breech presentation at birth. Every birth should be screened for CDH.

• **Management**

Treatment at Birth. Treatment with splint or harness (Pavlik) to hold the hips in an ab-ducted and forward-flexed position. Reduction is confirmed with radiographs and possibly arthrogram. Worn for 12 weeks.

Treatment at 2 Months. Managed with traction and plaster immobilization.

Treatment at 12 Months. Surgery is indicated to achieve a stable joint. Hip is never normal, however.

B. Legg-Calvé-Perthes Disease

• **H&P Keys**
Painful hip in child ages 2–11.

• **Diagnosis**
X-ray may be normal in early disease. Later x-rays will demonstrate increased femoral head density or subarticular fracture line.

• **Disease Severity**
Age is key to prognosis: Presentation after age 8 represents a poor prognosis.

• **Concept and Application**
Noninflammatory self-limiting deformity of the weight-bearing surface of the femoral head secondary to avascular necrosis of the femoral head. Increased incidence with a positive family history, low birth weight, and abnormal birth presentation.

• **Management**
Maintenance of the sphericity of the femoral head is most important factor for obtaining a good outcome. Treatment is to first obtain normal range of motion with bed rest, traction. This is followed with bracing or surgery to contain the femoral head in the acetabulum until revascularization and ossification occurs.

C. Slipped Capital Femoral Epiphysis

• **H&P Keys**
Presents as groin pain or as knee pain. Limp may be present with displacement. With complete displacement leg may be shortened and externally rotated.

• **Diagnosis**
Radiographic images, especially a lateral, are essential for showing displacement.

- **Disease Severity**

  Degree of displacement determines residual problems. Significant displacement may result in the development of avascular necrosis. Chondrolysis may occur with the resultant osteoarthritis.

- **Concept and Application**

  Adolescents with complaints of hip or knee pain should be considered to have a slipped capital femoral epiphysis. Occurs through the growth plate or epiphysis of the femoral neck during the adolescent growth spurt and is more common in boys than girls. The slip is probably caused by a weakening of the epiphyseal structures by hormonal changes of adolescence. Most often occurs in gynecoid boys.

- **Management**

  Slight to moderate displacement should be treated with percutaneous pinning to prevent further slip. Manipulation may disturb the blood supply and create avascular necrosis. For gross displacement, it is better to accept the deformity and correct it after growth has been completed with an osteotomy.

D. Intoeing

- **H&P Keys**

  Patient presents with an intoed gait. May complain of falling and tripping over feet.

- **Diagnosis**

  No diagnostic studies are necessary.

- **Disease Severity**

  Clinical evaluation of degree of intoeing.

- **Concept and Application**

  There are three causes of intoeing: (1) Anteversion of the femoral neck, (2) metatarsus adductus, and (3) outward-curved tibiae. Femoral anteversion allows for greater internal rotation of the hip than external rotation and is the major cause of intoeing. The condition corrects itself as growth continues. Most instances are corrected by age 10.

- **Management**

  No treatment other than reassurance is needed.

IV. METABOLIC AND NUTRITIONAL DISORDERS

A. Osteoporosis

Consider thyroid, hematologic, malignancy

- **H&P Keys**

  Progressive loss of height. Spontaneous, multiple vertebral body compression fractures. Development of thoracic kyphosis. Fractures of the hip and wrist. May complain of bone pain in the axial skeletal or in the long bones of the lower extremity.

- **Diagnosis**

  Plain radiographs may show osteopenia. Bone densitometry; single photon absorbtometry, dual energy x-ray absorptometry (DEXA), quantitative CT scan have technical limitations. DEXA is the most sensitive of the monitoring techniques. Complete lab evaluation should consider thyroid disease, hematologic disorders, and malignant disease.

- **Disease Severity**

  Loss of axial skeletal height, multiple compression fractures with thoracic kyphosis. Multiple fractures of hips, wrists, ribs, ankles.

- **Concept and Application**

  Decrease in bone mineral content leading to spontaneous fractures of the spine, hip, and wrist. Commonly postmenopausal women, other risk factors include hereditary, drug use (steroids, heparin, thyroid), nutritional factors, activity (sedentary), cigarette smoking, alcohol. Disuse osteoporosis results when bones are not stressed normally, eg, paralysis, prolonged bed rest or immobilization, space flight.

- **Management**

  Best treated with prevention, low-dose estrogen replacement in menopausal women. Calcitonin and bisphosphonates block bone resorption. Fluoride causes increases in bone density, but the bone is more brittle. Fall prevention education with avoidance of sedatives, alcohol use, slippery rugs, high-heeled shoes, unprotected bathrooms, and diuretics decrease incidence of fractures.

Tophus = Collection urate crystal masses surround by inflammatory cells c variable fibrosis

B. Gout

NEG BIFRINGENT
D/O purine metabolism
↑serum URIC ACID

- **H&P Keys**

Acute onset of painful, swollen, erythematous joints, deposition of crystals in soft tissue, tophi. Attacks may be preceded by trauma, alcohol, drugs, surgical stress, or acute medical illness. Great toe commonly involved; ankle, knee, tarsal bone may be affected. *Gr toe = PODAGRA*

Assoc c obesity DM HTN ↑Lipids Atherosclerosi

- **Diagnosis**

Aspiration of joint fluid for birefringent crystals. *NEG Bifrio ~ NEEDLE SHAPE Redc compensate polarized Lt.*

- **Disease Severity**

Polyarticular attacks, soft-tissue tophi formation, joint destruction, associated renal failure.

- **Concept and Application**

Tissue deposition of monosodium urate crystals from supersaturated extracellular fluids. Recurrent attacks of severe articular and periarticular inflammation: gouty arthritis. Accumulation of crystalline deposits in the soft tissue: gouty tophi. Renal impairment: gouty nephropathy. Causes: ①overproduction, 10%; ②underexcretion, 90%. Dehydration as a result of trauma, surgery, diuretics may precipitate attack.

OVERPROD UNDEREXCRETION

- **Management**

Treatment with anti-inflammatory medications, indomethacin (Indocin) 50 mg t.i.d. Aspiration and identification under polarized light microscopy diagnostic with birefringent crystals. If attacks reoccur, treatment with allopurinol is helpful.

1)Indocin 2)Allopurinol

C. Rickets

- **H&P Keys**

Brittle bones with ligamentous laxity, flattening of the skull, enlargement of the costal cartilages (rachitic rosary), dorsal kyphosis, bowing of long bones.

Rachitic Rosary

- **Diagnosis**

Radiographic evaluation: transverse radiolucent lines "Looser's lines," physeal cupping and widening. Laboratory evaluation: calcium levels are normal with low phosphate and high alkaline phosphatase levels.

Canc ↓phos ↑Alk P

- **Disease Severity**

Clinical evaluation: long-bone bowing, rachitic rosary.

- **Concept and Application**

Decrease in calcium and/or phosphorus affecting the mineralization of the epiphyses of long bones. Histology: Widened osteoid seams, distortion of the zone of maturation with poorly defined zone of provisional calcification. There are four causes for rickets:

1. Vitamin D deficiency resulting from inadequate diet or lack of exposure to sunlight.
2. Malabsorption of calcium secondary to steatorrhea.
3. Renal osteodystrophy caused by renal abnormality that affects the metabolism of vitamin D.
4. Hypophosphatemia resulting from defect in renal tubule (vitamin D-resistant rickets).

- **Management**

Vitamin D produces rapid improvement. Residual long-bone deformities may require surgical correction. Vitamin D-resistant rickets requires treatment with phosphate replacement and vitamin D_3.

V. INFLAMMATORY OR IMMUNOLOGIC DISORDERS

A. Polymyalgia Rheumatica

- **H&P Keys**

Occurs in men and women over 60, and occurs twice as often in men. Patients complain of abrupt onset of pain affecting the shoulders, neck, upper arms, lower back, and thighs. Morning stiffness and gelling are predominant features. Physical examination reveals only tenderness and restriction of motion.

- **Diagnosis**

Radiographs are normal. Rheumatoid factor and antinuclear antibodies (ANA) are normal, ESR is elevated. Diagnosis is by history and response to treatment with prednisone.

- **Disease Severity**
Elevated ESR, clinical impairment of activities.

- **Concept and Application**
Common syndrome of older patients, characterized by stiffness and pain in neck, shoulders, and hip lasting at least 1 month. Inflammation is present without joint destruction.

- **Management**
Responds rapidly to low-dose prednisone. If response is not seen in 1 week, diagnosis should be questioned. Start prednisone 10 to 20 mg/d with taper to 5 to 7.5 mg/d. Therapy may continue for longer than 1 year.

B. Lupus Arthritis   ANA ⊕

- **H&P Keys**
Disease of young females 14 to 40, with a 5 : 1 female : male ratio. The acute arthritis may involve any joint but usually involves the small joints of the hand, wrists, and the knee. It may be persistent and chronic or migratory. Soft-tissue swelling and effusion are mild.

- **Diagnosis**
Clinical symptoms of morning stiffness, myalgia, arthralgia. Serologic testing: 95% of ANA are positive.

- **Disease Severity**
Articular complaints are usually mild and reversible. They can become fixed deformities if untreated. Disease activity, however, can severely impair renal function and cause pulmonary and cardiac involvement. Neuropsychiatric manifestations may also be present.

- **Concept and Application**
Autoimmune disease characterized by the production of autoantibodies to components of the cell nucleus. Pathologic find-

ings are manifested by inflammation, vasculitis, and immune complex deposition disease (lupus kidney). Lupus arthritis is a polyarteritis characterized by low-grade synovitis without joint destruction. Joint distention may cause ligamentous laxity of the metacarpal phalangeal (MCP) and proximal interphalangeal (PIP) joints of the hand with resulting instability and deformity (swan-neck deformity, ulnar deviation of the fingers).

- **Management**
Treatment consists of periods of rest, avoidance of sun exposure, NSAIDs, and corticosteroids. Splinting may preserve function in weakened joints.

C. Polymyositis-Dermatomyositis

Polymoysitis + RASH = Dermatomy

- **H&P Keys**
Complaints of proximal hip weakness, with difficulty on stairs and getting out of cars. Arm symptoms with difficulty lifting above the horizontal. Physical examination will show diffuse symmetric muscle wasting and weakness. Affected muscles may be sore to palpation. Gait may be slow and wide-based.   Pt have problem combing HAIR

- **Diagnosis**
Clinical presentation of symmetric proximal muscle weakness. Elevated serum creatine kinase, aldolase, lactic dehydrogenase, and transaminase. Characteristic EMG abnormalities. Autoantibodies may be present. Muscle biopsy.   ↑CK LDH ALDOL. TRAN

- **Disease Severity**
Involvement may extend to the heart, gastrointestinal tract, lungs, peripheral joints.

- **Concept and Application**
This disease is an idiopathic inflammatory myopathy characterized by proximal limb weakness.

- **Management**
High-dose corticosteroid medication is the initial treatment. Graded exercise after inflammation is controlled restores some strength and range of motion. Methotrexate is used in patients not responding to corticosteroid.

D. Rheumatoid Arthritis (Juvenile, Adult)

- **H&P Keys**
  Characteristically presents with morning stiffness with symmetric painful swelling in the small joints in young women ages 15 to 35. It may involve other joints not seen in OA such as elbows, shoulders, ankles, hips, and spine. Fatigue may be present.

- **Diagnosis**
  Radiographs show juxta-articular erosions around the small joints of the hands and feet. Positive rheumatoid factor (RF), elevated ESR, and anemia are usually present.

- **Disease Severity**
  Functional impairment in activity of daily living. Systemic involvement of other organ systems such as the lung, heart, skin, eye, gastrointestinal and genitourinary systems.

- **Concept and Application**
  Etiology is unclear but is related to cell-mediated immune response (T cells) that incites an inflammatory response, initially against soft tissue and later cartilage, with subsequent bone loss secondary to periarticular bone resorption. Lymphokines and other inflammatory mediators initiate the cascade that leads to cartilaginous destruction.

- **Management**
  Aimed at controlling the inflammation with acetaminophen, NSAIDs, antimalarial, gold, penicillamine, and immunosuppressives. Corticosteroids may be used to improve patient functional levels. Severely affected joints can be protected with splints and braces to prevent destruction.

E. Ankylosing Spondylitis HLA B27

- **H&P Keys**
  Common in young men aged 15 to 30. Presents with complaint of diffuse low backache without radicular symptoms. Profound morning stiffness. Usually a rapid response to anti-inflammatory medication. May have painless effusions of large joints.

- **Diagnosis**
  History and physical examination are most important. Restriction of chest expansion and spine flexion. Elevated ESR. May be HLA-B27–positive. Radiographs of the sacroiliac joints show the earliest changes of sacroilliitis. Later the spine films demonstrate progressive ankylosis.

- **Disease Severity**
  Restriction of spine motion, chin-on-chest deformity, restriction of chest expansion.

- **Concept and Application**
  An inflammatory disease of the spinal joints and sacroiliac joints. If left untreated there can be complete loss of spinal motion from the occiput to the coccyx. Treatment is to preserve motion through exercise and control inflammation with medication.

- **Management**
  Initial flair is treated with rest and anti-inflammatory medication. Mobilization and flexibility exercises are started as the inflammation is controlled.

F. Bursitis

- **H&P Keys**
  Soft-tissue swelling that may be either painful or nonpainful, usually over a bony prominence. Swelling may occur spontaneously or as a result of trauma or an inflammatory disease (gout, rheumatoid arthritis).

- **Diagnosis**
  Clinical evaluation. Additional evaluation for underlying inflammatory diseases. Radiographs to evaluate for bony prominences and soft-tissue calcifications.

- **Disease Severity**
  Clinical evaluation.

- **Concept and Application**
  Bursae form wherever two tissue planes move in opposite direction or where tissues travel over a bony protuberance. Normal bursal locations are in the subacromial space

of the shoulder, over the olecranon of the elbow, and over the tibial tubercle, and in the prepatellar space. This normal structure allows skin and tendon and muscle to slide over each other easily. If the bursa becomes infected, injured, or inflamed, fluid will accumulate in the bursa and produce visible swelling. Fibrinous loose bodies may also be formed in the bursa. After the inflammation subsides, adhesions and fibrosis may occur in the bursa, resulting in crepitation and sometimes pain.

- **Management**
  Avoidance of repetitive motions and trauma will prevent bursal inflammation. Treatment of any underlying collagen vascular disease or crystalline arthritis will control the bursal swelling. Acute treatment consists of rest, ice, anti-inflammatory medication. Aspiration to identify crystals or elevated WBC and bacteria may be required. The use of protective padding, elbow and knee pads, can prevent recurrence. Surgical excision is sometimes needed if the size or the location interfere with activities of daily living.

G. Tendinitis

- **H&P Keys**
  Pain over tendon or at tendon insertion. May be acute in onset or as a result of repetitive overload, often seen after a sudden change in activity or sporting activity.

- **Diagnosis**
  Physical signs of localized inflammation with point tenderness over the tendon. Weakness may be present secondary to pain.

- **Disease Severity**
  Functional assessment of impairment.

- **Concept and Application**
  Tendinitis is an inflammation of the tendon secondary to overload. This may be due to acute overload with partial tearing of the tendon or as a result of repetitive stress. A sudden change in activity or sporting activity that exceeds the body's reparative capabilities will result in an "overuse" tendinitis.

- **Management**   *overload*
  Local treatment with ice massage and oral NSAIDs. Splinting to restrict motion and rest injury zone. Restoration of normal motion through a gentle stretching program followed by strength exercises and endurance training. Return to sport and activity is gradual. Assessment of work activity and sport intensity with adaptation of program will prevent recurrence. Training and equipment must also be adapted to prevent recurrence.

H. Fibromyalgia

- **H&P Keys**
  Patients present with diffuse achiness, stiffness, fatigue, associated with multiple areas of clinical tenderness. Seventy-five percent are female, with an age distribution of 20 to 60 years. Pain tends to be localized to axial locations such as the neck and lower back. The upper trapezius is a common location of pain. On physical examination tenderness is present with moderate pressure. Common locations: occiput, trapezius, supraspinatus at ridge of scapula, lower back, lateral epicondyle.

- **Diagnosis**
  Clinical examination makes the diagnosis. Laboratory evaluation to exclude collagen vascular diseases (ESR, RF, ANA, CBC) and infectious causes (Lyme disease). Thyroid functions are also valuable.

- **Disease Severity**
  Clinical examination.

- **Concept and Application**
  Etiology is unknown; fatigue is felt to be due to sleep disturbances, with loss of rapid eye movement (REM) sleep patterns.

- **Management**
  Patient education and reassurance. Aerobic exercise is more beneficial than stretching alone. NSAIDs are not effective as single agents but are effective in conjunction with bedtime dose of amitriptyline or cyclobenzaprine.

cyclobenzaprine - Flexeril

VI. NEOPLASMS

Painless mass [handwritten]

A. Osteosarcoma

- **H&P Keys**
  Most common in second and third decade of life. Presents often as a painless mass. Found after rather minor trauma on routine radiograph.

- **Diagnosis**
  Radiographs are diagnostic: demonstrate increased radiodensity with areas of radiolucency and permeative destruction and soft-tissue extension. Elevated periosteum (Codman's triangle) may be present. Bone scans and MRI will show extent of lesion and skip lesions.

  Codmans △ [handwritten]

- **Disease Severity**
  Extent of disease with involvement of multiple compartments.

- **Concept and Application**
  A malignant tumor of bone characterized by the production of osteoid directly from a malignant spindle cell stroma. The knee and proximal humerus are the most commonly affected locations. Early diagnosis is difficult because of the disease's painless nature. Secondary osteosarcomas can arise from Paget's disease of bone and post–radiation therapy fields.

  Knee [handwritten]
  Prox humerus [handwritten]

- **Management**
  Adjunctive chemotherapy pre- and postoperatively profoundly improves survival. Limb salvage surgery may be offered those patients who are good responders, with 95% tumor necrosis. Otherwise amputation and prosthetic fitting is the treatment of choice, with the best survival and lowest recurrence rates.

B. Metastases to Bone

- **H&P Keys**
  Presentation is usually with pain or with a pathologic fracture.

  lytic [handwritten]
  BLASTIC [handwritten]

- **Diagnosis**
  Radiographs demonstrate lytic and blastic lesions. Lesions involving greater than 50% of the cortex or that are greater than 2.5 cm

  Fx if 75 50% cortex [handwritten]
  72.5 cm [handwritten]

in diameter are at risk for spontaneous fracture. Bone scanning sensitive for detection of early metastatic disease. MRI will show accurately extent of metastatic tumor involvement of bone. Alkaline phosphatase is usually elevated.

Breast / PROSTATE / LUNG / KIDNEY / THYROID   Child / Wilms / neuroblastoma [handwritten]

- **Disease Severity**
  Lesions greater than 2.5 cm in diameter or greater than 50% of the cortex are at risk for spontaneous fracture and should be prophylactically stabilized.

- **Concept and Application**
  Metastatic tumors are the most common malignancies of bone. Spread to bone can be either arterial or venous. Classically, lytic lesions are found in the axial skeleton and long-bone diaphyses and usually multiply. Most common lesions are breast, prostate, lung, kidney, thyroid. Prostate and breast metastases are typically blastic. The most common metastases in children are Wilm's tumor and neuroblastoma.

- **Management**
  Radiation therapy is often helpful to control the pain and metastatic activity. For impending fractures, stabilization with load-sharing devices (intramedullary rods) is preferred. For collapse of bony support of joint surfaces, replacement arthroplasties may be useful procedures if survival is expected beyond 6 months.

C. Pulmonary Osteoarthropathy

- **H&P Keys**
  Clubbing of the fingers is the characteristic feature. In some patients, especially those with malignant lung tumors, severe bone pain may be present. Obtain family history of clubbing.

- **Diagnosis**
  Physical feature of bulbous deformity of the digits (clubbing). Periostitis and thickening of the bones is present radiographically.

- **Disease Severity**
  Clinical evaluation; evaluate for occult pulmonary tumor, especially if long-bone pain is present.

- **Concept and Application**
  Disease characterized by excessive proliferation of skin and bones at the ends of the digits (clubbing).

- **Management**
  A NSAID is useful in controlling the pain of the periostitis. Occult malignant tumor of the lung must be ruled out.

VII. OTHER DISORDERS

A. Shoulder-Hand (Frozen Shoulder) Syndrome

- **H&P Keys**
  Decreased range of motion in the shoulder often painful. May be associated with minor trauma. Associated with diabetes, hypothyroidism, surgery; and higher in females.

- **Diagnosis**
  Diagnosis is clinical; arthrogram will show decreased joint-space volume.

- **Disease Severity**
  Clinical evaluation of functional loss of shoulder motion.

- **Concept and Application**
  Adhesive capsulitis of the shoulder. Inflammatory condition with fibrosis and loss of normal joint space secondary to capsular contracture.

- **Management**
  Institution of early, aggressive range of motion exercises. Adjunctive treatment with NSAIDs and ice.

B. Dupuytren's Contracture

- **H&P Keys**
  Patients are usually males older than 40, of Northern European ancestry, with a family history of the condition. Alcohol, smoking, diabetes, and seizures are contributory. Forty percent are bilateral. Ulnar digits are more commonly involved.

- **Diagnosis**
  Clinical evaluation.

- **Disease Severity**
  Interference with hand function, inability to get the fingers out of the palm of the hand.

- **Concept and Application**
  Proliferative fibrodysplasia of the palmar subcutaneous tissue. Myofibroblast proliferation and increased type III collagen. Leads to progressive contracture from these nodules and cords of tissue.

- **Management**
  Surgical intervention for deformities of greater than 30° to 45° of the MCP or of any PIP involvement.

C. Carpal Tunnel Syndrome

- **H&P Keys**
  Patients usually complain of night symptoms with parasthesias in the median distribution (the front of the thumb, index and long finger, and the radial half of the ring finger).

- **Diagnosis**
  Other causes (thyroid disease, diabetes, pregnancy amyloidosis) need to be excluded. Physical examination is usually diagnostic. Diminished sensation in the median nerve distribution. Positive Tinel's sign of the carpal canal. Positive Phalen's test. Nerve conduction velocity delays across the carpal ligament.

- **Disease Severity**
  Progressive median nerve dysfunction with loss of two-point discrimination and weakness of thumb abduction. Thenar atrophy.

- **Concept and Application**
  The median nerve and common flexors pass through a common tunnel in the wrist, bounded volarly by the transverse carpal ligament. Any process that decreases the volume of the canal will compress the median nerve and create symptoms.

- **Management**
  Primary treatment is rest with a cock-up resting splint. Injection of hydrocortisone may be effective. Surgical decompression for those not responding to conservative treatment.

D. Paget's Disease of Bone

[handwritten: Spine, Pelvis, skull, Femur, TIBIA]

- **H&P Keys**

  The most common sites are the spine, pelvis, skull, femur, tibia. In most cases patients are asymptomatic. However, disease becomes clinically present with pain, progressive deformity, compression of neurologic structures, pathologic fractures.

- **Diagnosis**

  Laboratory evaluation: increased alkaline phosphatase, increased urinary hydroxyproline excretion. Radiographic appearance: initial lesion is a focal area of radiolucency (osteoporosis circumscripta of the skull). In the long bones, resorption is characterized by an advancing wedge of radiolucency. Attempts at repair create sclerotic-appearing bone with thickening of the cortex.

- **Disease Severity**

  [handwritten left margin:)SARCOMATOUS Δ]
  [handwritten left margin:) HIGH OUTPUT CHF]

  The major complication of Paget's disease is sarcomatous transformation. This occurs in less than 1% of cases. Presents with severe pain and extremely elevated serum alkaline phosphatase activity. Increased local circulation in hypervascular bone can create high-output congestive heart failure.

- **Concept and Application**

  Disorder of unknown etiology characterized by excessive bone resorption followed by excessive bone formation. Creates classic lamellar mosaic bone pattern.

- **Management**

  In most instances no treatment is necessary because of the paucity of clinical symptoms. In symptomatic patients, NSAIDs may suppress the discomfort. Calcitonin administered subcutaneously may decrease pagetoid bone activity. Etidronate will decrease bone resorption. With irreversible joint destruction, total joint arthroplasty offers relief of pain.

E. Eosinophil Granuloma

- **H&P Keys**

  [handwritten left margin: Pelvis Femur Spine]

  May present as progressive back pain, more often in the thoracic spine. Common locations: pelvis, femur, and spine. First and second decade of life. Lytic-appearing lesion characteristic. Periosteal thickening is common.

- **Diagnosis**

  Classically may cause vertebral flattening (vertebra plana), lytic lesions in long bones.

- **Disease Severity**

  Lesions that compromise the structural integrity of long bones or cause neurologic compromise.

- **Concept and Application**

  Bracing in children may be necessary to prevent progressive kyphosis.

- **Management**

  Treatment consists of observation (many lesions heal spontaneously), low-dose radiation for neurologic deficits. Curettage or excision may be indicated for persistent lesions.

VIII. ACUTE OR EMERGENCY PROBLEMS

A. Effusion of Joint

[handwritten: noninf, infl, Infectious]

- **H&P Keys**

  Swelling of the joint either spontaneous in onset or posttraumatic. Physical examination reveals loss of the normal joint contours and possibly a restriction in motion.

- **Diagnosis**

  Aspiration of the joint classifies the fluid as noninflammatory (WBC less than 2000/mm^3), inflammatory or infectious (WBC greater than 100 000/mm^3). Evaluation for crystals is essential to differentiate gout and pseudogout. Culture and Gram's stain are needed to rule out infection. A bloody effusion with the history of trauma is suggestive of a severe injury, either a fracture or ligament injury; 85% of hemarthroses of the knee are anterior cruciate injuries.

- **Disease Severity**

  High WBC indicate infectious etiologies until proven otherwise. They demand prompt

Hemarthrosis—Ant cruciate

treatment, or rapid joint destruction can occur as a result of proteolytic enzymes produced by the bacteria.

- **Concept and Application**
Any synovium-lined joint can have an effusion. The effusion is the production of excess synovial fluid in response to an inflammatory event. This event can be trauma, as in a hemorrhagic effusion, or inflammatory, as in gout or rheumatoid arthritis, or an infection.

- **Management**
Management depends on the etiology of the effusion. Treatment of the inflammatory condition with anti-inflammatory medications. Infectious effusions are treated with serial aspirations or surgical drainage in combination with antibiotics. Traumatic effusions resolve with rest, but treatment must address the injury pattern.

B. Spinal Stenosis

- **H&P Keys**
Elderly patients with complaints of back and buttock pain. Pain is made worse with walking and descending stairs and only relieved with prolonged rest. If activity continues, paresthesia and weakness may develop. Pain is increased with hyperextension of the spine and relieved with forward flexion of the spine. Sensory changes are described as water or candle wax dripping down the leg.

- **Diagnosis**
Radiographs often show degeneration of the facet joints. CT scan is best noninvasive test for bony stenosis. MRI underestimates the degree of stenosis. Myelogram and postmyelogram CT are useful to fully define the disease, especially stenosis of the lateral recesses of the neural foramina.

- **Disease Severity**
Clinical impairment of activities with neurogenic claudication. Pain increased with any activity that causes hyperextension of the spine. Acute trauma in the presence of stenosis may cause catastrophic neurologic symptoms with paraplegia and cauda equina

symptoms and demands prompt surgical decompression.

- **Concept and Application**
The maturing of the skeleton results in degenerative changes involving the disk margins and facet joints. The bony overgrowth constricts the nerve roots. This may be exacerbated by ligamentous thickening and diskogenic protrusions.

- **Management**
Adjustment to the limitations of the disease in conjunction with anti-inflammatory medications, ice or heat, and an exercise program. If symptoms are severely disruptive to the patient, surgery (laminectomy) to decompress the nerve roots will give relief.

C. Contusions

- **H&P Keys**
Contusions are a result of direct trauma. Localized erythema and swelling are present with palpable tenderness. There may be loss of adjacent joint motion if swelling is pronounced.

- **Diagnosis**
Diagnosis is by history and clinical examination. Radiographs rule out fracture or late myositis ossificans.

- **Disease Severity**
Clinical loss of function of the joint and affected extremity define severity. Large hematomas and contusions to a large area of the muscle mass will produce greater disability. Myositis ossificans, or calcification of the muscle, is a late sequela of a severe contusion or a result of repetitive contusions to the same muscle before primary healing has occurred.

- **Concept and Application**
Contusions are a result of direct trauma. Following the trauma there is local damage to blood vessels and muscle. As bleeding and swelling continue, there is increased muscle stiffness and loss of joint motion. Secondary agents of inflammation produced as response to the local tissue trauma

Contusions

produce the ache and stiffness that characterize the early period after a contusion.

- **Management**
Treatment consists of ice and compression to control the swelling and bleeding. Adjunctive use of NSAIDs is useful in controlling the secondary inflammation. Early therapy is provided to restore painless range of motion, followed by flexibility and strengthening exercises. Return to activity is allowed when there is full, painless range of motion and strength equal to the unaffected extremity.

D. Fractures and Dislocations

1. Cervical Spine

- **H&P Keys**
Fractures of the cervical spine are caused in four ways: (1) flexion, (2) extension, (3) vertical compression, and (4) rotation.

Flexion Injuries. Are the most common and usually involve the lower cervical spine. May be associated with compression of the vertebral body, rupture of the supraspinous ligament, dislocation of the posterior facets.

Low Cspine most comnu

Extension Injuries. Are generally less serious than flexion, with the most common being fractures of the odontoid; hyperextension injuries can result in damage to the anterior spinal artery, with the resultant anterior spinal artery syndrome. The hangman's fracture or fracture of the pedicles of C-2 and spondylolisthesis of C-2 on C-3 results from hyperextension during falls.

Ant spinal artery syndrome

HANGMAN C2-C3

Vertical Compression. Axial loading injuries cause vertical compression and result in fractures of the atlas or burst fractures.

- **Diagnosis**
Radiographs: anterior-posterior (AP), lateral, oblique, open-mouth odontoid view are the standard views. Flexion and extension lateral radiographs evaluate instability. CT scan and MRI are useful in determining the geometry of fracture fragments and evaluating the degree of cord compression.

- **Disease Severity**
Disease severity is based on clinical findings of neurologic compromise.

- **Concept and Application**
The pattern of injury is dependent on the mechanism of injury. Treatment is based on decompression of the neurologic elements and stabilization of the spine either surgically or with bracing.

- **Management**
Treatment is stabilization of the unstable elements with surgery or bracing. For neurologic compromise, prompt intervention to decompress the neural elements and stabilize the bony and ligamentous structures.

2. Thoracic Spine

- **H&P Keys**
Usually high energy is necessary to produce these injuries unless significant osteoporosis is present. The pattern of injury depends on the position of the axis of flexion and direction of the force at the time of injury. These result in compression fractures, burst fractures, flexion-distraction injuries (seat-belt) and fracture dislocations.

- **Diagnosis**
Radiographic evaluation with plane roentgenograms is usually adequate. CT scan is beneficial to define fracture geometry and neurologic compromise.

- **Disease Severity**
The degree of bony compression, displacement, and neurologic compromise defines the severity of the injury.

- **Concept and Application**
Compression fractures are common on falls from heights and falls onto the backsides by elderly osteoporotic patients. The injury occurs at the thoracic-lumbar junction where the thoracic kyphosis and lumbar lordosis meet. This results in loading forces on the anterior aspect of the vertebral body, with the resulting vertebral wedge fractures. Burst fractures are caused by pure axial loading and cause retropulsion of material, resulting in cord compression with neuro-

logic symptoms. The rapid deceleration injury of the seat-belted passenger results in the flexion-distraction fracture with a splitting of the vertebral body; displacement can be significant. Fracture dislocations are a result of a combination of flexion, compression, and rotation.

- **Management**
  Compression fractures of less than 50% are usually treated with a short period of rest with supportive bracing and restorative exercise. For those greater than 50%, surgical stabilization may be indicated. Persistent back pain may occur after even minor compression injuries. Burst fractures associated with neurologic symptoms require operative stabilization and may require decompression. Fracture dislocations often result in paraplegia; early operative stabilization will allow for early rehabilitation.

3. Lumbar Spine

- **H&P Keys**
  Mechanism of injury is usually flexion or a combination of flexion and rotation. Pain is present of the posterior elements of the spine, and neurologic compromise may be present. Compression fractures are caused by pure axial loading. Differentiating between cord and root lesion is essential for prognosis.

- **Diagnosis**
  Radiographs (AP, lateral, oblique), CT scan.

- **Disease Severity**
  Based on level of neurologic compromise.

- **Concept and Application**
  The cord ends at L-1 and therefore only the lower motor and sensory nerves are involved in this injury. There is greater room in the lumbar spine for displacement, and therefore greater displacement is necessary before neurologic compromise is present. The neurologic picture cannot be determined until spinal shock has passed, as exhibited by the return of the bulbocavernous reflex.

- **Management**
  Serial monitoring of the neurologic status and early stabilization and decompression of compressed neural elements provide for the best outcomes.

4. Closed Fracture of Hand Phalanges

- **H&P Keys**
  Fractures are usually caused by twisting or angular forces. With fracture there is loss of ability to use the hand fully, with associated pain and swelling. The location of the swelling and pain, as well as the pattern of altered motion, will suggest which of the phalanges has been injured. Loss of extension at the distal interphalangeal (DIP) joint is characteristic of a mallet finger or avulsion of the distal insertion of the extensor tendon onto the base of the distal phalanx and is the result of a sudden violent hyperflexion injury. Fractures of the phalanges may also present with acute angular deformities or rotation deformities, often seen with spiral fractures. Fractures of the distal phalanx are usually a result of a crushing blow.

- **Diagnosis**
  Clinical examination correlated with biplanar radiographs is usually diagnostic.

- **Disease Severity**
  Intra-articular comminution is associated with poor function outcomes. Spiral fractures may result in rotation residuals if great care is not taken in the treatment of the fracture. Fractures of the distal phalanx often result in injuries to the nail bed, which can result in nail deformities if not anatomically repaired.

- **Concept and Application**
  Fractures of the phalanges are caused by sudden, violent blows to the hand. They result in loss of joint function and angular deformities, accentuated by the pull of the tendons that act across the injured joints.

- **Management**
  Mallet fingers are treated with hyperextension splinting. Phalangeal fractures can be

treated with splinting and buddy taping. Care must be taken to ensure flexion at the MCP and gentle flexion of the PIP to prevent loss of motion secondary to contraction of the collateral ligaments seen with prolonged splinting in full extension. When there is loss of articular congruency, open reduction or percutaneous pinning is indicated. Unstable fracture geometries also require surgical stabilization. Distal phalangeal fractures that involve the nail bed require repair of the nail bed with suture.

5. Fracture of Neck of Femur

• H&P Keys

In the adolescent and early adult, femoral neck fractures occur as a result of high-energy accidents. In the elderly they may occur with relatively minor trauma secondary to osteoporosis. Fractures may occur as a result of a direct fall on the greater trochanter or from a rotational force along the shaft of the femur. Symptoms include groin pain, inability to bear weight with the hip held in mild adduction and external rotation. The pain is exaggerated by motion, especially rotation of the hip. In an impacted fracture in the elderly, the symptoms may consist of groin pain only with ambulation; the pain may be referred to the knee or thigh.

• Diagnosis

AP and lateral radiographs usually confirm the diagnosis. In the elderly with groin pain and osteopenia, CT and a bone scan may be necessary to confirm the diagnosis.

• Disease Severity

Displaced fractures of the femoral neck have a high rate of complications, with delayed unions and the development of avascular necrosis of the femoral head from disruption of blood supply to the femoral head by the circumflex vessels. In the young patients with axial loading fractures, posttraumatic chondrolysis may also be a complication. Even with minimal displacement, avascular necrosis and collapse of the femoral head may occur.

• Concept and Application

Femoral neck fractures should be considered in any elderly patient with groin pain. In younger patients, the diagnosis should be considered with high-energy trauma and associated groin pain. Displaced fractures of the femoral neck disrupt the blood supply to the femoral head and result in avascular necrosis.

• Management

In young patients, the fracture of the femoral neck should be promptly reduced and internally fixed. In the elderly, impacted and nondisplaced fractures may be pinned in situ. Because of the osteopenia, the fixation hardware may fail and require revision to a joint replacement. Displaced fractures in the elderly should be treated with hemiarthroplasty or total hip arthroplasty if degenerative arthritis is present.

6. Fractures of the Foot and Leg

• H&P Keys

Fractures are a result of trauma but may also occur as a result of repetitive stress that results in a stress fracture. Fractures usually present with acute pain and swelling. Ecchymosis develops secondary to the fracture hematoma. Inability to bear weight, or pain exacerbated with weight bearing is usually present. Obvious angular deformity may be present with severely displaced fractures.

• Diagnosis

Radiographs are usually diagnostic. AP and lateral films are standard. Special views are necessary to evaluate the ankle (mortise view) and the foot (oblique views) to fully assess the injury pattern. The mortise view evaluates whether there has been injury to the syndesmosis with widening of the ankle mortise. The oblique foot views evaluate Lisfranc's joint. Injury to this region is often missed with plain radiographs. When pain is present only with activity and there is no history of trauma, bone scan may be necessary to evaluate for a stress injury. The most common locations for stress fractures in the foot and leg are the metatarsal, tibia, and fibula.

- **Disease Severity**

  The location and the degree of comminution and displacement are predictive for rates of healing and complications of stiffness and lost joint motion. The distal third of the tibia is notorious for slow bony union, with a high percentage of delayed unions or nonunions. The fifth metatarsal in the diaphyseal region is also prone to nonunion, especially if weight bearing is allowed. Lisfranc's joint at the base of the second metatarsal is another region for complications following injury, with late arthritis and stiffness often present.

- **Concept and Application**

  Fractures of the lower extremity require definition of their location and fracture geometry to ensure proper treatment.

- **Management**

  Fractures of the lower extremity require immobilization for adequate healing. This may be provided with casting, fracture bracing, or internal fixation with plates and screws or intramedullary devices. Principles of treatment are restoration of joint congruity and bony length with correction of angular and rotation deformities.

7. Dislocations and Separations

- **H&P Keys**

  Any joint may suffer a dislocation. A dislocation occurs when a violent force applied to the joint results in the disruption of the supporting ligamentous structures. Pain is usually present, with ecchymosis over the injured ligamentous structures. Joint deformity and loss of motion may be present if the joint does not reduce spontaneously. There is joint instability with stress testing and a sense of insecurity with weight bearing.

- **Diagnosis**

  Radiographs are used to show displacement or associated fractures. Stress testing of ligamentous supports confirms damage to and instability of the joint.

- **Disease Severity**

  The residuals of joint dislocation depend on the joint injured. Hip dislocations have a high rate of complication with avascular necrosis. Dislocations of the knee may result in arterial injury to the popliteal vessels and loss of perfusion to the lower leg. Shoulder dislocations may result in injuries to the axillary or musculocutaneous nerves and persistent instability of the shoulder. Dislocations of Lisfranc's joint may result in persistent pain stiffness and ambulatory dysfunction.

- **Concept and Application**

  Joint dislocations are serious injuries. They result when the forces that are applied to the joint exceed the ligaments' ability to withstand the stress. Instability occurs as a result of the loss of the passive restraints provided by the ligaments. The displacement of the normal joint structures may result in secondary injury to adjacent structures. Chronic instability may be a result of the injury.

- **Management**

  Rapid reduction of the dislocation and assessment of secondary injury patterns are the mainstays of treatment. Fracture bracing and early protected motion programs may be useful in decreasing the morbidity associated with prolonged immobilization with rigid casting. Operative repair is indicated for irreducible dislocations and for stabilization of grossly unstable joints.

8. Rotator Cuff Syndrome

- **H&P Keys**

  Rotator cuff insufficiency may occur as an acute event after a fall into the shoulder. The injury usually occurs when the extremity is extended to break the fall and the weight of the body is suddenly applied to the tendon while it is under tension. The injury may result in sudden loss of shoulder function with inability to abduct the shoulder. The tear may occur by attrition in the older patient, with gradual deterioration of shoulder strength. Immediate symptoms are pain and swelling in the shoulder region. Pain may be increased with passive motion. There is weakness in shoulder abduction. Pain may be increased in activity above the horizontal and with resistance to abduction. There may be a positive drop arm test, with inability to hold the arm at the horizontal against any resistance.

- **Diagnosis**
Radiographs may be normal or may show superior migration of the humeral head, impinging on the inferior surface of the acromion. In an acute injury, the humeral head may be low in the glenoid fossa secondary to intra-articular hematoma. Arthrography and MRI will define the magnitude and location of the tear.

- **Disease Severity**
The degree of symptoms depends on the magnitude of the tear. Partial or small tears may result in only minimal dysfunction and present with the predominant feature of pain. Larger tears will result in loss of shoulder strength. Long-standing cuff tears will result in cuff arthropathy, arthritis characterized by a high-riding humeral head impinging on the acromion, with glenohumeral arthritis.

- **Concept and Application**
Rotator cuff tears may occur as a sudden failure or as a result of slow attrition. Loss of balance in the musculature of shoulder results in altered mechanics of the shoulder. The humeral head migrates superiorly and may herniate through the hole in the cuff to impinge on the acromion. The altered mechanics result in the late development of glenohumeral arthritis.

- **Management**
Initial treatment is with ice, rest, and anti-inflammatory medications. As the pain of the acute injury subsides, rehabilitation is started to increase strength in the cuff and restore muscle balance. If the shoulder does not improve with rehabilitation, surgery is indicated for repair of the cuff. In young patients and those who require overhead strength in the shoulder, early surgical repair is advised. Decompression of the subacromial space by partial acromionectomy is indicated to decrease the compressive forces on the shoulder. In older patients with irreparable tears, symptomatic relief may be obtained with debridement of the cuff and rehabilitation.

E. Other Orthopedic Emergencies

Other orthopaedic emergencies include compartmental syndrome, cauda equina syndrome, joint infections, open fractures, fractures and dislocations with vascular involvement.

1. Compartmental Syndrome

A rise in the interstitial compartment pressures as a result of bleeding or soft-tissue swelling that prevents the perfusion of the compartment. Presents first with severe pain, which increases with passive stretch of the compartment. Diagnosis with intracompartmental pressure assessment. Greater than 30 mm Hg warrants surgical decompression.

2. Cauda Equina Syndrome

Progressive loss of lower-extremity function, with loss of bowel and bladder control. Secondary to pressure on the cauda equina. Requires immediate surgical decompression.

3. Joint Infections

Painful inflammation with pain on passive motion of the joint. Serial aspiration or surgical lavage is needed promptly to prevent the destruction of the joint by chondrolytic enzymes.

4. Open Fractures

Fractures in which the bone is exposed through the skin surface either from within or without. Grading is dependent on the size of the wound and zone of injury and the degree of soft-tissue contamination. The greater the zone of injury and the greater the degree of contamination, the greater the increase in risk of infection and limb loss.

5. Vascular Compromise Following Fracture and Dislocation

Fractures and dislocations that cause loss of perfusion require prompt attention, with reduction usually restoring blood flow. Angiography is necessary if pulses are not restored. Knee dislocations mandate an angiogram because of the high rate of intimal injury to the popliteal artery and late thrombosis and subsequent limb loss.

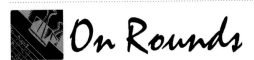

Musculoskeletal Disorders, Focus on Inflammatory/ Immunologic Conditions

Polymyalgia Rheumatica
- Women over age 60, more common in men
- Pain in the shoulders, neck, upper arms, low back, thighs; morning stiffness, gelling
- X-rays are normal, RF and ANA are normal, ESR is elevated
- Treat with prednisone

Ankylosing Spondylitis
- Common in men ages 15–30
- Low back pain, profound morning stiffness
- Elevated ESR, may be HLA-B27 positive, Sacroilliitis on x-ray.
- Treat with anti-inflammatory medication

Rheumatoid Arthritis
- Women ages 15–35
- Symmetric painful swelling in the small joints, morning stiffness, fatigue, may affect elbows, ankles, hips, spine and shoulders
- X-rays positive for erosions, Positive RF, elevated ESR, anemia

- Treat with acetaminophen, NSAIDs, antimalarial, gold, penicillamine and immunosuppressives

Lupus Arthritis
- Females 14–40 (5:1 female/male ratio)
- Acute arthritis most often affecting the small joints of the hand, wrists, and knee
- ANA positive in 95%
- Treatment includes NSAIDs and corticosteroids

Polymyositis-Dermatomyositis
- Symmetric proximal hip weakness, symmetric muscle wasting, weakness, slow gait, muscle tenderness to palpation
- Elevated serum creatine kinase, aldolase, LDH and transaminase. EMG abnormalities, may have autoantibodies.
- Treat with corticosteroids or methotrexate

BIBLIOGRAPHY

Ball GV. *Clinical Rheumatology.* Philadelphia: WB Saunders Co; 1986.

Birnbaum JS. *The Musculoskeletal Manual.* Orlando, FL: Academic Press; 1982.

Cailliet R. *Neck and Arm Pain.* 3rd ed. Philadelphia: FA Davis Co; 1991.

Callen JP. Cutaneous manifestations of collagen vascular disease and related conditions. *Med Clin North Am.* Philadelphia: WB Saunders Co; September, 1989.

Connolly JF. *The Management of Fractures and Dislocations: An Atlas.* 3rd ed. Philadelphia: WB Saunders Co; 1981.

D'Ambrosia RD. *Musculoskeletal Disorders.* 2nd ed. Philadelphia: JB Lippincott Co; 1986.

Dieppe PA. *Atlas of Clinical Rheumatology.* Philadlephia: Lea & Febiger; 1986.

Enneking WF. *Musculoskeletal Tumor Surgery.* New York: Churchill Livingstone Inc; 1983.

Morrissy RT. *Pediatric Orthopedics.* 3rd ed. Philadelphia: JB Lippincott; 1990; 1, 2.

Niwayama G, Resnick D. *Diagnosis of Bone and Joint Disorders.* 2nd ed. Philadelphia: WB Saunders Co; 1988.

O'Donoghue DH. *Treatment of Injuries to Athletes.* 4th ed. Philadelphia: WB Saunders Co; 1984.

Turek SL. *Orthopedics: Principles and Their Application.* 4th ed. Philadelphia: JB Lippincott Co; 1984; 1, 2.

10

Neurology

Jeffrey Greenstein, MD and Gerado R. Torres, MD

I. INFECTIOUS DISEASES OF THE CENTRAL NERVOUS SYSTEM

A. Viruses

1. Human Immunodeficiency Virus (HIV)

• **H&P Keys**

Risk factors include blood transfusion, needle sharing, unsafe sex; presentations include: headache and fever (meningitis) 1%, progressive dementia with impaired saccadic eye movements (15% to 20%), paraparesis (myelopathy) 20%, pain and numbness (neuropathy) 30%, focal deficits in central nervous system (CNS), lymphoma, toxoplasmosis, or progressive multifocal leukoencephalitis (PML).

• **Diagnosis**

HIV antibodies by enzyme-linked immunosorbent assay (ELISA) (if positive confirm with Western blot); magnetic resonance imaging (MRI) of affected area to exclude mass lesion in myelopathy, dementia, or focal deficits; cerebrospinal fluid (CSF) for pleocytosis; cultures in meningitis; CSF protein and electromyography (EMG) and nerve conduction velocities (NCV) in neuropathy; vitamin B_{12} level.

• **Disease Severity**

Total T4 lymphocyte count under 100; dementia, myelopathy, lymphoma, and PML carry poor prognosis.

• **Concept and Application**

Etiology of dementia and myelopathy unknown; direct invasion in meningitis; reduced immunocompetence in toxoplasmosis, lymphoma, neuropathy, or PML.

- **Management**
For parenchymal mass lesion, pyrimethamine and sulfadiazine for 2 weeks, biopsy if not better; radiation for CNS lymphoma; amphotericin for fungal meningitis; IV IgG if neuropathy is demyelinating; otherwise biopsy to rule out specific infectious or vasculitic etiologies and pain treatment with tricyclic antidepressants. Dementia and myelopathy have no specific therapy.

2. Herpes Simplex Virus (HSV)   PLEDS

- **H&P Keys**
In the CNS usually presents with encephalitic symptoms including clouding of consciousness, aphasia, fever, headache, seizures; exam denotes aphasia, hemiparesis, nuchal rigidity, confusion, and variable somnolence.

- **Diagnosis**
Computerized tomographic (CT) scan or MRI of head shows hypodense, ring-enhancing lesion, at times hemorrhagic in temporal lobes; EEG shows periodic epilepsylike discharges (PLEDS), CSF has increased protein and mild lymphocytic pleocytosis and, at times, xanthochromia; biopsy makes definitive diagnosis.

- **Disease Severity**
Sequelae directly related to duration of disease prior to therapy; often fatal if not treated; age greater than 30 associated with poor prognosis.

- **Concept and Application**
Virus accesses brain by reactivation from fifth cranial nerve; direct invasion causes necrosis, hemorrhage, edema; sporadic occurrence.

- **Management**
IV acyclovir when diagnosis suspected; biopsy of lesion, but therapy should not be delayed while waiting for biopsy; anticonvulsants for seizures; supportive care.

3. Spongiform Encephalopathy (Jakob-Creutzfeldt Disease)

- **H&P Keys**
Middle-aged patient with rapidly progressive change in behavior, intellectual function, and emotional responses, followed by startle myoclonic jerks, ataxia, and dysarthria. Stupor and coma follow.

- **Diagnosis**
Blood and CSF are normal. When advanced, EEG shows "burst suppression," which is synchronous with the myoclonus. Brain biopsy shows spongiform changes in the cortex, which is diagnostic.

- **Disease Severity**
Invariably fatal; mode of transmission unclear; may be transmissible iatrogenically; familial cases associated with mutations in prion protein gene.

- **Concept and Application**
The etiology is still unclear. Probably caused by abnormal prion protein, but transmissible.

- **Management**
No treatment available.

4. Poliomyelitis

- **H&P Keys**
Fever, anorexia, vomiting, followed in a week with asymmetric painful paralysis that involves any or all limbs and bulbar muscles; no sensory findings or levels.

- **Diagnosis**
CSF shows lymphocytic pleocytosis; viral cultures of feces; EMG and NCV show denervation of motor nerves.

- **Disease Severity**
Bulbar presentation, if severe, causes respiratory and vasomotor instability, leading to death in 25% of these cases.

- **Concept and Application**
Neurotropic virus affects anterior horn cells in spinal cord and motor nuclei of brain stem; also hypothalamus and thalamus.

- **Management**
Supportive, including mechanical ventilation and physical therapy; may develop

postpolio syndrome in 20 to 40 years, manifested by progressive weakness and fatigue; immunization with attenuated virus is now universal.

5. Rabies

- **H&P Keys**
  Rabid animal bite followed by anxiety, overactivity, difficulty swallowing fluids (hydrophobia) progressing to dysphagia, facial spasm, and seizures in 2 to 8 weeks; death occurs 4 to 10 days later.

- **Diagnosis**
  Obtain infected animal brain when bite occurs, test for Negri bodies.

- **Disease Severity**
  Lack of prior immunization is the largest risk factor for poor outcome.

- **Concept and Application**
  Viral particles seen as eosinophilic cytoplasmic inclusions (Negri bodies) throughout CNS.

- **Management**
  If the animal is rabid, treatment of patient with human rabies immunoglobulin or duck embryo vaccine (to offer passive immunity while active develops); if symptoms occur, supportive care.

B. Meningitis

1. Aseptic

- **H&P Keys**
  Preceding upper respiratory infection, exanthem, exposure to rat excreta; headache, fever, photophobia, nuchal rigidity.

- **Diagnosis**
  CT scan to rule out abscess; CSF examination shows pleocytosis, predominantly lymphocytic, mild protein elevation, normal glucose; negative bacterial cultures and Gram's stain; acute and convalescent viral titers helpful.

- **Disease Severity**
  Usually benign course, without sequelae; decreased mentation; focal neurologic signs, seizures suggest concurrent encephalitis and worse outcome.

- **Concept and Application**
  Meningeal infection with virus, most often enterovirus or mumps virus; initial infection with Lyme disease, HIV, leptospirosis, and syphilis may present similarly.

- **Management**
  Supportive management.

2. Bacterial (Septic)

- **H&P Keys**
  History of sinusitis, ear infection, epidemic meningitis, pneumonia; presents with headache, fever, photophobia, seizures, nuchal rigidity, and obtundation; suspect meningococcus with petechial rash, pneumococcus with pneumonia or sinus infection in adults, *Haemophilus influenzae* with similar symptoms in children.

  Dexamethasone in H infl ↓ Hearing loss

- **Diagnosis**
  Negative CT of head (if timely); CSF pleocytosis up to 10 000, mainly neutrophils; low (<40% of serum) glucose; protein elevation; positive bacterial cultures and Gram's stain; positive bacterial antigens if partially treated; positive blood cultures in 60%; elevated CSF pressure.

- **Disease Severity**
  Coma, focal neurologic signs, signs of herniation, seizures bear poor prognosis and may suggest abscess formation; sequelae and outcome directly related to time of institution of therapy.

- **Concept and Application**
  Pyogenic infection of meninges with prominent vascular changes (small to medium arteritis).

- **Management**
  Blood culture; CT of head, lumbar puncture (LP); do not delay antibiotics for LP or LP for CT; cefotaxime in adults and children over 3 months; ampicillin and cefotaxime in neonates and infants; steroids may lessen hearing loss in children; supportive care.

3. Fungal

- **H&P Keys**
  Progressive dementia, headaches, nuchal rigidity, lack of fever, cranial nerve involve-

ment, often immunosuppression or history of lymphoma or other malignant disease; exposure to birds; suspect *Cryptococcus* in the immunosuppressed, mucormycosis in diabetics.

- **Diagnosis**
CSF with predominantly lymphocytic and monocytic pleocytosis; positive cryptococcal antigen and positive India ink in cryptococcal meningitis; positive fungal cultures in weeks.

- **Disease Severity**
Hydrocephalus; arteritis, thrombosis, and infarction of the brain.

- **Concept and Application**
Granulomatous meningitis composed of fibroblasts, giant cells, and necrosis.

- **Management**
Amphotericin B; supportive care.

4. Tuberculous (TB)

- **H&P Keys**
Positive purified protein derivative (tuberculin) (PPD) in 75%; fever, malaise, headache; development of nuchal rigidity, decreased mental status, confusion, dementia, lower cranial nerve involvement.

- **Diagnosis**
Chest roentgenogram; PPD; CSF shows lymphocytic pleocytosis, elevated protein (often to several hundreds), low glucose (normal in 30%), positive acid-fast bacillus (AFB) stain or immunofluorescence; cultures take several weeks and often require multiple LPs.

- **Disease Severity**
Residual deficits depend on onset of therapy in relation to stage of disease; obtundation, seizures, hydrocephalus, or focal signs indicate poor prognosis.

- **Concept and Application**
Caseating granulomas surrounded by epithelioid cells, lymphocytes, and connective tissue; exudate results from fibrin, lymphocytes and areas of caseation necrosis; exudate spreads along pial vessels and invades underlying brain.

- **Management**
Isoniazid can cause peripheral neuropathy and seizures; daily addition of pyridoxine; addition of rifampin and pyrazinamide; use of streptomycin when resistance is suspected; careful observance for liver toxicity; use of steroids for treatment of all cases of TB meningitis; treatment of increased intracranial pressure; hydrocephalus treated with ventriculoperitoneal shunt.

C. Abscesses

- **H&P Keys**
History of sinus, ear, periodontal, pulmonary, or head wound infection, endocarditis; suspect congenital heart disease in children; presents with focal severe headache, nausea and vomiting, seizures; focal signs dependent on location.

- **Diagnosis**
MRI or CT with contrast of affected area shows ring-enhancing lesion with edema, mass effect, "daughter lesion"; LP shows "aseptic" pleocytosis but is usually not necessary and may be contraindicated because of possible herniation.

- **Disease Severity**
Untreated cases produce major disability or death; mortality rate in treated cases is 30%; 50% suffer neurologic sequelae.

- **Concept and Application**
Focal infection of brain parenchyma, usually without meningitis; encapsulated with central necrotic material and pus; solitary 75% of the time; usually caused by anaerobes or microaerophilic organisms, most commonly anaerobic streptococci or bacteroides.

- **Management**
Biopsy using stereotaxic CT guidance; steroids for management of intracranial pressure; mechanical hyperventilation and P_{CO_2} of less than 30 may be needed if severe; anticonvulsants for seizures; IV antibiotics include penicillin and metronidazole if pathogen is unknown; vancomycin for methicillin-resistant staphylococci and third-generation cephalosporin for gram-negative bacteria.

D. Spirochetes

1. Lyme Disease

- **H&P Keys**

  History of tick bite in about 50% of patients; history of erythema chronicum migrans in about 60% of patients; influenzalike symptoms; can present as an aseptic meningitis; weeks to months later neurologic involvement will happen in 15% of the cases; most common neurologic presentation is one of meningoencephalitis with cranial or peripheral neuritis; chronic symptoms include encephalopathy and axonal neuropathy; peripheral nervous system presentation include Bell's palsy, mononeuritis multiplex, myositis, and peripheral neuropathy.

- **Diagnosis**

  Lyme titers by ELISA, confirmed by Western blot; perform CSF examination in all neurologic cases; typical CSF abnormalities include mononuclear cell pleocytosis as high as 3000 and increased protein level up to 400; check for intrathecal production of Lyme-specific antibodies, which may cross-react with syphilis.

- **Disease Severity**

  Myelitis-causing quadriparesis, seizures, and dementia have infrequently been described but are likely to leave sequelae.

- **Concept and Application**

  Arthropod-borne infection. *Borrelia burgdorferi* is a spirochete inoculated into humans by the *Ixodes* or deer tick; endemic in northeastern United States.

- **Management**

  Treat erythema migrans or Bell's palsy with oral doxycycline or amoxicillin for 30 days; for any other neurologic symptoms or conditions treat with IV ceftriaxone 2 g daily for 14 days.

2. Neurosyphilis

- **H&P Keys**

  Sexually transmitted; develops a painless chancre in genital region; subsequently patient might complain of headaches, stiff neck, nausea, or vomiting that resolve within days to weeks and evolve within 6 to 12 years into a meningovascular disease with cerebrovascular accidents; within 15 to 20 years a progressive mental dissolution including dementia, dysarthria, myoclonic jerks, seizures, hyperreflexia, and Argyll Robertson pupils (general paresis); another presentation within the same time frame is tabes dorsalis, which includes the development of ataxia, lightning pains, urinary incontinence, and absent reflexes with impaired vibratory and position sense, Argyll Robertson pupils (90% of cases).

- **Diagnosis**

  Examine CSF for cells, protein, and Venereal Disease Research Laboratory (VDRL) in those patients who have a positive VDRL or rapid plasma reagin (RPR) test and whose past antibiotic therapy cannot be confirmed as adequate or have not had antibiotic therapy; CSF picture often consists of lymphocytic pleocytosis, elevated protein, and positive VDRL.

- **Disease Severity**

  Most late symptoms of neurosyphilis are unpredictable and often unresponsive to the treatment with penicillin; intraparenchymal gumma can develop in HIV-infected patients and behave like mass lesions.

- **Concept and Application**

  Syphilis is due to a treponemal disease that invades the CNS within 3 to 18 months of inoculation with the organism; after this time the chances of CNS infection are markedly reduced to a total of 1% if the CSF remains negative after 5 years.

- **Management**

  Treatment of choice is IV penicillin G 4 000 000 U q 4 h for 14 days; IV therapy should be started in the hospital because of possible Jarisch-Herxheimer reaction; lancinating pain treated with anticonvulsants; neuropathic joints treated with bracing; CSF examination repeated every 3 to 6 months; cells should clear first, then protein, then VDRL.

II. NEUROMUSCULAR DISORDERS

A. Carpal Tunnel Syndrome *assoc DM RA Lyme*

- **H&P Keys**
Nocturnal pain or numbness in first three digits of the hand, weakness on thumb opposition, wrist pain with rare shoulder pain; exacerbation with repetitive motion of wrist; positive Tinel's sign at median nerve at the wrist.

- **Diagnosis**
Wrist roentgenograms show bony deformities; MRI wrist demonstrates focal compression of median nerve; EMG and NCV will show focal median nerve conduction velocity slowing at the wrist, axonal loss; depending on history, check for diabetes, rheumatoid arthritis, Lyme disease, *hypothyroidism* *pregnancy + HNPP*

- **Disease Severity**
Severe atrophy of thenar muscles, marked thumb opposition weakness, permanent pain or numbness of first three digits, absent sensory or motor potentials on nerve conduction of the median nerve.

- **Concept and Application**
Compression of median nerve with intussusception of node of Ranvier or traumatic injury of nerve by repetitive motion; diabetes, rheumatoid arthritis, amyloidosis, and pregnancy increase risk of syndrome.

- **Management**
Mild cases will respond to wrist splint; recurrence of pain or numbness will respond to steroid injection; surgery offers excellent results in over 90% of cases of well-demonstrated carpal tunnel syndrome; reduction of repetitive activity; modification of work environment.

B. Guillain-Barré Syndrome (Acute Inflammatory Demyelinating Polyneuropathy)

- **H&P Keys**
Progressive ascending weakness a few weeks after an upper respiratory or gastrointestinal illness or surgery; back discomfort in 60%; no sensory level; areflexia; distal, but may be proximal, progressive weakness mainly in the legs; no fever on presentation; very symmetrical; maximum evolution of disease in 2 weeks in 50% of patients, in 4 weeks in 90% of patients.

- **Diagnosis**
CSF with high protein but less than 10 white blood cells (WBCs) (50 in HIV patients); low conduction velocities on EMG and NCV studies; check for Lyme, HIV, urine porphyrins, hepatitis; culture stools for *Campylobacter jejuni.*

- **Disease Severity**
Poor prognostic indicators include severe tetraparesis, hyperacute onset, assisted ventilation, low nerve amplitudes on EMG and NCV (suggesting axonal involvement and likely to result in prolonged sequelae), and abnormal phrenic nerve studies; autonomic instability may increase morbidity.

- **Concept and Application**
Proximal and later distal segmental demyelination with inflammatory cell infiltration in nerve.

- **Management**
Plasmapheresis in first week for quickly progressing cases (inability to stand) or ventilator dependence; supportive care; IV IgG may be beneficial but recently reported to cause relapsing syndrome in some cases.

C. Myasthenia Gravis

- **H&P Keys**
Diplopia, ptosis; symptoms worsen at end of day; young females; elderly males; demonstrable fatigue on examination, such as worsening of ptosis on prolonged upward gaze.

- **Diagnosis**
Dramatic improvement with IV edrophonium chloride (Tensilon) (test double blind); positive antibodies to acetylcholine receptors (80% in generalized, 50% in ocular only); decrement of motor nerve potential with repetitive stimulation; may need single-fiber analysis; thoracic MRI for thymoma.

- **Disease Severity**

  Bulbar weakness increases risk of aspiration; low pulmonary vital capacity indicates respiratory compromise; severe weakness; thymoma needs surgery.

- **Concept and Application**

  Antibodies that block or permanently bind to the acetylcholine receptors, presumably resulting from an immunologic aberration in the thymus; this prevents muscle excitation.

- **Management**

  Acetylcholinesterase inhibitor increases available acetylcholine; corticosteroids reduce the immunologic process; other immunosuppressants are used in severe cases; thymectomy, although controversial, can eliminate the need for medications in some cases or reduce the doses in others; acute worsening is best treated by discontinuation of medications and ventilatory support; plasmapheresis is useful for short periods to hasten improvement.

D. Myopathies and Dystrophies

- **H&P Keys**

  History of progressive proximal weakness in most cases; myalgias and cramps are more the exception than the rule; weakness is noted raising arms overhead and in related activities, or getting up from a chair; myotonic dystrophy will show myotonia on percussion of small muscles (eg, tongue); Duchenne's dystrophy shows calf muscle enlargement.

- **Diagnosis**

  Creatine kinase (CK) is elevated in most cases of myopathy and muscular dystrophy; EMG and NCV demonstrate small, brief (myopathic) potentials, with normal nerve conduction velocities; muscle biopsy is diagnostic in most cases; metabolic myopathies may require biochemical studies; ischemic exercise test is abnormal in some glycogen metabolic myopathies because of the inability to utilize energy substrate; electrocardiogram ECG needed because of high incidence of cardiac abnormalities.

- **Disease Severity**

  Severe weakness could be associated with respiratory compromise; high CK might cause myoglobinuria and renal failure in metabolic myopathies; many myopathies associated with life-threatening cardiac abnormalities; swallowing and respiratory difficulties could result in death.

- **Concept and Application**

  Duchenne's dystrophy is the result of lack of a protein prevalent in the myotendinous junction (dystrophin), which results in muscle membrane injury; a severe inflammatory process of the muscle results in polymyositis; other myopathies are the result of metabolic derangements (McArdle's), ion channel abnormalities (myotonic dystrophy), or intrinsic sarcomere dysfunction (congenital myopathies).

- **Management**

  Appropriate genetic studies facilitate diagnosis and genetic counseling along with prenatal diagnosis; corticosteroids in polymyositis and Duchenne's dystrophy; anticonvulsants in myotonic dystrophy to reduce cramps; orthoses and ambulatory aides might be helpful in activities of daily living.

III. NUTRITIONAL AND METABOLIC DISORDERS

A. Vitamin B$_{12}$ Deficiency

- **H&P Keys**

  Painful dysesthesias in feet and hands followed by difficulty ambulating; ataxia, leg weakness, spasticity, changes in mentation, visual loss.

- **Diagnosis**

  Vitamin B$_{12}$ levels can be obtained in most laboratories; because neurologic presentation does not necessarily parallel the hematologic picture, a high level of suspicion is needed; a few cases may have "normal" levels, and these may require measurement of methylmalonic acid and homocysteine, both of which are elevated in B_{12} tissue deficiency.

- **Disease Severity**
  Progressive leg weakness and spasticity leading to the need for ambulatory aids; in general symptoms lasting more than 3 months are unlikely to revert; the etiology for the deficiency should be established.

- **Concept and Application**
  White matter degeneration of the spinal cord and occasionally of the brain; changes begin in the posterior column of the lower cervical segment and spread downward, forward, and laterally.

- **Management**
  Initial management is emergent. Daily B_{12} (1000 μg) is needed in the first 7 days to replete stores. Subsequently, needs are supplied by 1000 μg of B_{12} monthly.

B. Thiamine Deficiency

- **H&P Keys**
  Usually undernourished alcoholics, but sometimes patients with gastric carcinoma or hyperemesis gravidarum, who present with ataxia of gait, gaze palsies, or nystagmus and mental confusion (Wernicke's encephalopathy); ocular abnormalities might include nystagmus that could be both horizontal or vertical, weakness or paralysis of conjugate gaze, or weakness of the external rectus muscle, which is always bilateral; the ataxia is one of stance and gait with no evidence of tremor, and the confusion could present as a global confusional state, stupor, and coma or as a hallucinatory state with overactivity; Wernicke's encephalopathy might progress to an amnesic syndrome with severe short-term memory impairment and confabulation (Korsakoff's psychosis).

- **Diagnosis**
  CSF is almost always normal; blood pyruvate may be elevated; red blood cell (RBC) transketolase activity is markedly reduced, but the diagnosis remains a clinical one.

- **Disease Severity**
  Transition to the Korsakoff state heralds poor outcome, even with therapy; other symptoms are likely to improve with treatment; concurrent septicemia, pneumonia, and liver disease result in about 15% mortality rate.

- **Concept and Application**
  Thiamine deficiency results in necrotic lesions of the mamillary bodies, periaqueductal region, thalamus, hypothalamus, and floor of the fourth ventricle.

- **Management**
  Administer IV thiamine 50 mg and IM 50 mg initially; and IM 50 mg daily subsequently until normal diet is resumed; avoid glucose infusion prior to thiamine administration; provide supportive care; evaluate for infections and other conditions.

C. Metabolic Encephalopathy

- **H&P Keys**
  Progressive clouding of consciousness in general without any focal symptomatology; history of medication overdose, infections, anoxia, hypo- or hyperglycemia, renal insufficiency, liver disease, alcohol intoxication; examination demonstrates normal pupillary reactions with small pupils, normal oculovestibular responses, normal corneal responses, and no focal deficits in a mentally obtunded patient.

- **Diagnosis**
  CT of the head is used to rule out mass lesions in patients with focal neurologic deficits (hypoglycemia, hypoxia, azotemia, and hepatic encephalopathies might cause focal neurologic signs); EEG to rule out nonconvulsive status epilepticus or postictal state; drug screen and metabolic parameters including sodium, glucose, oxygen, P_{CO_2}; chest roentgenogram and urine analysis (UA) to rule out infections.

- **Disease Severity**
  Prolonged hypoxia or hypoglycemia may result in permanent neurologic injury; ventilatory support might be needed in many instances of coma; fever should raise suspicion of meningitis or abscess.

- **Concept and Application**
Usually reversible; nonstructural injuries resulting in generalized cerebral dysfunction.

- **Management**
Correction of metabolic derangement.

IV. PAROXYSMAL DISORDERS

A. Seizures

- **H&P Keys**
History of abrupt stereotypic transitory loss or alteration of consciousness with or without involuntary movements; short or no warning (aura); confusional state after recovery of consciousness; bowel and bladder incontinence and tongue biting may happen, usually accompanied by bodily injuries; physical examination usually normal after the event; may have upgoing toes and abnormalities of tone immediately at the end of the episode; if witnessed, the event can start focally in one limb, with automatism or behavioral manifestations or generalized increase or decrease in tone; brief alteration of consciousness without postictal confusion happens in absence seizures in children.

- **Diagnosis**
CT or MRI of brain to rule out irritative lesion (stroke, tumor, abscess); routine EEG might be diagnostic in 20% or less of patients; prolonged EEG monitoring might be necessary in difficult cases; diagnosis remains a clinical one; cardiac evaluation might be needed to rule out convulsive syncope in selected cases.

- **Disease Severity**
Seizures, although most often idiopathic, can be the presentation of otherwise treatable conditions such as brain tumors, abscesses, arteriovenous malformations; repeated seizures during the day might result in severe functional and social disability along with bodily injuries; the disease carries a number of social limitations with it;

status epilepticus markedly increases morbidity and mortality.

- **Concept and Application**
Usually caused by an irritative lesion capable of causing abnormal neuronal discharges that can spread and perpetuate themselves.

- **Management**
Treatment depends on seizure type; when no seizures patients respond best to valproic acid; generalized and partial seizures respond to felbamate, phenytoin, and carbamazepine; febrile seizures do not require chronic anticonvulsant therapy; refractory cases may require surgery; status epilepticus (seizures lasting 20 minutes or more without stopping) are medical emergencies requiring immediate use of IV benzodiazepines followed by IV anticonvulsants and, if necessary, barbiturate coma with mechanical ventilation.

B. Trigeminal Neuralgia

- **H&P Keys**
Brief, sharp, lancinating pain mainly in the third or second division of the fifth cranial nerve. Precipitated by touch, cold, or chewing.

- **Diagnosis**
Normal neurologic exam; if abnormal, consider other conditions such as posterior fossa mass lesion; beware of young multiple sclerosis (MS) patients with similar symptoms; unless the examination is abnormal this condition does not require further diagnostic studies; any neurologic abnormality should cause a prompt investigation of the posterior fossa for cerebellar pontine angle tumors, tumors of the fifth nerve, and MS.

- **Disease Severity**
The condition is a painful disease that results in no permanent sequelae to the patient if untreated; however, the pain is severe enough to have caused some patients to commit suicide.

- **Concept and Application**
The specific etiology is unknown.

- **Management**
Medical management is highly satisfactory; oral carbamazepine is usually started at the beginning; refractoriness may require the addition of baclofen; monitoring for dizziness, unsteadiness, bone marrow suppression with carbamazepine; acute confusional state and seizures may occur with abrupt discontinuation of baclofen; microvascular decompression of the nerve might result in long-standing relief.

C. Headaches

- **H&P Keys**
History of intermittent or persistent head pain with or without associated vegetative symptoms; migraines are usually unilateral, pulsating headaches and if classic are associated with visual scotomata, hemisensory disturbances, nausea and vomiting, and photophobia; cluster headaches are retro-orbital, occurring in the adult smoker associated with lacrimation; ipsilateral Horner's syndrome usually lasts 90 minutes, may occur at the same time of the day; tension headaches are chronic, bandlike headaches with no other symptomatology; examination should be normal.

- **Diagnosis**
CT or MRI of the head to rule out intracranial mass lesion; early generalized, pulsating headaches might mean nocturnal hypoxemia and may require oximetry; LP should be done on patients with nuchal rigidity or fever; sinus roentgenography should be done on patients with percussion tenderness.

- **Disease Severity**
Headaches might be the initial and sole presentation of intracranial lesions such as brain tumors, abscesses, hydrocephalus, and other space-occupying lesions; otherwise these are benign conditions.

- **Concept and Application**
Migraines are secondary to intracranial vasospasm with secondary reflex vasodilation; chronic tension headaches are secondary to self-perpetuating muscle tension; cluster headaches could be paroxysmal parasympathetic discharges through the superficial petrosal nerve.

- **Management**
Abortive therapy can be provided by means of nonsteroidal anti-inflammatory drugs (NSAIDs); sumatriptan, a serotonin-1 agonist, can be given subcutaneously for quick effect; oral and rectal ergotamines can be used except in patients with known vascular disease or hypertension; migraine prophylaxis can be achieved by using β-receptor blockers, calcium channel blockers, or tricyclic antidepressants; cluster headaches respond well acutely (over 70% of cases) to oxygen inhalation; ergotamine orally and intranasal lidocaine can provide abortive therapy also; prophylaxis is achieved by oral corticosteroids or verapamil.

V. CEREBROVASCULAR DISORDERS

A. Ischemic Thrombotic Strokes

- **H&P Keys**
Predisposing risk factors include diabetes, hypertension, hypercholesterolemia, smoking; acute onset of fixed neurologic deficit, usually while sleeping; possible prior history of short-lived deficits or unilateral visual loss (transient ischemic attacks); contralateral hemiparesis and aphasia in middle cerebral or carotid distribution; contralateral leg and shoulder weakness in anterior cerebral territory; dense visual field cut in posterior cerebral territory.

- **Diagnosis**
CT or MRI of head to further localize lesion and exclude bleeding; carotid noninvasive or magnetic resonance angiogram (MRA) study to assess for stenosis; blood count and chemistry for risk factors; antinuclear antibodies (ANA), sedimentation rate, RPR, coagulation factor deficiency studies, homocysteine; arteriography in young individuals.

- **Disease Severity**
Large clinical or radiologic deficits correlate with large areas of infarction and have increased risk of edema and herniation or hemorrhagic conversion; rehabilitation is also limited.

- **Concept and Application**
Predisposing factors reduce resilience of large arteries; atherosclerosis at branching and curves of cerebral arteries cause stenosis with subsequent embolization or narrowing of lumen. Migraines and oral contraceptives increase risk of infarction.

- **Management**
Includes reduction of risk factors, management of stroke complications, secondary prevention with antiplatelet or anticoagulant agents, surgery in carotid arteries if stenosis over 70%, discontinuation of oral contraceptives, physical therapy, periodic follow-up for recurrences.

B. Cardioembolic Strokes

- **H&P Keys**
History of rheumatic fever, cardiac dysrhythmias; in younger patient, abrupt onset, hemorrhagic strokes, or multifocal distribution. Evidence of cortical signs including aphasia, seizures, more than one arterial distribution in addition to findings similar to thrombotic strokes.

- **Diagnosis**
CT or MRI of head, ECG, transthoracic and transesophageal echocardiogram if ECG is normal and suspicion for cardiac source still high, Holter monitor, blood cultures if endocarditis suspected.

- **Disease Severity**
Embolic strokes tend to be larger and more commonly hemorrhagic, higher incidence of edema with mass effect and seizures increase morbidity and mortality.

- **Concept and Application**
Sources of embolization include atrial fibrillation (with or without valvular disease), prosthetic valves, endocarditis, left ventricular hypokinesis or thrombus, cardiac tumors (myxomas).

- **Management**
With the exception of myxoma and recent heart attack, long-term anticoagulation is needed. Anticoagulation with heparin can be started within a few hours if stroke is not too large or there is no hemorrhage. Switch to warfarin (Coumadin) when therapeutic and follow International Normalized Ratio (INR) recommendations depending on cause of stroke.

C. Intracerebral Hemorrhage

- **H&P Keys**
Usually history of uncontrolled hypertension or coagulation deficits, sudden apoplectic onset, severe headache, nausea, vomiting, and focal neurologic deficits; exam shows hemiparesis, obtundation, sensory deficits, conjugate eye deviation contralateral to hemiparesis (toward hemiparesis if brain stem), rapidly developing coma in pontine or cerebellar hemorrhage, elevated blood pressure.

- **Diagnosis**
CT or MRI of head to assess extent of bleeding, LP may be bloody but nonspecific and may induce herniation.

- **Disease Severity**
Both pontine and cerebellar hemorrhages carry increased risk; cerebellar hemorrhage is usually amenable to surgery.

- **Concept and Application**
Hypertensive hemorrhages are due to aneurysmal dilatation (Charcot-Bouchard syndrome) of small-caliber arteries as a result of lipohyalinosis.

- **Management**
Supportive therapy, management of intracranial hypertension, careful control of systemic hypertension; lobar and cerebellar hemorrhages may be amenable to surgical resection.

D. Subarachnoid Hemorrhage

- **H&P Keys**
Acute onset of worst headache of patient's life, nausea, vomiting, variable loss of consciousness, may have had previous "warn-

ing" headaches; nuchal rigidity, obtundation, hemiparesis in middle cerebral territory, third cranial nerve palsy in posterior communicating artery distribution, leg weakness, confusion in anterior cerebral artery territory. Two thirds of ruptured aneurysms occur in anterior circulation.

- **Diagnosis**
  CT of head positive in about 90% of cases; MRI may miss initial picture; LP shows elevated pressure, markedly bloody and xanthochromic, protein elevated, leukocytosis in 48 hours. Arteriography is mandatory for definitive diagnosis; if initially negative (vasospasm) repeat in 6 to 12 weeks. Delay study if severe vasospasm present.

- **Disease Severity**
  Outcome depends on mental status at time of ictus. Lethargic or obtunded patients have poorer outcome. Vasospasm and seizures add to morbidity. Disease associated with polycystic kidneys. Multiple aneurysms in many cases.

- **Concept and Application**
  Hypertension, arteriosclerosis cause weakness of large-artery walls at bifurcations, leading to saccular dilatation. Rupture of this dilatation with associated arterial pressure results in symptoms. Reflex vasospasm causes oligemia and in severe cases, infarcts. Arteriovenous malformation can also rupture.

- **Management**
  Control of hypertension; reduction of Valsalva with stool softeners, quiet room; reduction of vasospasm with nimodipine; reduction of increased intracranial pressure with osmotic agents; hyperventilation and ventriculostomy if necessary; treatment of seizures with anticonvulsants; surgery when stable.

E. Venous Thrombosis

- **H&P Keys**
  History of sinus or ear infection, cyanotic heart disease, sickle cell anemia, or hypercoagulable state. Headache, papilledema, nausea, and vomiting; seizures with cortical vein involvement. Cranial nerves IX, X, XI involved in transverse sinus thrombosis; proptosis, periorbital ecchymosis and edema with cranial nerves II, IV, VI in cavernous sinus thrombosis; visual field defects, crural monoplegia in sagittal sinus thrombosis.

- **Diagnosis**
  MRA (angiogram) and MRV (venogram) are preferred. Arteriography with venous phase will show thrombosis also; LP shows raised intracranial pressure and xanthochromia but may be contraindicated because of risk of herniation.

- **Disease Severity**
  Because many thrombi are caused by septic infection, abscesses and meningitis may appear concurrently.

- **Concept and Application**
  Thrombosis of venous drainage resulting from infection or inappropriate coagulation impedes venous flow, causing increased intracranial pressure, infarction of tissue.

- **Management**
  Antibiotics if septic, anticoagulants otherwise; supportive management; treatment of seizures.

VI. TOXIC DISORDERS

A. Heavy Metals

1. Lead

- **H&P Keys**
  In adults, exposure occurs from burning lead batteries, water ingestion (lead pipes), "moonshine" ingestion, gasoline fumes. Colic (usually precipitated by alcohol intoxication), anemia, and neuropathy presenting as wrist drop or predominantly motor polyneuropathy. In children, exposure occurs from ingestion of lead paint. Clinical presentations include anorexia, colic, ataxia, followed by drowsiness, stupor, seizures, and coma (most frequently in summer if ingestion continues).

- **Diagnosis**
Basophilic stippling in RBCs, urine porphyrins elevated, increased blood levels of lead. Lead lines along metaphysis in children.

2. Mercury

- **H&P Keys**
History of mercury exposure in thermometer manufacturing plants, mirrors, x-ray machines. Presents with tremor of arms, lips, tongue, and legs, ataxia, and chorea.

- **Diagnosis**
Elevated mercury levels in blood.

3. Arsenic

- **H&P Keys**
Usually suicidal (intentional ingestion) attempts with herbicides or rat poison. Headaches, drowsiness, confusion, and seizures if acute, associated with hemolysis, weakness, and myalgia if chronic.

- **Diagnosis**
Transverse (Mees') white lines on the fingernails, scaly desquamation, and gastrointestinal (GI) symptoms. Elevated arsenic levels in hair and urine.

4. Manganese

- **H&P Keys**
History of exposure in miners separating ore from manganese. Present with a parkinsonlike syndrome including marked drooling, tremors, rigidity, and retropulsive gait.

- **Diagnosis**
Elevated levels of manganese in blood.

- **Disease Severity**
Improvements in symptoms depend on timing of initiation of therapy in relation to onset. Manganese poisoning in children can be fatal or result in mental deficiencies.

- **Concept and Application**
Calcarine neuronal loss, cerebellar granule cell loss in mercury; diffuse punctate hemorrhages in arsenic; endothelial damage and swelling in lead poisoning; pallidal and striatal neuronal loss in manganese poisoning.

- **Management**
Chelation with dimercaprol (BAL) for lead and arsenic poisoning, *N*-acetylpenicillamine for mercury poisoning; L-dopa for manganese poisoning; mannitol for edema and anticonvulsants for seizures for lead poisoning in children.

B. Medications

1. Opioids

- **H&P Keys**
High incidence of addiction; inadvertent poisoning or suicidal attempts, results in varying degrees of obtundation followed by decreased ventilation, miosis, bradycardia, and hypothermia.

2. Barbiturates

- **H&P Keys**
High incidence of addiction; suicide attempts or accidental poisoning result in progressive unarousal, respiratory depression; pupillary response present and pulmonary edema.

3. Benzodiazepines

- **H&P Keys**
Similar to barbiturates.

4. Antipsychotic Drugs

- **H&P Keys**
Use of phenothiazines and butyrophenones, treatment of schizophrenia; side effects are parkinsonian syndrome, buccolingual involuntary movements (tardive dyskinesias), inability to sit still (akathisia), and a syndrome of severe rigidity, fever, and confusion (neuroleptic malignant syndrome), which can prove fatal in 20% of cases even when treated.

5. Cocaine

- **H&P Keys**
History of dependency; can be administered nasally, intravenously, or smoked; symptoms of intoxication include tremor, myoclonus, seizures, and psychosis. Stroke, seizures, and subarachnoid hemorrhages have been described.

VII. NEOPLASMS

A. Glioblastoma

- **H&P Keys**
  Most common type of tumor in adults; history of hemiparesis or other focal neurologic signs, also seizures, confusion, obtundation, and late headache. No clear predisposing factors; most common cause of new-onset seizures in middle age. Exam correlates with complaints.

- **Diagnosis**
  Contrast CT or MRI will show characteristic ring-enhancing lesion; rarely may be multicentric or across corpus callosum. Other studies are negative, including search for a metastatic origin. Biopsy shows typical pseudopallisading, hemorrhage, pleomorphism, and hypercellularity, and necrosis and endothelial hyperplasia.

- **Disease Severity**
  Younger patients have better prognosis than older ones. Less than one fifth of all patients survive more than a year.

- **Concept and Application**
  Likely arises from anaplasia of astrocytes. Secondary characteristics of the tumor lead to further tissue invasion and mass effect.

- **Management**
  Radiation accompanied by use of corticosteroids (vasogenic edema) and anticonvulsants is routine because of patients symptoms. Chemotherapy can be offered to patients under 55.

B. Meningioma   *Psammoma bods*

- **H&P Keys**
  Benign tumor, causes symptoms by compression or irritation. Convexity tumors present with hemiparesis, seizures, and headaches; parasagittal with bicrural asymmetric weakness and spasticity, with sphincter disorder. Can happen in spinal canal (mainly females) or on optic nerve. Exam relates to complaints and presentation.

- **Diagnosis**
  CT of head will show a usually rounded dural lesion with mass effect; MRI may only show lesion clearly with contrast enhancement. It may calcify and show on plain roentgenograms.

- **Disease Severity**
  Location of the tumor and potential for surgical resection determine outcome. Usually tumor recurs if not completely resected.

- **Concept and Application**
  Arise from arachnoid cells and may attain great size prior to development of symptoms. Usually cause exostosis rather than bone erosion. Some have estrogen receptors and enlarge because of this. Psammoma bodies can be seen microscopically.

- **Management**
  Surgical resection when accessible, radiation otherwise if symptomatic. Incidental tumors can be observed because of slow growth. Corticosteroids for edema, anticonvulsants for seizures.

C. Metastases

- **H&P Keys**
  History of smoking, breast cancer, or other predisposing factors. Usually presents with focal neurologic signs, behavioral changes, headaches, or seizures. May be apoplectic if it bleeds.

- **Diagnosis**
  MRI or CT scan shows single or multiple lesions with surrounding edema and enhancement. Physical examination including breast, gynecologic and rectal exam, chest roentgenography, blood count may lead to diagnosis of primary. Biopsy of lesion if primary unknown will lead to separation from other etiologies.

- **Disease Severity**
  Choriocarcinoma, melanoma, thyroid carcinoma, and hypernephroma may present with high incidence of bleeding. Solitary lesions have better prognosis and can be resected in some cases. Final outcome is relative to the primary disease itself.

- **Concept and Application**
  Most commonly arises from lung, breast, or melanoma.

- **Management**
  Radiation, steroids, and anticonvulsants. Chemotherapy in appropriate cases.

VIII. DEGENERATIVE DISEASES

A. Alzheimer's Disease

- **H&P Keys**
  Onset in late fifties or sixties; presents initially with deficit in retentive memory followed by dysnomia, spatial disorientation, personality changes, and gait disorder. The mental status examination shows findings related to these complaints. Seizures, paraparesis, and abulia can be seen in advanced cases.

- **Diagnosis**
  CSF is normal, EEG is diffusely slow late in the disease, and the CT or MRI show atrophy; single-photon emission computed tomography (SPECT) scan shows biparietal perfusion defects. Efforts are being made to develop a biologic marker.

- **Disease Severity**
  Progressive dementia leads to both physical and mental dissolution and eventually death.

- **Concept and Application**
  The etiology is unknown, but a relationship exists with chromosome 21 in familial cases, the same chromosome involved in Down syndrome. The latter condition has pathologic similarities to Alzheimer's disease. Possible linkage with mutations in amyloid precursor protein or apolipoprotein E.

- **Management**
  No known treatment.

B. Amyotrophic Lateral Sclerosis

- **H&P Keys**
  Progressive weakness, usually asymmetrically, involving all voluntary muscles except extraocular ones. Prominent cramps, fasciculations, accompanied by "stiffness," dysarthria, and dysphagia. Exam shows mainly distal weakness with atrophy and fasciculation. Reflexes are exaggerated, tone is increased (spastic), toes are extensor. Combination of weak limb with atrophy and hyperreflexia is very suggestive.

- **Diagnosis**
  Do MRI of cervical spine if exam shows atrophy and weakness of arms with hyperreflexia of legs to rule out cervical lesion. EMG shows denervation and reinnervation as does the muscle biopsy. CK is minimally elevated in some cases. Do lead blood levels, hexosaminidase A, serum protein electrophoresis to exclude conditions that will mimic it, particularly when upper motor neuron signs are absent or mild.

- **Disease Severity**
  The disease is fatal; bulbar forms have a shorter course. Respiratory failure and malnutrition are causes of death.

- **Concept and Application**
  Neuronal loss in the anterior horn and motor cortex. Etiology unknown. Familial cases associated with mutation of calcium or zinc superoxide dismutase gene.

- **Management**
  No treatment known.

C. Parkinson's Disease

- **H&P Keys**
  Progressive tremor, slowness, festinating gait, stooped posture. Early on, symptoms may be nonspecific ("arm discomfort"). Exam shows a resting tremor of 4 to 6 Hz, difficulty with passive motion (rigidity) evenly through the full range, decreased expression, paucity of movements (bradykinesia), and difficulty with posture. When tremor is added to the rigidity, "cogwheeling" results. Dementia occurs in 30% of cases.

- **Diagnosis**
  No routine diagnostic studies exist; have decreased basal ganglia dopamine activity on positron emission tomography (PET) scan.

Exclude medications, progressive supranuclear palsy, olivopontocerebellar degeneration.

- **Disease Severity**
  The disease eventually leads to disability in spite of therapy. Swallowing can be markedly affected.

- **Concept and Application**
  Neuronal loss of the substantia nigra and other pigmented nuclei. Reduced dopamine levels. Similarity to a syndrome caused by the designer drug MPTP has raised question of environmental factor.

- **Management**
  Replace dopamine with L-dopa; added carbidopa (Sinemet) reduces peripheral effects. This medication can cause variations in clinical state not associated with dosing (on–off phenomenon). Dopamine receptor stimulators are also helpful; anticholinergics improve tremor but can worsen dementia. Selegiline, a selective monoamine oxidase (MAO)-B inhibitor, is used to slow down the disease progression.

D. Huntington's Disease

- **H&P Keys**
  Progressive mental deterioration; becoming irritable, impulsive, exhibiting poor self-control. Hand and face chorea develops and eventually all muscles follow. The exam shows chorea, dementia, oculomotor disturbances.

- **Diagnosis**
  The CT or MRI shows caudate head atrophy; genetic studies can define the patient at risk and the subject with overt disease.

- **Disease Severity**
  The disease is transmitted as autosomal dominant with complete penetrance. It is also fatal. Childhood cases present with rigidity and seizures also. Mode of transmission leads to anticipation (subsequent generations show earlier and more severe signs).

- **Concept and Application**
  Autosomal dominant inheritance; gene located on the short arm of chromosome 4; multiple erroneous repeats of nucleic acid triplets (CGA) results in defective Huntington's gene.

- **Management**
  No known treatment. Genetic counseling available for receptive individuals. Since there is no cure, patients or individuals at risk may commit suicide.

IX. TRAUMA

A. Subdural Hematoma

- **H&P Keys**
  History of head trauma with progressive change in mentation, focal neurologic signs, often loss of consciousness but not always, hemiparesis, large unreactive pupil with ophthalmoplegia if acute; seizures, headache, progressive change in mentation if chronic.

- **Diagnosis**
  CT of head, if performed without contrast, may miss an isodense (chronic) subdural hematoma. MRI of head with contrast (gadolinium) is the study of choice. Both will show crescentic lesion with signal compatible with blood.

- **Disease Severity**
  Progressive focal neurologic deficit, progressive obtundation, requires quick intervention. Mass effect and shift of intracranial contents in radiologic studies also are usually suggestive of increased severity.

- **Concept and Application**
  Ruptured bridging superficial cortical veins are responsible for blood accumulation. Chronic subdural may have recent rebleeding. Mass effect and cortical irritation are responsible for symptoms.

- **Management**
  Subdural hematomas with rapidly or incapacitating symptoms are best treated with

surgical evacuation of the clot. Prudent observation or corticosteroids can be used for small, incidental, or symptom-free subdurals.

B. Epidural Hematoma

- **H&P Keys**
Severe head trauma accompanied by loss of consciousness, transient recovery of consciousness followed by progressive obtundation, posturing, shallow respirations, seizures, focal neurologic signs, coma.

- **Diagnosis**
CT of head or MRI will show concave blood clot, white on CT, bright on T1- and T2-weighted images on MRI. Skull roentgenograms will show fracture through area of middle meningeal artery or, less commonly, across venous sinus.

- **Disease Severity**
If untreated, the condition is lethal; timing is of the essence.

- **Concept and Application**
Tear of middle meningeal artery or venous sinus results in accumulation of blood at great pressure in a potential space.

- **Management**
Emergent surgical evacuation; supportive.

C. Contusion

- **H&P Keys**
History of moderate severe head trauma (unconscious for more than 5 minutes); returns to alertness with confusion and mild mutism. Exam shows extensor plantar reflexes, mild hemiparesis, elevated blood pressure and heart rate.

- **Diagnosis**
CT or MRI may show focal parenchymal swelling or delayed hemorrhage.

- **Disease Severity**
Degree of alertness at the time of evaluation, time unconscious, degree of retrograde amnesia determine severity of injury if otherwise uncomplicated. Temporal lobe herniation is main cause of morbidity and mortality.

- **Concept and Application**
Sustained head trauma results in neuronal swelling and axonal shearing, often maximal 24 to 48 hours after event.

- **Management**
Control of intracranial pressure with hyperventilation, ventriculostomy; barbiturate coma may lessen neuronal injury. Delayed physical and cognitive deficits may occur and will require therapy.

X. DEMYELINATION

A. Multiple Sclerosis

- **H&P Keys**
History of arm, leg, hand, or foot numbness (50% of patients), visual loss (25%), diplopia, incoordination, weakness, bladder dysfunction. Exam shows sensory loss in spinal distribution, afferent pupillary deficit, ataxia, dysarthria, hyperreflexia, internuclear ophthalmoplegia.

- **Diagnosis**
MRI will show periventricular white matter demyelination or lesion in the spinal cord or optic nerve. LP shows lymphocytic pleocytosis (<100), increased protein (<100), normal glucose, increased IgG intrathecal production, and oligoclonal bands. The last two are present in more than 85% of acute exacerbations. Large myelinated pathways can be assessed with evoked potentials (visual, auditory, sensory). The disease can be mimicked by syphilis, Sjögren's syndrome, systemic lupus erythematosus, sarcoidosis, and Lyme disease. The diagnosis remains clinical and depends on finding different lesions on separate occasions.

- **Disease Severity**
Pure spinal forms, chronic progressive, and early presentation are correlated with worst outcome. Elevation of body temperature (Uhthoff's phenomenon), stress, and infection can cause exacerbation.

- **Concept and Application**
The etiology of the disease is multifactorial, with environmental factors, increased incidence in temperate regions, and, prior to age 15, immunogenetic factors such as certain HLA-Dw or DR antigens, followed by an aberrant immunologic response against CNS myelin.

- **Management**
Acute attacks respond to IV corticosteroids; chronic prophylaxis can be obtained with interferon beta. The tremor responds to isoniazid; baclofen orally or intrathecally reduces spasticity. Fatigue responds to amantadine or pemoline; gait disability, bladder disorders require appropriate care.

XI. SPINE DISEASE

A. Spinal Stenosis

1. Cervical

- **H&P Keys**
Neck pain; gait difficulty; progressive leg and arm weakness; spasticity of weak limbs; hyperreflexia; Babinski's and Lhermitte's signs.

- **Diagnosis**
CT or MRI of cervical spine confirms diagnosis, usually due to spondylitic "bars"; EMG and nerve conductions document root involvement; post myelography CT scan delineates questionable stenosis.

- **Disease Severity**
Bowel and bladder disorder; progressive paresis; clonus; anterior-posterior diameter of spinal canal under 8 mm of circumference.

- **Concept and Application**
Repeated trauma on flexion-extension; spinal vascular insufficiency.

- **Management**
Conservative therapy may be of some help (NSAIDs, therapy). Surgery may be necessary.

2. Lumbar

- **H&P Keys**
Progressive pain and weakness in lower extremities on exertion; back pain; weakness of the legs.

- **Diagnosis**
As in cervical area.

- **Disease Severity**
As in cervical area.

- **Concept and Application**
Vascular insufficiency.

- **Management**
In the cervical area, immobilization has been advocated; NSAIDs or epidural analgesic injections help reduce pain. Surgery remains the most definitive method of treatment to decompress.

B. Radiculopathy

- **H&P Keys**
Pain and weakness in the distribution of a root, shoulder pain, deltoid and biceps weakness, absent biceps reflex (C-5); arm, forearm, and first-digit pain, brachioradialis and biceps weakness, absent brachioradialis reflex (C-6); more commonly in cervical area. Hip, lateral thigh, anterior leg, and big-toe pain, foot and big-toe extensor weakness (L-5); posterior leg and thigh, small-toe pain, absent ankle jerk, foot extension weakness (S-1).

- **Diagnosis**
Cervical or lumbar roentgenogram if history includes trauma; MRI of appropriate level to assess intervertebral disk herniation; EMG and NCV in 3 to 4 weeks to assess distribution of radiculopathy.

- **Disease Severity**
Severe weakness correlates with prominent nerve involvement. Prolonged deficits will improve slowly or not at all.

- **Concept and Application**
Root compression leads to axonal injury.

- **Management**
Mild and moderate deficits can be treated conservatively with physical therapy. Sur-

gery may be used if physical therapy does not improve symptoms over 6 to 12 weeks or for severe deficits (drop foot).

XII. SLEEP DISORDERS

A. Sleep Apnea

- **H&P Keys**
  Heavyset build, short neck, large tongue, large tonsils in children, myxedema, acromegaly, myotonic dystrophy in obstructive type; poliomyelitis, syringobulbia, and brainstem infarct in central type; history of heavy snoring, daytime sleepiness, fatigue, early morning headache, impotence.

- **Diagnosis**
  Thyroid studies to rule out hypothyroidism; polysomnogram to exclude other etiologies of daytime sleepiness and to assess apneas and differentiate between central or obstructive type; multiple sleep latencies to assess the degree of nocturnal disturbance.

- **Disease Severity**
  Six or more apneas per hour; oxygen desaturation; nocturnal cardiac arrhythmias. Sleep apnea is associated with cerebrovascular accidents, heart attacks.

- **Concept and Application**
  Upper airway laxity and collapse on inspiration; reduced nocturnal respiratory drive in central type.

- **Management**
  Weight reduction of as small as 5 lb may reduce symptoms. Continuous positive airway pressure (CPAP) for obstructive type, repeat studies and adjust settings; protriptyline for central apnea.

B. Narcolepsy

- **H&P Keys**
  Present with excessive daytime sleepiness; multiple daytime naps; paralysis with strong emotions in 70% (cataplexy); sleep paralysis; hypnagogic hallucinations; normal examination.

- **Diagnosis**
  Sleep study (polysomnogram) is normal and will exclude other pathologies; multiple sleep latencies show rapid eye movement (REM) sleep onset; same abnormality can be seen with use of drugs, drug withdrawal, or sleep deprivation; therefore need good clinical correlation.

- **Disease Severity**
  Most patients have narcolepsy and cataplexy by history; there could be milder cases; few have all symptoms.

- **Concept and Application**
  The etiology of the disease is unknown.

- **Management**
  Nondrug therapy consists of short naps, avoidance of heavy meals. Drug therapy (often needed) consists of pemoline, and if unsuccessful, methylphenidate (Ritalin). Imipramine may be useful in controlling cataplexy.

XIII. DEVELOPMENTAL DISORDERS

A. Tay-Sachs Disease

- **H&P Keys**
  Mostly Jewish infants of Eastern European background; presents in early infancy with startle to noises, irritability, and subsequent developmental delay or regression of acquired milestones. Initial hypotonia is followed by spasticity, blindness, and retinal cherry-red spots and seizures. Death occurs in 3 to 4 years.

- **Diagnosis**
  Exclude other cause of a similar syndrome, such as embryologic abnormalities or infections and other systemic diseases. The enzyme abnormality is the lack of hexosaminidase A, which can be measured in fibroblasts, WBCs, or serum. This enzymatic assay allows the recognition of the heterozygote asymptomatic carrier and permits genetic counseling.

- **Disease Severity**
  Other variants of this disease are recognized, including one mimicking motor neuron disease in adults. The disease is invariably fatal.

- **Concept and Application**
  Hexosaminidase A is needed for the cleavage of *N*-acetylgalactosamine, and its absence leads to ganglioside accumulation.

- **Management**
  No treatment is available, and prevention depends on preconceptual identification of parents at risk and genetic counseling.

DEFINITIONS

APHASIA   Language deficits of several types acquired after the acquisition of normal speech and reading skills. Often caused by a left hemispheric lesion. The type and degree of involvement of language depend on the localization of the injury.

COMA   Alteration of consciousness in which the subject appears asleep but is incapable of any response to external or internal stimuli. Degree may vary, and various vegetative functions may be absent or present, including breathing, pupillary response, corneal response, tendon reflexes, and reflex ocular movements. Coma can be reversible if caused by metabolic injuries (eg, hypothermia, drug intoxication).

BRAIN DEATH   Medical and legal term that refers to complete absence of any brain activity with preserved cardiac or pulmonary function without reversible causative factor. Legally, the diagnosis allows the discontinuation of life-support measures, and its definition depends on finding no evidence of any neurologic function other than spinal reflexes. This includes absent corneal reflexes, reflex eye movements to caloric stimulation, pupillary responses, or significant response to pain. The absence of a respiratory drive is tested by oxygenating the patient through a cannula without mechanical assistance. Absent electroencephalogram (EEG) potentials larger than 2 µV, absent brain-stem–evoked potentials, or lack of cerebral circulation on arteriography are supportive of but often not absolutely required for the diagnosis.

DEMENTIA   Defined as a loss of various intellectual functions including memory (often the earliest), language, and abstract reasoning. In addition, behavioral and personality changes (such as paranoia) often accompany the intellectual dissolution.

DYSLEXIA   Reading or reading and spelling disability that is unexpected based on development and general aptitude. Often associated with attention deficit disorders in the child.

SYNCOPE   Transitory loss of consciousness secondary to hypoperfusion of the brain. Often secondary to a vasovagal reflex (eg, during blood donation), can also be the presentation of cardiac arrhythmias, inability to sustain adequate blood pressure, etc. It is in the differential diagnosis of seizure but different from it because it is often preceded by prolonged warnings, is of short duration, is not accompanied by tongue biting or sphincter disorder, and consciousness is recovered quickly with supine position.

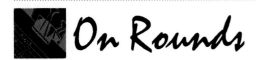

Neurology

Meningitis CSF Findings

- **Aseptic:** Pleocytosis, predominantly lymphocytic, mild protein elevation, normal glucose, negative bacterial cultures
- **Bacterial:** Pleocytosis up to 10 000, mainly neutrophils, low glucose, elevated protein, positive culture
- **Fungal:** Lymphocytic and monocytic pleocytosis, positive fungal culture in weeks
- **TB:** Lymphocytic pleocytosis, elevated protein, low glucose, positive acid-fast bacillus stain

Degenerative Diseases

- **Alzheimer's**

  Onset late 50s or 60s

  Retentive Memory deficit, personality changes, gait disorder

  Normal CSF, CT/MRI may show atrophy

  No treatment

- **Amyotrophic Lateral Sclerosis**

  Progressive asymmetric weakness of voluntary muscles

  Due to neuronal loss in the anterior horn and motor cortex

  No treatment

- **Parkinson Disease**

  Resting tremor 4–6 Hz, cogwheel rigidity, bradykinesia

  No diagnostic tests available

  Results from neuronal loss of the substantia nigra, reduced dopamine levels

  Treatment: L-dopa, carbidopa, anticholinergics, MAO-B inhibitor

- **Huntington's Disease**

  Progressive mental deterioration, hand and face chorea, dementia

  CT or MRI positive for caudate head atrophy

  Transmitted as an autosomal dominant with complete penetrance, gene on the short arm of chromosome 4

  No treatment

BIBLIOGRAPHY

Adams RD. *Principles of Neurology.* 2nd ed. New York: McGraw-Hill Book Co; 1981.

Aminoff MJ. *Neurology and General Medicine.* New York: Churchill Livingstone; 1989.

Glaser JS. *Neuroophthalmology.* 2nd ed. Philadelphia: JB Lippincott; 1990.

Pryse-Phillips W. *Essential Neurology.* 4th ed. New York: Medical Examination Publishing Company; 1992.

Samuels MA. *Manual of Neurology.* 4th ed. Boston: Little Brown and Company; 1991.

Smith DB. *Epilepsy: Current Approaches to Diagnosis and Treatment.* New York: Raven Press; 1991.

Weiner WJ. *Emergent and Urgent Neurology.* Philadelphia: JB Lippincott; 1992.

Weiner WJ. *Neurology for the Non-Neurologist.* 2nd ed. Philadelphia: JB Lippincott; 1989.

11

Male and Female Reproduction

Samuel L. Jacobs, MD

I. UTERUS

A. Malignant Neoplasm

I Endometrium
II cervix
III pelvic
IV bowel, bladder mets

Endometrial Cancer

- **H&P Keys**
  Obesity, nulliparity, chronic anovulation, diabetes, hypertension, postmenopausal bleeding, median age 61, early menarche, late menopause.

- **Diagnosis**
  Fractional dilatation and curettage, endometrial biopsy, hysteroscopy.

Advanced Disease. Chest roentgenogram, intravenous pyelogram (IVP), computerized tomographic (CT) scan, barium enema, cystoscopy.

- **Disease Severity**
  International Federation of Gynecology and Obstetrics (FIGO) stage I endometrium, stage II cervix, stage III pelvic organs, stage IV, bowel mucosa, bladder, distant metastases.

- **Concept and Application**
  Relationship between estrogen production and endometrial proliferation; overgrowth of the endometrium in response to unopposed estrogen.

- **Management**

Early Disease. Total abdominal hysterectomy and bilateral salpingo-oophorectomy; otherwise radiation or both.

Stage III & IV. Chemotherapy.

B. Leiomyoma of Uterus

- **H&P Keys**
  Present in 20% of whites, 50% of blacks by 30 years of age; pain, abnormal uterine bleeding, pressure, infertility (repeated pregnancy loss), uterine enlargement.

- **Diagnosis**
  Complete blood count (CBC) with differential, pelvic ultrasound, IVP, magnetic resonance imaging (MRI).

- **Disease Severity**
  Severity of pain, anemia, urinary frequency or retention, hydronephrosis, uterine size beyond 12 weeks.

- **Concept and Application**
  Localized proliferation of smooth muscle cells, estrogen-dependent, shrinkage after menopause.

- **Management**

Observation. Pelvic examinations, serial ultrasonograms, monitoring hydronephrosis.

Medical. Gonadotropin-releasing hormone (Gn-Rh) agonists.

Surgical. Myomectomy (via hysteroscopy, laparoscopy, or laparotomy), total abdominal hysterectomy.

C. Other Disorders

Endometriosis

- **H&P Keys**
  Dysmenorrhea, dyspareunia, infertility, chronic pelvic pain, retroverted uterus, uterosacral nodularity, nonmobile uterus.

- **Diagnosis**
  History and physical examination, bimanual examination, CA125 (questionable), pelvic ultrasonography (for presence of endometrioma), laparoscopy (gold standard of diagnosis), biopsy (histology shows endometrial glands and stroma).

- **Disease Severity**
  American Fertility Society stages I to IV (minimal through severe), extent of pelvic pain, duration of infertility.

- **Concept and Application**
  Retrograde menstruation, hematogenous spread, lymphogenous spread, genetic and family predisposition, coelomic metaplasia, estrogen-dependent growth of endometriosis, resolves after menopause.

- **Management**
  Depends on age of patient, duration of infertility, severity of symptoms, extent of disease. Expectant therapy. Medical therapy consists of Gn-RH agonist, progestogens, oral contraceptives, nonsteroidal anti-inflammatory drugs (NSAIDs), danazol (androgenic side effects). Conservative surgery, radical surgery via laparoscopy, laparotomy.

II. OVARY

A. Malignant Neoplasm

Ovarian Cancer

I ovary
II pelvic
III intraperitoneal
IV met

- **H&P Keys**
  Asymptomatic more than two thirds of the time; leading cause of gynecologic cancer deaths in United States. Ascites, abdominal distention, pelvic mass in advanced stages.

- **Diagnosis**
  History and physical exam, pelvic ultrasonography, CA125, CT scan, barium enema, chest roentgenogram, surgical staging.

- **Disease Severity**

  Surgical Staging. Stage I limited to the ovaries; stage II pelvic extension; stage III intraperitoneal metastases outside the pelvis; stage IV distant metastases.

Main Histologic Types. Epithelial tumors (80%), sex-cord stromal tumors (3%), germ-cell tumors (5%).

- **Concept and Application**
  Spread to adjacent peritoneal surfaces; most common death result of bowel obstruction.

- **Management**
  Total abdominal hysterectomy, bilateral salpingo-oophorectomy, omentectomy, adjunctive chemotherapy, radiation therapy, second-look laparotomy. Overall 5-year survival rate: 30%.

B. Ovarian Cysts

- **H&P Keys**
  Anovulation, irregular bleeding, irregular periods, abdominal pain; reproductive age group; usually unilateral, bimanual exam.

- **Diagnosis**
  CBC and differential, pelvic ultrasonography (size, loculations, unilaterality versus bilaterality, calcifications), β-human chorionic gonadotropin (β-hCG).

- **Disease Severity**
  Amount of pain, cyst size, presence of loci, fluid in the peritoneal cavity.

- **Concept and Application**
  Most common is functional cyst related to anovulation. Follicular cyst continues to develop and enlarge without ovulation, thereby causing pain, possibly intraperitoneal rupture, and irregular menses. Eighty-five percent will resolve by 9 weeks.

- **Management**
  Observation, serial ultrasonograms, serial CBC with differential; if suspicion of intraperitoneal bleeding; surgery. If danger of torsion, possible laparotomy, ovarian cystectomy, or oophorectomy.

III. CERVIX

A. Malignant Neoplasm

- **H&P Keys**
  Multiple sexual partners, cigarette smoking, early intercourse, high-risk sexual be-

Cervix CC haviors, abnormal Pap smears, mean age 45 years, postcoital bleeding, abnormal discharge, occasional pelvic pain.

- **Diagnosis**
  Pap smear, colposcopy, cone biopsy, endocervical curettage (ECC), chest roentgenogram, IVP, barium enema, cystoscopy, proctosigmoidoscopy, MRI (optional).

- **Disease Severity**

Stage I. Confined to cervix.

Stage II. Upper vagina, not pelvic sidewall.

Stage III. Extending to pelvic sidewall.

Stage IV. Beyond pelvis: distant organs.

- **Concept and Application**
  Associated with sexually transmitted diseases: Herpes simplex virus type II, human papilloma virus, metaplasia of the cervical transformation zone (where squamous epithelium merges into columnar epithelium).

- **Management**
  Total abdominal hysterectomy (cure rate 95%). Stage IB–IIA: Radical hysterectomy or radiotherapy. Recurrence of advanced stage: chemotherapy, radiotherapy; possible pelvic exenteration. Death eventually from uremia.

B. Cervicitis and Sexually Transmitted Diseases

- **H&P Keys**

Herpes. Inguinal nodes, fever, multiple tender vesicles.

Gonorrhea. Discharge, abdominal pain, asymptomatic.

Syphilis. Chancre, fever, secondary skin rash, condyloma latum.

Chlamydia. Asymptomatic or endocervicitis, inguinal lymphadenopathy.

Chancroid. (*Haemophilus ducreyi*) ulcerative disease: soft, painful ulcers.

Human Papilloma Virus (HPV). Multifocal fleshy warts.

Lymphogranuloma venereum (LGV). "Groove sign" (line between lymph nodes), buboes.

- **Diagnosis**

Herpes. Clinical examination; viral culture.

Gonorrhea. Culture on Thayer-Martin medium.

Syphilis. VDRL, fluorescent treponemal antibody (FTA), rapid plasma reagin (RPR).

Chlamydia. Culture.

Chancroid. Biopsy, LGV, complement fixation.

- **Disease Severity**

Herpes. Primary lesions 2 to 3 weeks, recurrent lesions.

Gonorrhea. Severity of symptoms; advanced stages: arthritis.

Syphilis. Primary, secondary, tertiary syphilis.

Chlamydia. Primary, secondary, tertiary stages.

Chancroid. Severity of symptoms.

HPV. Severity of warty infection.

HPV type 6,11. Low-risk oncoviruses.

HPV type 31,33,35,42. Intermediate-risk oncoviruses.

HPV type 16,18. High-risk oncoviruses.

LGV. Severity of symptoms.

- **Concept and Application**
  Transmitted sexually via oral, vaginal, and anal contact; also associated with specific microorganism; also with body fluid contact.

Herpes. Herpes simplex virus.

Gonorrhea. *Neisseria gonorrhoeae.*

Syphilis. *Treponema pallidum.*

Chlamydia. *Chlamydia trachomatis.*

Chancroid. *Haemophilus ducreyi.*

HPV. Human papilloma virus.

LGV. *Chlamydia trachomatis.*

• Management

Herpes. Acyclovir.

Gonorrhea. Tetracycline, amoxicillin, probenecid, cefoxitin, ceftriaxone.

Syphilis. Benzathine penicillin.

Chlamydia. Doxycycline, tetracycline.

Chancroid. Oral sulfonamides, tetracycline.

HPV. Chemical destructive techniques (podophyllin), cryotherapy, electrocautery, laser vaporization, 5-fluorouracil, interferon, bichloroacetic acid.

C. Cervical Dysplasia and Management of Abnormal Pap

• **H&P Keys**
Early age of coitus, sexual promiscuity, multiple sexual partners, cigarette smoking, high-risk male partner, abnormal Pap, HPV infection, cervical discharge, postcoital bleeding.

• **Diagnosis**
Pap smear, colposcopy, colposcopic biopsy, ECC, cone biopsy.

• **Disease Severity**
Cervical intraepithelial neoplasia (CIN) I, CIN II, CIN III, carcinoma in situ (CIS).

• **Concept and Application**
Oncogenic agents such as sexually transmitted viruses help induce malignant transformation of the cervical transformation zone.

• **Management**
Electrocautery, cryotherapy, cold coagulation, diathermy loop, laser vaporization, cone biopsy, chemotherapy agents (5-fluo-

rouracil, bichloroacetic acid), repeat Pap smear in 3 months, then 6 months; annual colposcopy for 2 years.

IV. VAGINA AND VULVA

A. Malignant Neoplasms

1. Vulvar Carcinoma

• **H&P Keys**
Chronic vulvar irritation, labial lesion, history of condyloma; age range 60 to 80 years.

• **Diagnosis**
Toluidine blue stain of vulva. Incisional or excisional biopsy.

• **Disease Severity**
Clinical assessment of tumor size (T), node assessment (N), metastases (M).

• **Concept and Application**
Little known; may be associated with HPV 16 and 18.

• **Management**
Wide local incision for microinvasive carcinoma. Radical vulvectomy for stages I and II; adjunct radiation therapy or exenteration for advanced stages III and IV.

2. Vaginal Cancer

• **H&P Keys**
Vaginal discharge, urinary symptoms; very rare, may be associated with a history of diethylstilbestrol (DES) ingestion in mother (clear cell adenocarcinoma).

• **Diagnosis**
Pap smear, colposcopy, biopsy.

• **Disease Severity**
Staging: Stage I limited to the vaginal mucosa, stage II to subvaginal tissue involvement, stage III to extension to pelvic sidewall, stage IV beyond true pelvis.

• **Concept and Application**
Squamous cell carcinoma: Most commonly in upper vagina, possibly of sexually transmitted disease origin.

- **Management**
  Radiation therapy, surgery, chemotherapy.

B. Candidiasis of the Vulva and Vagina

- **H&P Keys**
  Thick whitish discharge, cottage cheesy, itching, no odor, burning, swelling, dysuria.

- **Diagnosis**
  Microscopic specimen examination including potassium hydroxide (KOH) and saline wet mount; hyphae on wet-mount exam; no odor.

- **Disease Severity**
  Severity of symptoms.

- **Concept and Application**
  Candida albicans.

- **Management**
  Clotrimazole, miconazole, terconazole, avoidance of perfumed soaps and douches, cotton underwear, avoidance of tight-fitting clothing. Recurrent with severe yeast infections, oral agents required.

C. Vaginitis and Vulvovaginitis

- **H&P Keys**

  Trichomoniasis. May be asymptomatic, greenish-gray, frothy, malodorous discharge, strawberry spots on cervix and vagina, vaginal pH between 5 and 6.

  Bacterial Vaginosis. Watery malodorous discharge, pH 5.0 to 5.5.

- **Diagnosis**

  Trichomonas. Saline wet mount and KOH prep show trichomonad organisms intermixed with clumps of white blood cells (WBCs).

  Bacterial Vaginosis. Clue cells (squamous cells with coccobacilli bacteria obscuring the sharp borders and cytoplasm), fishy odor, positive "whiff" test.

- **Disease Severity**
  Severity of symptoms.

- **Concept and Application**

  Trichomonas. *Trichomonas vaginalis.*

  Bacterial Vaginosis. *Gardnerella vaginalis.*

- **Management**

  Trichomonas. Metronidazole.

  Bacterial Vaginosis. Metronidazole, sulfonamide, ampicillin.

D. Prolapse of Vaginal Walls

- **H&P Keys**
  Varies, based on structure or structures involved and the degree of prolapse, pressure, heaviness, urinary (stress) incontinence, frequency, hesitancy, incomplete voiding, recurrent infections, painful or incomplete defecation.

- **Diagnosis**
  Cystourethrocele: Q-tip test; evaluation of urinary function, urodynamic testing, anoscopy, sigmoidoscopy.

- **Disease Severity**
  First degree, second degree, third degree; procidentia (uterus completely outside vagina).

- **Concept and Application**
  Weakening of the pelvic musculature, levator muscles, fascia (urogenital diaphragm), and ligaments (uterosacral and cardinal), associated with aging and multiple childbirth.

- **Management**
  Bladder training, biofeedback, anticholinergic drugs, β-sympathomimetic agonists, antidepressants, estrogen replacement therapy, Kegel exercises, pessaries, surgery: colporrhaphy, obliteration of the rectovaginal space (Moschowitz procedure), vaginal hysterectomy.

V. MENSTRUAL DISORDERS

A. Dysmenorrhea

- **H&P Keys**
  Pelvic pain with menses; nausea, diarrhea, headache, ovulatory menstrual cycles.

- **Diagnosis**
  Ovulatory menses, menstrual pain history.

- **Disease Severity**
  Severity of symptoms.

- **Concept and Application**
  Result of uterine contractions, caused by prostaglandins.

  Primary Dysmenorrhea. No associated pelvic pathology.

  Secondary Dysmenorrhea. Associated with pelvic pathology: endometriosis, fibroids, etc.

- **Management**

  Primary Dysmenorrhea. NSAIDs to inhibit prostaglandin synthetase, combination oral contraception to inhibit ovulation. If no relief, laparoscopy may be needed to rule out pelvic pathology (eg, secondary dysmenorrhea).

B. Premenstrual Syndrome

- **H&P Keys**
  Anxiety, breast tenderness, crying spells, depression, fatigue, irritability, weight gain around the luteal phase of the cycle; prior to the onset of menses, usually relieved with the onset of bleeding.

- **Diagnosis**
  Basal body temperature charts; symptom-recording diaries; daily weight recordings.

- **Disease Severity**
  Severity of symptoms. PMS is classified into 4 major groups by symptoms: Group A—anxiety group; group C—carbohydrate group; group H—edema group; group D—depression group.

- **Concept and Application**
  Unknown.

- **Management**
  No good, double-blind, placebo-controlled, crossover studies have shown any specific treatment to be effective. Treatments include exercise, vitamin B_6, progesterone, diuretics, oral contraceptives.

C. Disorders of Menstruation

Amenorrhea

- **H&P Keys**
  Primary amenorrhea is defined by no menses by age 16. *Secondary* is 3 months or longer of amenorrhea in a normally cycling individual. Possible sexual ambiguity or virilization; possible absence of secondary sex characteristics.

- **Diagnosis**
  History and physical examination, β-hCG, prolactin, follicle-stimulating hormone (FSH), luteinizing hormone (LH), progesterone withdrawal test. If virilization, testosterone, dehydroepiandrosterone (DHEA)-S. *Primary:* Karyotype, FSH, estradiol.

- **Disease Severity**
  Presence or absence of secondary sex characteristics; no breast development by age 15.

- **Concept and Application**

  Primary. Müllerian agenesis, testicular feminization (androgen insensitivity), Turner's syndrome.

  Secondary. Pregnancy, Asherman's syndrome (intrauterine synechiae), polycystic ovarian disease, adrenal hyperplasia, hyperandrogenism, hypothyroidism.

  Hypothalamic. Associated with weight loss, chronic anxiety, excessive exercise, marijuana, tranquilizers, head injury, chronic medical illness, central nervous system (CNS) tumor.

  NOTE. In the absence of all the above, diagnosis is dysfunctional uterine bleeding.

- **Management**

  Primary. If abnormal karyotype, phenotypic female: estrogen replacement therapy for completion of secondary sex characteristics. Müllerian agenesis requires surgery.

Secondary. Requires cyclic menstrual function to prevent endometrial hyperplasia: cyclic combination oral contraceptive therapy or monthly progestin therapy.

Hypothalamic. Hormone replacement therapy to prevent osteoporosis and maintain normal physiologic status.

Asherman's Syndrome. Amenorrhea not responsive to estrogen-progesterone cycle; hysteroscopic surgical intervention.

VI. MENOPAUSE

A. Menopausal Symptoms

- **H&P Keys**
Changes in menstrual cycle regularity, decreased cycle interval, finally cessation of menses; mean age 51.4 years; atrophy of estrogen-dependent tissue (uterus, breasts, vagina), vasomotor symptoms (hot flashes), osteoporosis, urethral changes, increased frequency of cystitis.

- **Diagnosis**
FSH; estradiol; if osteoporosis severe, bone scan. Menopause prior to age 40 means premature ovarian failure; if menopause prior to age 30, check karyotype.

- **Disease Severity**
Serum lipid profile, elevation of FSH, decrease in serum estradiol, severity of symptoms, fractures, overt cardiovascular disease.

- **Concept and Application**
Sequelae of decreased estrogen result of loss of all remaining follicles. Estrone is principle estrogen in menopause, produced from androgen precursor androstenedione.

- **Management**
Estrogen replacement therapy; if uterus present, must add progestin; if uterus absent, progestin equivocal; increase calcium intake; increase exercise; decrease fat intake. Daily Ca requirements 1500 mg/day. Bisphosphonates may be helpful.

VII. BREAST

A. Malignant Neoplasm

- **H&P Keys**
Family history the most important epidemiologic factor, long history of unopposed estrogen exposure, nulliparity, first child born after age 30, early menarche, late menopause; discrete lump, retracted nipple, puckering of breast skin (peau d'orange), axillary lymphadenopathy, nipple bleeding or discharge.

- **Diagnosis**
Mammography, physical examination, fine-needle aspiration, thermography (not as useful).

- **Disease Severity**
Stated by T (tumor size), N (regional lymph nodes), and M (distant metastases). Evaluations done for hormone receptors reflect tumor responsiveness to chemotherapy.

- **Concept and Application**
Unknown, possibly related to hormones; surgical menopause appears to be protective; complex combination of environmental and genetic influences.

- **Management**

Surgery. Lumpectomy, simple mastectomy, radical mastectomy.

Hormonal Therapy. If positive hormone receptors, progestins.

B. Fibroadenoma

This is a benign breast neoplasm.

- **H&P Keys**
Younger women, peak age 21 to 25, single breast mass, smooth, well-circumscribed, firm, mobile, and rubbery nodule. Intraductal papilloma most common cause of unilateral bloody nipple discharge.

- **Diagnosis**
Sonography, fine-needle aspiration, cytologic smear of discharge.

- **Disease Severity**
Severity of symptoms.

- **Concept and Application**
  Unknown.

- **Management**
  Fine-needle aspiration to make diagnosis, subsequent observation.

C. Inflammatory Disease of the Breast

- **H&P Keys**

Mastitis. Usually in nursing women; pain, fever, erythema.

Breast Abscess. Fluctuant lesions, well-localized, difficult to palpate.

Superficial Thrombophlebitis. Acute pain, redness, upper outer quadrant.

- **Diagnosis**
  Diagnosed by history, CBC with differential, fever.

- **Disease Severity**
  Elevation of WBCs, fever, severity of symptoms.

- **Concept and Application**

Mastitis. Penicillin-resistant *Staphylococcus aureus* from the infant's nose and throat; organism enters the breast through fissure or abrasion in nipple.

- **Management**

Mastitis. Dicloxacillin.

Breast Abscess. Incision and drainage.

Superficial Thrombophlebitis. Warm compresses, non-narcotic analgesics.

D. Fibrocystic Disease

- **H&P Keys**
  Cyclic bilateral pain (mastalgia) and breast engorgement, may radiate to shoulders or upper arms, diffuse bilateral nodularity, "lumpy-bumpy" pattern.

- **Diagnosis**
  Mammography, physical examination, history.

- **Disease Severity**
  According to symptoms.

- **Concept and Application**
  May be hormone-related; initially with proliferation of stroma, especially in the upper outer quadrant, followed by adenosis, leading to cyst formation, then marked proliferation of the ducts and alveolar cells.

- **Management**
  Diet therapy, avoidance of caffeine and tobacco; occasionally medical therapy is helpful; progestins, diuretics, danazol, bromocriptine, tamoxifen, regular breast exams.

VIII. OTHER PROBLEMS

A. Infertility, Male and Female

- **H&P Keys**

Primary Infertility. Never having conceived, despite 12 months of having unprotected intercourse.

Secondary Infertility. Previous history of conception but currently unable to establish a subsequent pregnancy despite 12 months of unprotected intercourse.

- **Diagnosis**
  Complete history and physical on both partners, semen analysis, postcoital test, hysterosalpingogram, progesterone level (midluteal phase), endometrial biopsy.

- **Disease Severity**
  Directly proportional to the duration of the infertility; worse prognosis with longer duration of infertility.

- **Concept and Application**
  45% male factor, 45% female factor; 10% unexplained.

Male Factor. Most commonly associated with varicocele (etiology of infertility uncertain).

Female Factor. Blocked tubes, ovulatory dysfunction, peritoneal factor (pelvic adhesive disease, endometriosis, etc).

• **Management**

Ovulatory Dysfunction. Ovulation-induction agents.

Tubal Factor. Surgery, in vitro fertilization (IVF), gamete-intrafallopian transfer (GIFT).

Cervical Mucus Factor. Intrauterine insemination, bicarbonate douching.

Peritoneal Factor. Treat condition as indicated, surgical or medical.

Male Factor. Intrauterine insemination, in vitro fertilization.

B. Pelvic Inflammatory Disease

• **H&P Keys**
  Pain, adnexal tenderness, fever, nausea and vomiting, dysuria, vaginal discharge, adnexal masses.

• **Diagnosis**
  Cervical Gram's stain (for gonorrhea), gram negative intracellular diplococci, culdocentesis, laparoscopy, ultrasound, β-hCG, CBC with differential, sedimentation rate.

• **Disease Severity**
  Depends on extent of signs and symptoms, multiple episodes of pelvic inflammatory disease (PID) may result in infertility, chronic pelvic pain, increased ectopic pregnancy rate.

• **Concept and Application**
  Infection of the upper genital tract, usually polymicrobial consisting of *Neisseria gonorrhoeae, Chlamydia trachomatis,* endogenous aerobes (*Escherichia coli, Proteus,* etc), and endogenous anaerobes (*Bacteroides, Peptostreptococcus*), *Mycoplasma hominis.*

• **Management**
  Individualized treatment; hospitalization may be necessary.

Outpatient. Aqueous procaine penicillin G, ampicillin with probenecid, tetracycline, ceftriaxone.

Acute PID. Doxycycline plus intravenous cefoxitin, clindamycin plus gentamicin, doxy-cycline plus metronidazole. Patient may require surgery with colpotomy or actual laparotomy with total abdominal hysterectomy and bilateral salpingo-oophorectomy.

IX. HEALTH MAINTENANCE

A. Gynecologic Examination and Screening

• **H&P Keys**

Menstrual History. Age at menarche, cycle length, duration of flow; vaginal discharge; pelvic pain; sexual history; history of abnormal cervical cytology; obstetrical history (gravidity and parity).

Review of Systems. Gastrointestinal, urinary, endocrine, metabolic, cardiovascular, hematologic.

Physical Examination. Vital signs, breast exam (sitting and supine), axillary lymph nodes, abdomen, hair distribution.

Pelvic Examination. External genitalia, speculum examination, cervical cytology, evaluation of vaginal contents.

Bimanual Examination. Cervix, uterine fundus, adnexal masses.

Rectal Examination. Rectovaginal exam, uterosacral nodularity, Guaiac test.

• **Diagnosis**
  CBC with differential, gonorrhea culture (GC), chlamydia culture, Pap smear, lipid profile, rubella status (if interested in conception), RPR.

NOTE. General gynecologic exam should be done annually along with counseling about tobacco, alcohol, caffeine, exercise, and diet.

B. General Counseling for Contraception

Types. Natural family planning; spermicides and barrier contraceptives (spermicide, condoms, diaphragms, sponges, cervical caps); intrauterine devices (IUDs) (Progesta-Sert, Paraguard); steroid oral contraceptives: progestin-only contraceptives; injectable and implantable contraceptives (medroxyprogesterone acetate, Levonorgestrel implants (Norplant); postcoital contraception (mifepristone [RU-486], stilbestrol).

Effectiveness (Given as Failure Rate). Oral contraceptives: less than 1% to 2%; Norplant: less than 1% to 3%; IUD: 2% to 4%; diaphragm with spermicide: 10% to 20%); condom: 5% to 15%.

Surveillance of Prescribed Contraceptives. Oral contraceptives: regular pelvic examinations, initial blood pressure check; IUD: string check 6 weeks after insertion.

C. Sterilization

Most frequent method of controlling fertility in United States.

Male Sterilization. Vasectomy failure rate 1%.

Female Sterilization. Postpartum failure rate 1 in 250; interval (between pregnancies) failure rate 1 in 500.

Counseling must include permanent nature of procedure, operative risk, failure rate. Despite careful counseling, approximately 1% of patients undergoing sterilization subsequently request reversal. Most common reason, new sexual partner.

D. Genetic Counseling

Assessment of risk for developing disease and providing information to the patient regarding appropriate screening or diagnostic tests. Chromosome abnormalities account for 50% to 60% of first-trimester spontaneous abortions, 5% of stillbirths, and 2% to 3% of couples experiencing repeated pregnancy loss. Overall, 6% of live-born infants have a chromosomal abnormality.

- **H&P Keys**
  Data forms, questionnaires, pedigree construction, and patient interviews, family medical history, parental exposure to harmful substances.

- **Diagnosis**
  Karyotype, extensive family history, pedigree. If patient pregnant, chorionic villus sampling, amniocentesis.

Indications for Prenatal Cytogenetic Analysis. Advanced maternal age, previous child with chromosome abnormality, parental chromosome abnormality (balance translocation).

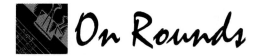

Vaginitis

Candidiasis

- Thick white discharge, itching, swelling, no odor
- Diagnosis by KOH preparation, saline wet mount
- Treatment—chlortrimazole, miconazole, terconazole

Trichomoniasis

- Green-gray discharge, frothy, bad odor, strawberry spots on cervix
- Diagnosis by wet mount (trichomonads)
- Treatment—metronidazole

Bacterial Vaginosis

- Watery discharge, bad odor
- Diagnosis by "clue cells," fishy odor, "whiff" test
- Treatment—metronidazole, sulfonamide, ampicillin

BIBLIOGRAPHY

Beck WW. *Obstetrics and Gynecology.* The National Medical Series for Independent Study. 3rd ed. Philadelphia: Harwal Publishing; 1993.

Beckmann CRB, Ling FW, et al. *Obstetrics and Gynecology for Medical Students.* 2nd ed. Baltimore: Williams & Wilkins; 1995.

Gant NF, Cunningham FG. *Basic Gynecology and Obstetrics.* Norwalk, CT: Appleton & Lange; 1993.

Jacobs AJ, Gast MJ. *Practical Gynecology.* Norwalk, CT: Appleton & Lange; 1994.

12

Obstetrics

R. Douglas Ross, MD

I. UNCOMPLICATED PREGNANCY

A. Health and Health Maintenance

Prenatal Care

- **H&P Keys**
Accurate dating! Presumptive of pregnancy: amenorrhea with nausea and breast tenderness and bluish vaginal mucosa. Probable: positive pregnancy test (β-human chorionic gonadotropin [β-hCG]), uterine change, and outlining of fetus. Diagnostic: fetal imaging (ultrasonography, etc), auscultation of the fetal heart.

- **Diagnosis**
Complete blood count (CBC), urine analysis (UA), urine culture and sensitivity (C&S), blood type and Rh factor, antibody screen, hepatitis B surface antigen, rubella titer, syphilis serology, Pap smear (GC), and chlamydia cultures at first visit. Maternal serum-alpha fetoprotein (MS-AFP) at 15 to 18 weeks and 50-g glucose screening at 24–28 weeks.

- **Disease Severity**
Surveillance for complications: preeclampsia, low birth weight, malnutrition, pre- and post-term delivery, anemia, and common infections, abnormal lab tests.

- **Concept and Application**
Prevention and early treatment of pathologic change.

- **Management**

Initial Care. Accurate dating and diagnosis, education.

Emergency Care. Refer to specific problems.

Continued Care. Routine education, surveillance, and maintenance.

B. Rh Immunoglobulin Prophylaxis

- **H&P Keys**
Rh-negative, Du-negative mother of an Rh-positive or unknown fetus.

- **Diagnosis**
Rh antibody screen to rule out preexisting sensitization.

- **Disease Severity**
Kleihaurer-Betke test to determine quantity of fetal cells in the maternal circulation if large feto-maternal transfusion is suspected.

- **Concept and Application**
Rh immune globulin (RhIg) removes Rh-positive red blood cells (RBCs) prior to maternal sensitization. Three hundred micrograms neutralizes 15 mL of Rh-positive RBCs.

- **Management**

Initial Care. Give at 28 weeks; invasive fetal diagnostic procedures, termination, or delivery at any gestation may result in feto-maternal transfusion. Administer to all with indications within 72 hours of exposure.

Emergency Care. Same.

Continued Care. Same.

C. Prenatal Diagnosis

- **H&P Keys**
Exposure to teratogens, pedigree, accurate pregnancy dating, exam looking for expression of genotype.

- **Diagnosis**
Specific for condition evaluated: biochemical screening tests: MS-AFP, unconjugated estriol, and β-subunit hCG abnormal patterns are associated with aneuploidy. Ultrasound screening: major structural anomalies, thickened nuchal fold, growth lag, and abnormal amniotic fluid volume.

- **Disease Severity**
Specific for condition evaluated.

- **Concept and Application**
Hundreds of biochemical, chromosomal, and genetic disorders can be diagnosed by condition-specific tests including: ultrasonography, identified structural change, karotyping, DNA analysis technologies, fetal tissue enzyme activity, and metabolic product accumulation in fetal cells obtained by chorionic villous sampling (CVS), amniocentesis, percutaneous umbilical blood sampling, or fetal biopsy.

- **Management**
Specific for the condition evaluated. Nondirective counseling is used.

D. Teratology

- **H&P Keys**
Exposure of potential teratogens and gestational age of fetus. Examination of fetus is limited to high-resolution ultrasonography.

- **Diagnosis**
Specific for the condition evaluated.

- **Disease Severity**
Specific for the condition evaluated.

- **Concept and Application**
Three percent of all pregnancies have a major congenital anomaly, and another 3% will have a minor one. There are very *few known teratogens:* viruses (rubella), parasites (toxoplasmosis), bacteria (syphilis), heavy metals (mercury), cancer chemotherapeutics (folic acid antagonists), antiepileptics (most), maternal conditions (phenylketonuria [PKU]), anticoagulants (warfarin), antibiotics (tetracycline), as well as ethanol and radiation.

- **Management**
Specific to the exposure and evaluation.

E. Immediate Care of the Newborn

- **H&P Keys**
Prenatal history, labor history. Assess the dry baby for neonatal depression, anomalies, respirations, heart rate, and meconium while under the warmer.

- **Diagnosis**
Heel stick blood sugar if mother is diabetic.

- **Disease Severity**
Apnea, heart rate < 100, central cyanosis.

- **Concept and Application**
Resuscitation based on Apgar score alone results in a 45-second delay. A chilled baby requires more oxygen.

- **Management**
Initial care: Intubate and aspirate if meconium stained; dry and stimulate; apneic or heart rate <100: bag and mask; <60: closed chest cardiac massage.

F. Postpartum Care of the Mother

- **H&P Keys**
Childbirth in the preceding 6 weeks. Lochia changes from red to brown to serous over first 2 weeks. Episiotomy heals rapidly. Uterus is in pelvis at 2 weeks and normal size at 6 weeks.

- **Diagnosis**
Pap smear at postpartum visit.

- **Disease Severity**
Infection: endomyometritis (mixed aerobic and anaerobic flora), mastitis (*Staphylococcus aureus*), breast abscess. Depression: <50% will have a week of "the blues," 10% will be depressed, and 0.05% suicidal. See section on postpartum hemorrhage and lactation.

- **Concept and Application**
Fifty percent of nonlactating women ovulate between 28 and 90 days postpartum. Cardiac output normalizes in several hours. Glomerular filtration rate (GFR) is down to normal in a few weeks.

- **Management**

  Initial Care. Evaluation, support, and problem-specific therapy. Rh immune globulin if indicated.

  Emergency Care. Problem-specific.

G. Lactation

- **H&P Keys**
  Absence of pain, erythema, localized induration, abscess, nipple fissures or cracks. Prefeeding engorgement and discomfort is common in the first couple weeks. Limit medications to those necessary and not contraindicated.

- **Diagnosis**
  None.

- **Disease Severity**
  Same as history and physical examination.

- **Concept and Application**
  Human breast milk best nutrition and immunologic stimulation for the baby. Prolactin is essential. Suckling stimulates the neurohypophysis to release oxytocin, which contracts the breast's myoepithelial cells, allowing milk "let-down." Less than 1% of most medications is found in breast milk. Nipple fissures and cracks allow ingress of bacteria, causing cellulitis to abscess.

- **Management**

  Initial Care. Encourage relaxation and hydration to facilitate breast feeding.

  Emergency Care. Treat mastitis with antibiotics effective against *S. aureus,* and continue breast feeding. Abscess may require surgical drainage.

H. Normal Labor and Delivery

- **H&P Keys**
  Progressive uterine contractions associated with cervical change; progressively intense, about every 3 minutes and lasting 60 seconds.

- **Diagnosis**
  Normal latent phase lasts a maximum of 20 hours in the nulligravida and 14 hours in the multipara. Normal active phase dilatation is at least 1.2 cm/h in the nulligravida and 1.5 cm/h in the multipara.

- **Disease Severity**
  Failure of acceptable progress.

- **Concept and Application**
  Increased prostaglandins cause an increased number of myometrial gap junctions that allow cells to communicate and rhythmically depolarize in labor.

- **Management**

  Initial Care. Make diagnosis by serial examinations and initiate management.

  Continued Care. When cephalopelvic disproportion is diagnosed, a cesarean section is used for delivery. Hypotonic dysfunction is treated with oxytocin augmentation.

II. COMPLICATED PREGNANCY

A. Adolescent Pregnancy

- **H&P Keys**
  Nineteen years old and younger, sexually transmitted disease surveillance, nutritional deficiency, substance abuse, sexual abuse.

- **Diagnosis**
  Same for pregnancy; assist with social support network.

- **Disease Severity**
  Disease-specific.

- **Concept and Application**
  Seventeen percent have *Chlamydia trachomatis,* and 3% *Neisseria gonorrhoeae* per year; increased need for calcium (1600 mg/d) and calories (2700 c/d); 89% of 10th graders have alcohol exposure, and 8% have cocaine, up to 38% have had nonvoluntary sexual activity.

- **Diagnosis**
Clinical diagnosis, CBC, platelet count, fibrin split products, fibrinogen and prothrombin time (PT) and partial thromboplastin time (PTT) for disseminated intravascular coagulation (DIC). Ultrasonography is of limited value.

- **Disease Severity**
Shock out of proportion to the observed blood loss, especially if concealed hemorrhage. Fetal demise if >50% abruption.

- **Concept and Application**
Bleeding into the decidua basalis. Couvelaire uterus is caused by blood extravasating into the myometrium (ecchymosis). Abruptio may be caused by hypertension, cocaine, smoking, uterine decompression, and trauma.

- **Management**

Initial and Emergency Care. Hemodynamic stabilization, observation for complications, and delivery of the mature fetus; vaginal delivery is attempted if the patient is stable hemodynamically and the baby's monitoring is reassuring; immature fetus may be expectantly managed in mild abruptions.

H. Preeclampsia

- **H&P Keys**
Hypertension (>140/90 mm Hg and proteinuria (>300 mg/24 h) after 20 weeks.

- **Diagnosis**
Careful blood pressure (BP) measurement, 24-hour urine for protein and creatinine clearance, CBC with platelets, and uric acid. Aspartate aminotransferase (AST, formerly SGOT), bilirubin, and lactate dehydrogenase (LDH) may be elevated. Fetal growth and well-being assessment.

- **Disease Severity**
Mild preeclampsia is without symptoms and signs of severe preeclampsia. Severe preeclampsia if BP >160/110 mm Hg, >5 g of proteinuria in 24 hours, visual disturbances, headache, pulmonary edema, cyanosis, epigastric pain, right upper quadrant pain, liver dysfunction, oliguria, thrombocytopenia, intrauterine growth restriction or oligohydramnios.

- **Concept and Application**
Diffuse multiorgan vasospastic disease starting months before diagnosis, characterized by decreased sensitivity to angiotensin II and increased thromboxane: prostacyclin ratio. Delivery is the only specific therapy.

- **Management**

Initial Care. Gestational age, fetal, and maternal assessment.

Term. Delivery.

Preterm. Weighing the risks and benefits of expectant management for the baby and the mother. Bed rest is the mainstay of expectant care.

Emergency Care. Magnesium sulfate (4- to 6-g load and 2 g/h) is used for seizure prophylaxis. Monitoring blood pressure, respiration, reflexes, and urinary output. Diastolic blood pressures over 110 mm Hg are treated with hydralazine (5-mg boluses).

I. Eclampsia

- **H&P Keys**
Preeclampsia with tonic-clonic seizures of no other etiology.

- **Diagnosis**
Same as preeclampsia.

- **Disease Severity**
Same as preeclampsia.

- **Concept and Application**
Same as preeclampsia.

- **Management**

Initial and Emergency Care. Same as preeclampsia. Treatment of seizures with magnesium sulfate.

J. Premature Labor

- **H&P Keys**

  Uterine contractions with cervical change <u>prior to 37 weeks</u>. Symptoms: cramps, backache, pressure, and uterine contractions.

- **Diagnosis**

  Monitor, rule out rupture of membranes, check for cervical change, culture vagina for group B *Streptococcus*, evaluate for urinary tract infection, confirm dating if indicated.

- **Disease Severity**

  No tocolysis if: rupture of membranes, advanced cervical dilatation (5+ cm), fetal distress, fetal anomalies, mature fetus, in utero infection, and conditions made worse by tocolysis.

- **Concept and Application**

  Preterm labor associated with: premature rupture of membranes (PROM), incompetent cervix, infection, uterine overdistention, abnormal placentation, dehydration, and idiopathic causes. Prostaglandin activation is a common final pathway. β-Sympathomimetics (ritodrine and terbutaline), magnesium sulfate, prostaglandin synthetase inhibitors (indomethacin), and calcium channel blockers (nifedipine) have been used to treat preterm labor (PTL). All tocolytics are associated with serious complications.

- **Management**

  Emergency Care. Monitoring, hydrating, and evaluation of the patient; administration of tocolytic (usually SQ terbutaline 0.25 mg × 6 doses or incremental increases from IV 0.050 mg/min or IV MgSO4 6-g load and 2 to 3 g/h) and monitoring for complications (pulmonary edema, etc). Penicillin for group B *Streptococcus* prophylaxis. Betamethasone IM 12 mg × two doses to hasten pulmonary maturity and decrease hemorrhagic disorders and necrotizing enterocolitis.

  Continued Care. Outpatient on oral β-sympathomimetics.

K. Infections of the Genitourinary Tract

- **H&P Keys**

  Asymptomatic bacturia (>100 000 colony-forming units per milliliter (CFU) progresses to pyelonephritis in 1% to 3% of gravidas. Increased nocturia, urgency, frequency, dysuria are common symptoms. Pyelonephritis is associated with a significantly elevated temperature, flank pain, costovertebral angle (CVA) tenderness.

- **Diagnosis**

  Urinalysis positive for leukocyte esterase, nitrate, white blood cells (WBCs), RBCs. 10 000 CFU/mL is significant in the symptomatic patient.

- **Disease Severity**

  Pyelonephritis: evaluate for intrauterine infection, sepsis in 2% of patients, rarely associated with septic shock and adult respiratory distress syndrome (ARDS).

- **Concept and Application**

  Urinary stasis (decreased tone, mechanical ureteral or bladder compression) and glucosuria facilitate bacterial (*Escherichia coli*) overgrowth; 8% have asymptomatic bacturia.

- **Management**

  Initial Care

  Lower Tract. Antibiotic therapy by local sensitivities (usually 7 to 10 days of ampicillin or nitrofurantoin).

  Pyelonephritis. IV, then oral therapy. Monitoring for preterm labor.

  Continued Care. Reculturing monthly.

L. Hepatitis Complicating Pregnancy

- **H&P Keys**

  Malaise, jaundice 15 to 50 days following exposure to infected blood or body secretions; high-risk groups (patients and partners) include IV drug users, multiple sexual partners, and health care workers.

- **Diagnosis**
  Bilirubin, AST (SGOT), alaninine amino-transferase (ALT, formerly SGPT), hepatitis B surface antigen (HBsAg), antibody to hepatitis B core antigen (HBcAb), antibody to hepatitis Be antigen (HBeAb), and hepatitis Be antigen (HBeAg).

- **Disease Severity**
  Fewer than 10% develop chronic infection. Hepatic failure, coma, and death. Vertical transmission is highest (80%) in HBeAg-positive.

- **Concept and Application**
  Major cause of jaundice in pregnancy, 80% HBV, 10% HAV, and 10% HCV, HDV, and HEV. Well-nourished patients usually tolerate the disease.

- **Management**

  Initial Care. Uninfected at-risk pregnant patient may be vaccinated. Supportive and serial liver function evaluation.

  Emergency Care. Treatment of newborn with hepatitis B immune globulin and hepatitis B vaccine.

M. Incompetent Cervix

- **H&P Keys**
  Painless preterm (second trimester) effacement and dilatation of the cervix. Patient complains of several days of vaginal or pelvic pressure, watery-to-pink vaginal discharge, or backache prior to rupture of the membranes.

- **Diagnosis**
  Internal os dilated >1 cm or painless passage of a #8 Hegar dilator.

- **Disease Severity**
  Associated with deep lacerations or conizations and cervical amputations.

- **Concept and Application**
  Cervix is not able to maintain closure pressure against the expanding gestation.

- **Management**

  Initial Care. Prophylactic transvaginal cerclage at 12 to 16 weeks.

  Emergency Care. An emergency cerclage may be placed after PTL is ruled out.

  Continued Care. Physical and coital activities may be restricted.

N. Central Nervous System Malformation in the Fetus and Neural-Tube Defect

- **H&P Keys**
  Fifteen percent have a positive family history; multifactorial inheritance; 1% recurrence risk. Preconceptional poor glycemic control increases risk in diabetics. Presents in the United States as an incidental ultrasonographic finding and during the evaluation of an elevated MS-AFP.

- **Diagnosis**
  Elevated MS-AFP, amniotic fluid (AF)-AFP, elevated AF acetylcholinesterase. Directed scan.

- **Disease Severity**
  Anencephaly (failure of development of the forebrain) occurs in 50% of neural-tube defects (NTDs). Spina bifida or meningomyelocele may occur at any level.

- **Concept and Application**
  Failure of closure of at least a portion of the neural tube prior to the 28th day postconception. Prepregnancy folic acid decreases the risk.

- **Management**

  Initial Care. Diagnosis, nondirective genetic counseling and option counseling.

  Emergency Care. Delivery by cesarean section.

  Continued Care. If pregnancy is maintained, monitoring for hydrocephalus.

O. Trisomy

- **H&P Keys**

  Advanced maternal age, previous history, balanced translocation, low MS-AFP.

- **Diagnosis**

  Fetal sampling via CVS, amniocentesis, or percutaneous umbilical blood sample (PUBS) is definitive.

- **Disease Severity**

  Babies with a mosaicism may not fully express the typical phenotype.

- **Concept and Application**

  Aneuploidy results from nondisjunction in the first meiotic division or from an unbalanced translocation. Trisomy 21 is most common, followed by trisomy 18 and trisomy 13.

- **Management**

  Initial Care. Nondirective counseling, support of the patient's decision within the legal and ethical framework.

P. Rh Incompatibility or Isoimmunization

- **H&P Keys**

  Inadequate or no RhIg after Rh-positive RBC exposure in Rh-negative woman; Kell-negative recipient of Kell-positive transfusion.

- **Diagnosis**

  Serial maternal antibody titering; amniocentesis or PUBS once greater than the critical titer.

- **Disease Severity**

  Delta OD450 (a measure of bilirubin in amniotic fluid) in zone III is associated with imminent fetal death from erythroblastosis fetalis. PUBS is used for both diagnosis (hemoglobin and hematocrit and antigen determination) and treatment (transfusion).

- **Concept and Application**

  Maternal hemolytic IgG antibody formation to fetal red cell antigens (Rh, Kell, Duffy, Kidd, etc), extramedullary hematopoiesis in the fetal liver, decreased oncotic protein production and edema, anasarca (erythroblastosis fetalis). Rh-negative woman has a 15% risk of sensitization in the first exposed Rh-positive, ABO-compatible pregnancy.

- **Management**

  Initial Care. Serial measurement of the indirect Coombs' and antibody titering. Amniocentesis or PUBS (diagnostic and therapeutic) is performed once critical titer is reached.

  Emergency Care. PUBS or delivery.

  Continued Care. Serial studies and therapy are determined by previous results.

Q. Multiple Gestation

- **H&P Keys**

  High index of suspicion when size greater than dates, positive family history, ovulation induction; 1 of 80 black women, 1 of 100 white women.

- **Diagnosis**

  Ultrasonogram, elevated MS-AFP.

- **Disease Severity**

  Serial ultrasonographic evaluation for growth and polyhydramnios.

- **Concept and Application**

  Thirty percent are monozygotic; 70% of monozygotic are monochorionic diamniotic (division day 3 to 8). Risks: 15% perinatal mortality, preterm labor, intrauterine growth retardation, malformations, preeclampsia, anemia, abruption, polyhydramnios.

- **Management**

  Initial Care. Increased calories and iron, preterm labor education, a management program of maternal and fetal surveillance.

  Emergency Care. Treatment of specific complications.

  Continued Care. Following through on the management plan.

R. Gestational Trophoblastic Disease

- **H&P Keys**
  Size–date discrepancy (usually greater size than norm); hyperemesis gravidarum; preeclampsia before 20 weeks; hyperthyroidism, and bleeding.

- **Diagnosis**
  β-hCG, ultrasonography, and histology.

- **Disease Severity**
  Malignant gestational trophoblastic disease (GTD) with a poor prognosis has pretreatment β-hCG >40 000 mIU/mL, more than 4 months' duration, brain or liver metastases, failed chemotherapy, or antecedent term pregnancy. Complete moles increase risk of serious complications.

- **Concept and Application**
  Incidence is 1/1000 pregnancies. Complete moles are paternal in origin (46, XX > 46, XY) and are histologically distinct (absence of fetus and blood vessels, diffuse villous edema, and variable trophoblastic proliferation). Partial moles may coexist with a normal pregnancy and are 69, XXX or XXY.

- **Management**

Initial Care. After diagnosis, chest roentgenogram and labs. Suction curettage.

Continued Care. Serial β-hCG every 1 to 2 weeks until normal, then every month for the remainder of a year; serial pelvic exams; contraception.

S. Maternal Mortality

- **H&P Keys**
  Self-evident.

- **Diagnosis**
  Self-evident.

- **Disease Severity**
  Self-evident.

- **Concept and Application**
  Causes: embolism (24%), hypertensive disease (20%), hemorrhage (16%), and infection (10%) are the most common. Rates have been declining since the mid-1970s.

- **Management**
  Initial care: Prevention.

T. Depression

- **H&P Keys**
  Mean age 40 years; disturbance of mood, intense anguish, and loss of a sense of control; predisposing factors include: victim of abuse, childhood loss of a parent, genetic predisposition, deprivation, and lifestyle stress.

- **Diagnosis**
  High index of suspicion: a high score on the Beck Depression Inventory.

- **Disease Severity**
  Suicide threats and attempts.

- **Concept and Application**
  Most common psychiatric disorder in women.

- **Management**

Initial Care. Mild to moderate depression is treated with psychotherapy. Severe, chronic, recurrent depression is treated with antidepressants and psychotherapy.

Emergency. Hospitalization and psychotherapy for suicidal ideation.

U. Preterm Premature Rupture of Membranes

- **H&P Keys**
  Leakage of amniotic fluid (AF) from vagina prior to term.

- **Diagnosis**
  Demonstration of ferning and Nitrazine-positive fluid. Culture the cervix for gonorrhea, group B *Streptococcus* and *Chlamydia trachomatis*. Quantitative AF volume. Vaginal pool specimen for maturity studies.

- **Disease Severity**
  Chorioamnionitis or fetal distress.

- **Concept and Application**
  Rupture allows bacteria access to the fetus. If less than 24 weeks, risks of pulmonary hypoplasia, contractures, and limb anomalies increase.

• **Management**

Initial Care. Observation for symptoms and signs of infection (uterine tenderness or irritability, fever, maternal or fetal tachycardia, leukocytosis, purulent fluid).

Emergency Care. Delivery if mature lungs or fetal or maternal indications.

Continued Care. Initial care plus periodic fetal assessment.

V. Hyperemesis Gravidarum

• **H&P Keys**
Intractable morning sickness associated with significant weight loss, dehydration, electrolyte imbalance, or ketonemia.

• **Diagnosis**
Rule out other causes: gastroesophageal reflux, pancreatitis, hepatobiliary disease, etc.

• **Disease Severity**
Protracted negative protein balance and ketonemia adversely affect fetal growth.

• **Concept and Application**
Etiology unknown.

• **Management**

Initial Care. Frequent small, bland meals with liquids at separate intervals, antiemetics.

Emergency Care. Intravenous hydration. Hyperalimentation is used rarely.

W. Abnormalities of Labor, Dystocia

• **H&P Keys**
Patient in labor with abnormal progress based on graphic analysis.

• **Diagnosis**
Graphic analysis of labor, assessment of pelvis and fetal attitude, position, and presentation.

• **Disease Severity**
Prolonged latent phase: no progress from latent to active phase (nulligravidas >20 hours, multiparas >40 hours. Protracted active phase dilatation: nulligravidas <1.2 cm/h, multiparas <1.5 cm/h. Arrest of dilatation: no change in 2 hours. Arrest of descent: no descent in >1 hour.

• **Concept and Application**
Reason for over one quarter of all cesarean sections. Uterine contractions may be ineffective when associated with mechanical factors.

• **Management**
Initial and continuing care: Prolonged latent phase, therapeutic rest or augmentation. Protracted dilatation, augmentation if no disproportion. Arrest of dilatation, same. Arrest of descent, same or obstetric forceps if indicated.

X. Postpartum Hemorrhage

• **H&P Keys**

Uterine Atony. Predisposing factors: prolonged labor, precipitous labor, infection, uterine overdistention, multiparity, fibroids, oxytocin augmentation, and magnesium sulfate.

Genital Tract Laceration. Predisposing factors: instrumented vaginal delivery, precipitous delivery, macrosomic infant, previous genital tract laceration, and in utero manipulation.

Retained Placental Fragments. From incomplete removal of normal placenta, retained accessory lobe, or partial placenta accreta.

• **Diagnosis**
Vital signs, CBC, blood product availability, and search for the source of the bleeding.

• **Disease Severity**
Normal blood loss: singleton, vaginal, 500 mL; twin, vaginal, 1000 mL; cesarean section, 1000 mL. Normal parturient can lose 900 mL without any symptoms; 1500 mL is associated with tachycardia, narrowed pulse pressure, positive blanch test; 2000 mL is associated with hypotension; 2400 mL is associated with profound hypotension and vasoconstriction.

• **Concept and Application**
Uterine blood flow is 500 to 600 mL/min. Interference with the normal mechanisms of hemostasis may result in significant blood loss.

- **Management**

Emergency Care. Uterine massage, oxytocin, methylergonine maleate (Methergine) or 15-methylprostaglandin $F_{2\alpha}$; transfusion if hemodynamically unstable; determination of etiology of the hemorrhage; definitive treatment. Hysterectomy is last resort.

Y. Postpartum Sepsis

- **H&P Keys**
Predisposing factors: cesarean section, prolonged rupture of membranes, chorioamnionitis, prolonged labor, multiple pelvic exams, internal monitors, obesity, and anemia. Febrile morbidity: temperature of >100.4°F on two occasions at least 6 hours apart 24 hours postpartum.

- **Diagnosis**
Endomyometritis presents with uterine tenderness and fever; cultures are not reliable. Wound infection presents with fever, pain, tenderness, erythema, and swelling; wound cultures are helpful. Pyelonephritis, pneumonia, and atelectasis should be ruled out.

- **Disease Severity**
Evaluate for septic pelvic thrombophlebitis, which presents as persistent fever and tachycardia after presumed effective antibiotic treatment; responds to the addition of heparin.

- **Concept and Application**
Uncontrolled sepsis results in physiologic instability, organ failure, and death.

- **Management**

Initial Care. Endomyometritis: broad-spectrum antibiotics until afebrile for 24 hours and patient is asymptomatic.

Wound Infection. Probe for fascial integrity; drainage and broad-spectrum antibiotics until resolved.

Emergency Care. Same.

Z. Obstetric Forceps and Vacuum Extractor

- **H&P Keys**
Adequate anesthesia, empty bladder (if not outlet), full cervical dilatation, known fetal attitude, position, and station.

- **Diagnosis**
Clinical assessment of fetal size and pelvis.

- **Disease Severity**
Mid: Station engaged but <-2. Low: Station is at least $+2$ but not on the pelvic floor, and rotations of >45 degrees. Outlet: Fetal head is at or on the perineum and the rotation is <45 degrees.

- **Concept and Application**
Shortening of the second stage for a variety of fetal and maternal reasons.

- **Management**
After prerequisites are met, apply instruments, check application, and apply traction with contractions. Inspect genital tract for injury after delivery.

AA. Diabetes, Gestational

- **H&P Keys**
Universal screening or screen if risk factors are present (prior history, obesity, macrosomia, hydramnios, family history, excessive weight gain).

- **Diagnosis**
50-g glucola screen >140 mg/dL, 3-hour oral glucose tolerance test (GTT); abnormal if any 2 values exceed fasting blood sugar (FBS) >105, >190 at 1 hour, >165 at 2 hours, or >145 at 3 hours.

- **Disease Severity**
Start on diet of 30 to 35 kcal/kg of ideal body weight (IBW). If FBS is >105 or 2-hour postprandial levels are >120, evaluate for insulin. Fifteen percent of patients progress to insulin. Monitor for preeclampsia, bacterial infection, macrosomia, and hydramnios.

- **Concept and Application**
Pregnancy is diabetogenic. Prevalence 2%. hPlacental Lactogen induces peripheral insulin resistance.

• **Management**

Initial. Initiate diet, monitor BS, culture urine monthly, fetal well-being.

Continued. As in initial management, normalize blood sugar in labor. Test for diabetes at 6 weeks postpartum.

BB. Diabetes, Overt

• **H&P Keys**

PRISCILLA WHITE CLASSIFICATION

Class	Age at Onset		Duration	Vascular Disease	Therapy
A	Any		Any	None	Diet
B	Over 20	OR	Under 10	None	Insulin
C	10–19	OR	10–19	None	Insulin
D	Before 10	OR	Over 20	Benign Retinopathy	Insulin
F	Any		Any	Nephropathy	Insulin
R	Any		Any	Proliferative Retinopathy	Insulin
H	Any		Any	Heart disease	Insulin

• **Diagnosis**
Hemoglobin A1c, home glucose monitoring, ultrasound, 24-hour urine for protein and creatinine clearance, blood pressure, MS-AFP.

• **Disease Severity**
Elevated hemoglobin A1c increases risk of congenital anomalies (neural tube defect [NTD] and heart), maternal and fetal risks increase with duration of disease, presence of small-vessel disease (retino-pathy, nephropathy, and intrauterine growth retardation [IUGR]).

• **Concept and Application**
Impaired insulin secretion and insulin resistance. Prone to ketoacidosis at lower blood sugar levels.

• **Management**
Education, diet, exercise, normalization of blood sugar (FBS >70 or <105, 2-hour postprandial <120). Monitor for complications. Tight control of blood sugar in labor.

CC. Asthma

• **H&P Keys**
Acute dyspnea, wheezing, cough. One-third become better, one-third stay the same, one-third experience a worsening of the condition in pregnancy. Patients usually tolerate labor well.

• **Diagnosis**
Peak flow monitoring.

• **Disease Severity**
Accessory muscle usage, respiratory rate, pulse oximetry, arterial blood gases (ABGs).

• **Concept and Application**
Bronchospasm in response to allergens, antigens or irritants, infection.

• **Management**

Acute. Beta agonist inhalers, parenteral glucocorticoids.

Continuing. Beta agonists, inhaled glucocorticoids, cromolyn. Peak flow monitoring.

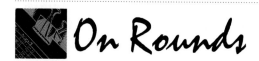 On Rounds

Problems in Obstetrics

Preeclampsia

- Hypertension and proteinuria or edema after 20 weeks
- Diagnosis by blood pressure measurement, 24 hour urine for protein
- Treatment includes bed rest (if pre-term) and delivery (if term). Magnesium sulfate to prevent seizures

Eclampsia

- Preeclampsia with tonic-clonic seizures
- Diagnosis as in preeclampsia
- Treatment as in preeclampsia

Abruptio Placenta

- Vaginal bleeding, tender uterus, shock
- Clinical diagnosis, ultrasound no help
- Treatment includes hemodynamic stabilization and delivery (with mature fetus)

Placenta Previa

- Painless third trimester vaginal bleeding, often at night
- Diagnosis by ultrasound
- Treatment for asymptomatic cases:
  - –education
  - –hematinics
  - –serial ultrasounds
  - –coital restriction in 3rd trimester

  urgent cases: Hemodynamic stabilization

BIBLIOGRAPHY

Gabbe SG. Obstetrics: *Normal and Problem Pregnancies.* 2nd ed. New York: Churchill Livingstone; 1993.

Martin DH. Sexually Transmitted Diseases. *The Med Clin North Am.* Philadelphia: WB Saunders Co; 1990.

Niswander KR. *Manual of Obstetrics, Diagnosis and Therapy.* 4th ed. Boston: Little, Brown & Co; 1991.

Pernoll ML. *Current Obstetric and Gynecologic Diagnosis and Treatment.* 7th ed. Norwalk, CT: Appleton & Lange; 1991.

Pritchard JA. *Williams Obstetrics.* 19th ed. Norwalk, CT: Appleton & Lange; 1993.

Sweet RL. *Infectious Disease of the Female Genital Tract.* 2nd ed. Baltimore: Williams & Wilkins; 1990.

13

Ophthalmology

Andrea M. Saxon, MD, Guy H. Chan, MD, and Richard Rubin, MD

I. CONJUNCTIVITIS

Hyperemia of conjunctival blood vessels. Types: allergic, bacterial, viral; common, often not serious.

- **H&P Keys**

Red eye, usually without blurred vision, pain, photophobia, or colored halos. Exudation is more severe in bacterial, moderate in viral, and least in allergic. Itching is pronounced in allergic. Ciliary flush is absent. Conjunctival injection is prominent in bacterial, moderate in viral, and least in allergic. Corneal disturbance may be present in viral, absent in bacterial and allergic. Pupil, anterior chamber depth, and intraocular pressure are normal. Preauricular lymph node may be present in viral but absent in bacterial and allergic (Tables 13–1, 13–2).

- **Diagnosis**

Correct diagnosis for cause of red eye determines effectiveness of treatment and reduces complications. Aside from conjunctivitis, other causes of red eye must be ruled out. Differentiate from acute glaucoma, acute iridocyclitis, and keratitis corneal lesions (Tables 13–3, 13–4).

TABLE 13–2. SIGNS OF CONJUNCTIVITIS

Signs	Bacterial	Viral	Allergic
Conjunctival injection	+++	++	+
Discharge	+++	++	+
Preauricular lymph node	0	+	0
Corneal opacification	0	0/+	0
Corneal epithelial disruption	0	0/+	0
Ciliary flush	0	0	0
Pupil	N	N	N
Anterior chamber depth	N	N	N
Intraocular pressure	N	N	N

N, normal; +, present; 0, absent.

Most cases are managed without laboratory studies. Smear of exudates. Conjunctival scrapings for culture and sensitivities studies.

1. Allergic conjunctivitis: Eosinophils.
2. Bacterial conjunctivitis: Polymorphonuclear cells and bacteria.
3. Viral conjunctivitis: Lymphocytes.

- **Disease Severity**

Assess vision, amount of pain, and sensitivity to light. Rule out red eye caused by acute glaucoma, corneal lesions, or iridocyclitis.

TABLE 13–1. SYMPTOMS OF CONJUNCTIVITIS

Symptoms	Bacterial	Viral	Allergic
Exudation	+++	++	+
Itching	0	0	++
Blurred vision	0	0	0
Colored halos	0	0	0
Pain	0	0	0
Photophobia	0	0	0

+++, severe; ++, moderate; +, present; 0, absent.

TABLE 13–3. SYMPTOMS OF RED EYE

Symptoms	Acute Conjunctivitis	Acute Iritis	Acute Glaucoma	Corneal Lesions
Exudation	+/+++	0	0	0/+++
Itching	0/++	0	0	0
Blurred vision	0	+/++	+++	+++
Colored halos	0	0	++	0
Pain	0	++	++/+++	++
Photophobia	0	+++	+	+++

+++, severe; ++, moderate; +, present; 0, absent.

TABLE 13–4. SIGNS OF RED EYE

Signs	Acute Conjunctivitis	Acute Iritis	Acute Glaucoma	Corneal Lesions
Conjunctival injection	+/+++	++	++	++
Discharge	+/+++	0	0	0/+
Preauricular lymph node	0/+	0	0	0
Corneal opacification	0/+	0	+++	0/+++
Corneal epithelial disruption	0/+	0	0	+/+++
Ciliary flush	0	++	+	+++
Pupil	N	Mid-dilated irregular	Small/irregular	N/small
Anterior chamber depth	N	N	Shallow	N
Intraocular pressure	N	Low	High	N

+, present; ++, moderate; +++, severe; N, normal; 0, absent.

Allergic Conjunctivitis. Itching, watery discharge, history of allergies, edematous lids, and no preauricular nodes.

Bacterial Conjunctivitis. Severe purulent discharge; may have subconjunctival hemorrhage and chemosis. Eyelid sticking, worse in the morning. Red eye subconjunctival hemorrhage. Gram's stain for causative bacteria.

Viral Conjunctivitis. History of recent upper respiratory tract infection or contact with someone with a red eye. Usually gets worse the first few days after onset and may last for 2 to 3 weeks. Watery or mucous discharge, red and edematous eyelids. May have subconjunctival hemorrhages and corneal irritations. Palpable preauricular lymph nodes suggests viral cause.

• **Concept and Application**
  Viral conjunctivitis associates with systemic problems, upper respiratory infection and fever, pharyngoconjunctival fever, adenovirus type 3 or type 7. Allergic conjunctivitis associates with seasonal rhinitis of hay fever, erythema multiforme, serious systemic disorders with ocular involvement, Stevens-Johnson syndrome, allergic reaction to medication (Table 13–5).

• **Management**
  (See Table 13–6.)

Allergic Conjunctivitis

1. Detection and removal of source of irritants.

2. Cold compress for comfort during waking hours.
3. Topical steroids to the affected eyes four times a day or as often as needed for comfort. Improvement should be noted immediately or within 2 to 3 days.
4. Persistent irritation requires consultation and further investigation.

Bacterial Conjunctivitis

1. Appropriate topical antibiotic drops during the waking hours of the day and ointment at night.
2. Washing away exudates and warm soaks of eyes for comfort.
3. Avoidance of topical steroids.

Viral Conjunctivitis. Usually subsides after its natural course. It is very contagious about 2 weeks after onset. Patients with red and weep-

TABLE 13–5. ASSOCIATED SYSTEMIC DISEASES IN CONJUNCTIVITIS

Systemic Diseases	Bacterial Conjunctivitis	Viral Conjunctivitis	Allergic Conjunctivitis
Pharyngoconjunctival fever (adenovirus type 3, type 7)	0	+	0
Seasonal rhinitis of hay fever	0	0	+
Erythema multiforme (Stevens-Johnson syndrome)	0	0	+

+, present; 0, absent.

TABLE 13–6. MANAGEMENT OF CONJUNCTIVITIS

	Bacterial Conjunctivitis	Viral Conjunctivitis	Allergic Conjunctivitis
Topical antibiotics	Sulfa, neomycin, polymixin B, erythromycin	0	0
Topical steriods	0	0	+++
Antihistamines (oral)	0	0	±
Isolation precaution	0	++	0
Remove irritants	+	++	+++

+, of some benefit; ++, moderate benefit; +++, treatment of choice; ±, may or may not help; 0, no benefit.

ing eyes should avoid spreading to other people.

1. Isolation from group gatherings.
2. Artificial tears and cold compresses as often as needed for comfort.

II. DISORDERS OF THE EYELIDS

A. Blepharitis

Chronic bilateral inflammation of the lid margins.

- **H&P Keys**
  Itching, irritation, burning of lid margins, red rims, scales of lashes, ulcerated areas along lid margins.

- **Diagnosis**
  Lid margin ulceration or no ulceration, scales oily or dry.

- **Disease Severity**
  Check scalp, brows, ears for seborrhea. Smear and stain of scraping from lid margins. Stain cornea. Evaluate for ulceration.

- **Concept and Application**

Seborrheic Blepharitis. Associated with seborrhea of scalp, brows, ears. Nonulcerative lid margin, scales oily, *Pityrosporum ovale* present.

Staphylococcal Blepharitis. *Staphylococcus aureus* or *Staphylococcus epidermidis,* coagulase-

negative, ulcerative lid margin, hordeola, chalazia, epithelial keratitis lower one third of cornea, marginal infiltrates, recurrent conjunctivitis.

- **Management**

Seborrheic Blepharitis. Soap-and-water shampoo of scalp. Removal of scales from lid margins with damp cotton applicator, baby shampoo.

Staphylococcal Blepharitis. Daily antibiotic ointment against staphylococcus. Long-term low-dose systemic antibiotic therapy.

B. Stye

External hordeolum (glands of Zeis or Moll, hair follicles).

- **H&P Keys**
  Recent onset; localized red, swollen tender area of the lid, frequently preceded by diffuse edema of the lid.

- **Diagnosis**
  Red, swollen gland with pore opening can be seen at the lid margin. Tender area can be identified with a cotton tip.

- **Disease Severity**
  Pain is related to the amount of swelling. Pus tends to point to the skin surface of the lid margin.

- **Concept and Application**
  Common staphylococcal infection of Zeis's or Moll's glands of the lids. A small abscess sometimes is formed.

- **Management**

1. Warm compresses over affected lids 10 minutes three times a day after application of antibiotic ointment.
2. Incision and drainage of pus when needed.

C. Chalazion

Internal hordeolum (meibomian gland).

- **H&P Keys**
  Persistent nontender lump palpable or visible along the margin of upper or lower eyelid. Inflammation and swelling develop

over a period of days and can remain for months.

- **Diagnosis**
  When the lid is everted, the nodules usually point toward the conjunctival side and can be detected as reddened, elevated areas. Absence of acute inflammation is seen in fully developed chalazion.

- **Disease Severity**

  1. Evaluate for malignancy if recurrent at same site.
  2. Assess visual disturbance caused by the lump on the lids.
  3. Perform biopsy if recurrent.

- **Concept and Application**
  A granulomatous inflammation of the meibomian gland. Seldom subsides spontaneously. Langhans' giant cells, yellowish, fatty content. Large chalazion pressing on the eyeball, can cause astigmatism. Recurrence at same site after excision suggests malignant disease.

- **Management**

  1. Warm compresses.
  2. Topical antibiotics.
  3. Local steroid injection.
  4. Excision if large and disturbs vision.
  5. Biopsy if recurrent.

D. Entropion

Turning inward of the lid margin, usually affects the lower lid.

- **H&P Keys**
  Tearing, irritation of the cornea. Eyelashes turn inward, touching cornea.

- **Diagnosis**
  Check the lid margin, position of the eyelashes, and the integrity of the cornea. Early detection of corneal ulcer.

- **Disease Severity**
  Entropion can cause trichiasis, the turning inward of the lashes so that they rub on the cornea. Irritation of the cornea can predispose to corneal ulcer.

- **Concept and Application**
  Senile type caused by degeneration of fascial attachments in the lower lid. *Cicatricial* type caused by scarring of the palpebral conjunctiva and the tarsus. Common in trachoma.

- **Management**

  1. Temporary taping to evert lid.
  2. Corrective surgery.

E. Ectropion

Turning outward of lower lid.

- **H&P Keys**
  Tearing, irritation. Sagging and eversion of lid margin.

- **Diagnosis**
  Test closure of lids and integrity of cornea.

- **Disease Severity**
  Exposure keratitis. Fluorescein stain for corneal integrity.

- **Concept and Application**
  Bilateral. Older persons. Relaxation of orbicularis oculi. Present in aging and seventh cranial nerve palsy.

- **Management**

  1. Protection of cornea.
  2. Lubrication with artificial tears or ointment.
  3. Surgical correction of deformed lid.

F. Epicanthus

Wide nasal folds.

- **H&P Keys**
  Vertical folds of skin over medial canthi; in Asians and most children of all races.

- **Diagnosis**
  Corneal light reflex test is normal. So-called esotropia, or turning in of the eye, appears present on side gaze.

- **Disease Severity**
  Prominent epicanthal folds in children becomes less obvious as child grows older.

• **Concept and Application**

The large skin fold covers the nasal sclera and causes pseudoesotropia. Frequent concern as strabismus. A common cause for referral.

• **Management**

Explanation and understanding. No treatment needed.

G. Blepharoptosis

Droopy eyelids.

• **H&P Keys**

May be noted at birth; congenital or acquired. Drooping of upper lids when both eyes are open. Unilateral or bilateral. Constant or intermittent.

• **Diagnosis**

Determine amount of movement of upper lid and severity in blocking of vision. Assess cosmesis and skin position.

• **Disease Severity**

Degree of upper lid movement and occlusion of pupillary axis for vision. Concern with visual development in children.

• **Concept and Application**

Congenital. Developmental failure of levator muscle of the lid, anomalies of superior rectus muscle, complete external ophthalmoplegia. Dominant transmission.

Acquired

Mechanical Factors. Edema of lids, swelling, tumor, fat.

Myogenic Causes. Muscular dystrophy, myasthenia gravis.

Neurogenic (Paralytic). Weakness of cranial nerve III.

• **Management**

1. Conservative: No cosmetic or visual acuity disturbance.
2. Myasthenia gravis: Neostigmine.
3. Special spectacle frames.
4. Surgery for improvement of vision or cosmesis: frontalis sling for no action of levator, to lift upper lid; levator strengthening for partial weakness of levator.

III. DISORDERS OF THE LACRIMAL SYSTEM

A. Undersecretion

Dry-eye syndrome, Sjögren's disease.

Dry-eye Syndrome (Keratoconjunctivitis Sicca) ~~assoc lymphone Sjogren~~

• **H&P Keys**

Dry, irritative conjunctiva. Dry, sore mouth. Foreign-body sensation, scratchy and sandy feeling of the eyes. Itchy, burning, photosensitivity, excessive mucus, redness, pain, dry lids. Grossly, normal-looking eyes.

• **Diagnosis**

Dry undersecretion is confirmed by Schirmer's test with strip of blotting paper (4 mm × 30 mm). The strip is inserted onto the lower lid margin so that the strip protrudes forward from the eye. The rate of lacrimation is measured. By the end of 5 minutes the strip should be moistened for at least 15 mm in a normal response. In Sjögren's disease, the moistening rarely extends beyond 5 mm along the strip, suggesting inadequate tear production.

• **Disease Severity**

Undersecretion of tears. Evaluation studies for corneal epithelium and conjunctival defects with vital stain such as rose bengal (1%). The affected areas will be colored bright red. Rheumatoid arthritis should be investigated, if not yet diagnosed.

• **Concept and Application**

Dryness of eye may be of many causes. Hyposecretion, excessive evaporation, mucin deficiency are predisposing factors.

Sjögren's disease is a general glandular atrophy. It affects the lacrimal and salivary glands and associates with rheumatic diathesis. Postmenopausal women. Dryness affects conjunctiva, cornea, mouth, trachea.

• **Management**

1. Search for cause.
2. Artificial tears, methyl cellulose, are used frequently.

B. Acute Dacryocystitis

- **H&P Keys**

  Infection of lacrimal sac. Common acute or chronic. Infants or in patients over 40. Tearing and discharge. Swelling lump, pain, tenderness over tear sac area.

- **Diagnosis**

  Persistent tearing. Purulent material can be expressed from tear sac. Nasolacrimal duct is blocked. Staining of conjunctival smear to identify infectious organisms.

- **Disease Severity**

  Tearing in mild cases. Purulent discharge in moderate to severe blockage of nasolacrimal ducts.

- **Concept and Application**

  Blockage of nasolacrimal duct is the cause of infection. May be developmental.

- **Management**

  In children, forceful massage of the tear sac is tried initially. Irrigation and probings of nasolacrimal duct are usually effective.

  1. Acute: Warm compresses. Appropriate antibiotics. Incision and drainage if necessary.
  2. Chronic: Surgical removal of obstruction of nasolacrimal duct (dacrocystorhinostomy).

IV. DISORDERS OF THE OPTIC NERVE

A. Elevation of the Disc

1. Congenital Anomalous Disc Elevation

Blurred optic disc since birth, caused by developmental anomaly.

- **H&P Keys**

  No symptoms, blurred disc margin, elevated disc substance, obliterated cup, no edema, no hemorrhage.

- **Diagnosis**

  Dilated ophthalmoscopy; document with optic disc photography, pseudopapilledema, intravenous fluorescein angiography (Tables 13–7, 13–8).

- **Disease Severity**

  Benign, nonprogressive; rule out true papilledema.

- **Concept and Application**

  Hyperopia, glial tissue, persistent hyaloid remnants, drusen of the disc.

- **Management**

  Detection and follow-up through serial examinations to monitor possible progression.

TABLE 13–7. SYMPTOMS OF BLURRED OPTIC NERVE HEAD

Symptoms	Papilledema	Papillitis	Pseudopapilledema
Etiology	Acute swelling of optic disc • Increased intracranial pressure • Brain tumor • Hypertension • Pseudotumor cerebri	Acute blurred disc margin • Ischemia • Inflammation • Multiple sclerosis	Blurred disc • Congenital, developmental anomalies • Hyperopia
Acute loss of vision	+	+++ (Severe)	0
Headaches	+++	0/+	0
Retrobulbar pain on eye movement	0	+/+++	0

+, present; ++, moderate; +++, severe; 0, absent.

TABLE 13–8. SIGNS OF BLURRED OPTIC NERVE HEAD

Signs	Papilledema	Papillitis	Pseudopapilledema
Hyperemia of disc	+++	+++	0
Hemorrhages	+++	+	0
Tortuosity of veins, capillaries	+++	++	+
Disc margin			
blurred,	+++	+++	+++
elevated	+++	0/+	++
One eye affected	Rare	+++	++
Both eyes affected	+++	Rare	Rare
Afferent pupillary defect	0	+++	0/+
Visual field defect	0/+	+++	0/+

+, present; ++, moderate; +++, severe; 0, absent.

2. Papilledema

Swelling of optic disc caused by increased intracranial pressure.

- **H&P Keys**
  Symptoms of brain tumor, hyperemia of optic disc, tortuosity of veins and capillaries, blurring and elevation of disc margin, hemorrhages on and surrounding nerve head.

- **Diagnosis**
  Studies for brain lesions, computed tomographic (CT) scan, magnetic resonance imaging (MRI), intravenous fluorescein angiography.

- **Disease Severity**
  Brain tumor, pseudotumor cerebri, severe systemic hypertension.

- **Concept and Application**
  Swelling of optic disc secondary to increased intracranial pressure, brain tumor 50%.

- **Management**
  Detection and referral for evaluation by neurologists or neurosurgeons.

3. Papillitis

Anterior optic neuritis. Inflammatory edema of the optic nerve head visible by ophthalmoscope.

- **H&P Keys**
  Sudden loss of central vision, usually in one eye. Pain behind the eyeball on movement of the affected eye. Reduced vision. Swinging light test for relative afferent pupillary defect.

- **Diagnosis**
  Ophthalmoscopy. Visual field test for central scotoma. CT of orbits and chiasm.

- **Disease Severity**
  Search for multiple sclerosis, lyme disease, and neurosyphilis. Rule out compressive lesions of optic nerve and chiasm.

- **Concept and Application**
  Inflammation of optic nerve. Idiopathic. Associated with multiple sclerosis, lyme disease, and neurosyphilis. Prognosis for return vision after single attack is good. Spontaneous resolution can follow in weeks to months.

- **Management**
  IV corticosteroid versus no treatment for acute phase. Oral prednisone treatment is contraindicated in the treatment of idiopathic optic neuritos.

B. Pallor of the Disc, Optic Atrophy

Optic nerve degeneration.

- **H&P Keys**
  Decreased vision, visual field loss, relative afferent pupillary defect, fixed dilated pupil, pale optic disc.

- **Diagnosis**
  Vision, pupillary reaction to light, swinging light test, ophthalmoscopy; compare both discs for asymmetry of color, cupping, fine-vessels pattern.

- **Disease Severity**
  Intraocular pressure for glaucoma, orbital mass compression of nerve. Intravenous fluorescein angiography of disc.

- **Concept and Application**
  History of diseases that damage nerve fiber layer of retina, optic nerve, optic chiasm, optic tracts. Common causes: optic neuritis, long-standing papilledema, compression of

the nerve by a mass, meningioma, ischemic optic neuropathy, glaucoma.

- **Management**
Detection and referral for investigation and treatment.

V. DISORDERS OF THE VISUAL PATHWAYS

A. Monocular Defects (Central Scotomas)

(Anterior to chiasm.)

- **H&P Keys**
Loss of central vision in one eye. Reduction of visual acuity (Fig. 13–1).

- **Diagnosis**
Visual acuity testing. Pupillary reaction to light. Swinging light test for relative afferent pupillary defect. Ophthalmoscopy. Visual field testing. Red-color appreciation. Amsler grid.

- **Disease Severity**
Ophthalmoscopy for macular and optic nerve diseases. Rule out retinal detachments, vascular occlusions, such as central retinal artery occlusion, branch retinal artery occlusion, central retinal vein occlusion. Intravenous fluorescein angiography.

- **Concept and Application**
Prechiasmal lesions mean monocular loss of vision. Optic nerve lesions. Scotoma is a blind or partially defective area in the visual field. Central scotoma means central vision is affected. Optic neuritis. Ischemic optic neuropathy. Multiple sclerosis.

- **Management**
Detection and referral.

B. Bitemporal Defects

(At the chiasm.)

- **H&P Keys**
Visual field defect affects both eyes, bitemporal hemianopsia, side vision defect of both eyes (see Fig. 13–1). Confrontation testing with red object.

- **Diagnosis**
Vision. Visual fields testing. CT scan, MRI.

- **Disease Severity**
CT scan. Check out enlarged sella turcica for pituitary tumor.

- **Concept and Application**
Bitemporal visual field defects means chiasmal lesions; suspect pituitary tumor.

- **Management**
Detection and referral.

C. Homonymous Defects

(Posterior to chiasm.)

- **H&P Keys**
Loss of visual fields of both eyes on the same side (see Fig.13–1). Visual field defects on the right or left side. Confrontation testing with red object.

- **Diagnosis**
Visual field testing. Intracranial studies. CT scan. MRI.

- **Disease Severity**
Check out neurologic symptoms and signs for brain tumor and cerebral vascular lesions, stroke.

- **Concept and Application**
Defects indicate lesions behind the chiasm. Lesions affect optic tract opposite the defects, extending to occipital cortex. The more posterior the lesion, the more similar in shape, size, and severity the damage in the two eyes. Check out tumor, cerebral vascular diseases.

- **Management**
Detection and referral.

VI. AMBLYOPIA

Defective vision, uncorrectable by glasses, in an otherwise normal eye.

- **H&P Keys**
Eye fixation pattern, vision test, ophthalmoscopy.

- **Diagnosis**
Refraction, check out anisometropia.

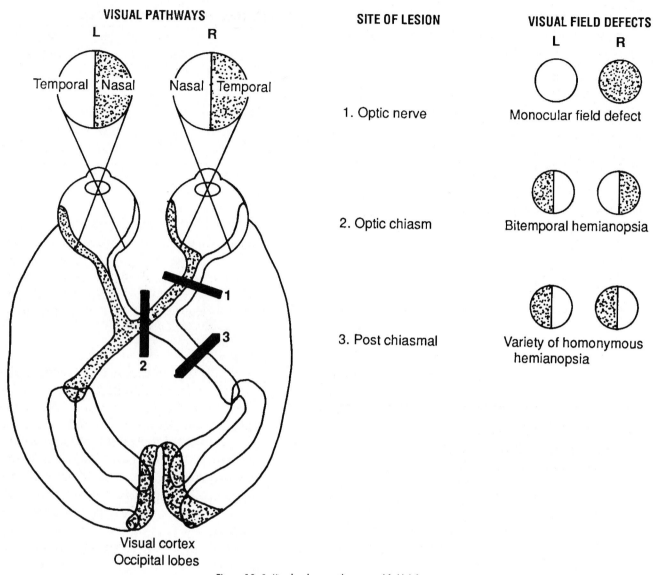

Figure 13–1. Visual pathways with associated field defects.

Within the figure:

VISUAL PATHWAYS
L   R

Temporal Nasal   Nasal Temporal

Visual cortex
Occipital lobes

SITE OF LESION

1. Optic nerve

2. Optic chiasm

3. Post chiasmal

VISUAL FIELD DEFECTS
L   R

Monocular field defect

Bitemporal hemianopsia

Variety of homonymous
hemianopsia

• **Disease Severity**
  Check out visual loss caused by organic diseases, congenital cataracts, retinoblastoma.

• **Concept and Application**
  Preventable blindness. Strabismus in 50% of patients with amblyopia. Amblyopia secondary to strabismus. Organic visual loss causes strabismus. Predisposing factors: strabismic amblyopia, refractive amblyopia, form-deprivation and occlusion amblyopia.

• **Management**
  Early detection. Early treatment before age 5.

VII. STRABISMUS

Misalignment of two eyes so that both eyes cannot be directed toward the object of fixation.

- **H&P Keys**
Family history, head trauma, systemic disease, neurologic disorder.

- **Diagnosis**
General inspection, corneal light reflex, cover test, dilated ophthalmoscopy.

- **Disease Severity**
Check for intraocular lesions, cataract, retinoblastoma, other retinal abnormalities. Examine for neurologic disorder.

- **Concept and Application**
Early detection (Tables 13–9, 13–10). Delayed diagnosis affects vision, eye, and systemic problems.

- **Management**

1. Detection early to allow diagnosis and treatment.
2. Search for serious organic conditions that cause strabismus.

VIII. DIABETES WITH OPHTHALMOLOGIC MANIFESTATIONS

- **H&P Keys**
Decreased vision often a late symptom that may not be evident until ocular damage is severe. The longer a patient is diabetic, the more likely the retinopathy and visual loss. Age of onset, type of diabetes, history of hypertension, and presence of obesity are relevant to disease severity and management. Changes in refraction of lens, decreased or abnormal

TABLE 13–10. TYPES OF IMBALANCE OF THE TWO EYES

	Tropia (Visible Turning)	Phoria (Tendency to Turn)
Horizontal		
Inward turning	Esotropia	Esophoria
Outward turning	Exotropia	Exophoria
Vertical		
Upward turning	Hypertropia	Hyperphoria
Downward turning	Hypotropia	Hypophoria

pupillary responses, extraocular muscle palsy, cataract, iris neovascularization, optic neuropathy, or retinopathy. Diabetic retinopathy progresses in severity from nonproliferative or background retinopathy to preproliferative and proliferative changes (Table 13–11).

- **Diagnosis**
Direct ophthalmoscopy detects most ophthalmic clinical manifestations of diabetes, including retinopathy, optic neuropathy, blockage of the red reflex by cataract. Indirect ophthalmoscopy: wider, stereoscopic view of retina. Biomicroscopy with a slit lamp: useful in evaluating for diabetic changes in anterior segment including cataracts and iris neovascularization. Pupillary dilation for easier, more thorough examination of retina and lens. Ultrasonography for internal structure (eg, tractional retinal detachment),

TABLE 13–9. CLASSIFICATION OF STRABISMUS

	Comitant (Nonparalytic) Strabismus	Noncomitant (Paralytic) Strabismus
Onset	Childhood (under 6 y)	Later in life
Angle of misalignment *varies* with direction of gaze	0	+
Extraocular muscles palsy	0	+
Associated neurologic disease*	0	+

* Blowout fracture; palsy of cranial nerve III; orbital diseases; thyroid.

+, present; 0, absent.

TABLE 13–11. PROGRESSION OF DIABETIC RETINOPATHY

Nonproliferative retinopathy
    Microaneurysms
    Hemorrhages (dot and blot, flame)
    Hard exudates
    Retinal edema
Preproliferative retinopathy
    Retinal nerve fiber layer infarcts (cotton-wool patches)
    Venous dilation, loops, and beading (irregularities of the vein caliber)
    Telangiectasias (intraretinal microvascular abnormalities)
Proliferative diabetic retinopathy
    Neovascularization of the retina, optic disc, or vitreous
    Preretinal and vitreous hemorrhages
    Fibrous proliferation
    Tractional retinal detachment

when blood, debris, or membranes impede direct visualization of retina.

- **Disease Severity**
Biomicroscopy with a contact lens system provides stereoscopic, detailed view of structures of retina; especially valuable in diagnosis of macular edema. Fluorescein angiography to assess extent of disease, such as leakage from abnormal vessels in suspected neovascularization, and in guiding laser photocoagulation treatment of clinically evident macular edema by revealing characteristic lesions and pathologic processes of retinopathy, eg, microaneurysms, capillary leakage, and nonperfusion areas.

- **Concept and Application**
Cellular edema, pericyte destruction, endothelial damage and dysfunction from increased intracellular sorbitol and hypoxia lead to capillary hyperpermeability. Abnormal retinal vascular permeability leads to macular edema, which threatens vision and may be an indication for laser therapy. Increased hemoglobin A_{1c} oxygen affinity impairs oxygen release, resulting in retinal hypoxia. Basement membrane thickening and increased platelet and red blood cell aggregability predispose to regions of microvascular occlusions, retinal hypoxia, and release of vasogenic factors with subsequent neovascularization of the retina, optic nerve, or iris. Widespread panretinal laser photocoagulation reduces release of vasogenic stimuli and therefore neovascularization.

- **Management**
Tight medical control with long-term near-normalization of blood sugar level slows the progression of diabetic retinopathy. Laser photocoagulation for diabetic retinopathy with clinically significant macular edema and high-risk proliferative retinopathy. Vitrectomy may be indicated for severe vitreous or preretinal hemorrhages, or tractional retinal detachment.

IX. DISORDERS OF THE CORNEA

(See Table 13–12.)

A. Corneal Ulcers

- **H&P Keys**
Pain, photophobia, blepharospasm, lacrimation, discharge and decreased vision often present. The lesion begins as a dull, grayish, circumscribed superficial infiltration of the cornea that subsequently ulcerates. Conjunctival and limbal injection is usual and blood vessels may grow in from the limbus in long-standing cases (pannus). Pus may appear in the anterior chamber (hypopyon). Corneal perforation with iris prolapse may occur.

- **Diagnosis**
The ulcer stains green with fluorescein. Bacterial and fungal cultures from corneal scrapings should be obtained prior to starting antibiotic treatment.

- **Disease Severity**
Slit-lamp biomicroscopy may be used to determine the extent of corneal thinning and infiltration and the presence of hypopyon.

TABLE 13–12. DISEASES OF THE GLOBE

A. Cornea
  1. Ulcers
  2. Herpes simplex keratitis
  3. Ophthalmic herpes zoster
  4. Dry eye (keratoconjunctivitis sicca)
  5. Interstitial keratitis
B. Sclera
  1. Scleritis
C. Uvea
  1. Uveitis
    a. Anterior
    b. Posterior
D. Retina
  1. Retinal detachment
  2. Vascular occlusions
    a. Arteriolar
    b. Venous
  3. Hypertensive retinopathy
  4. Retinitis pigmentosa
  5. Age-related macular degeneration
E. Penetrating injuries

• **Concept and Application**

Bacterial or fungal infection following trauma, corneal foreign body, contact lens wear, or previous corneal disease. Assume bacterial until proven otherwise.

• **Management**

Cycloplegia (scopalamine), broad-spectrum or fortified topical antibiotics, subconjunctival antibiotics, eye shield if corneal thinning, pain medication (acetaminophen).

B. Herpes Simplex Keratitis

• **H&P Keys**

Red eye, foreign-body sensation, photophobia, tearing, decreased vision, skin vesicles. Decreased corneal sensation. Dendritic corneal branching lesion. Possible recent topical steroids, systemic steroids, or immune deficiency state.

• **Diagnosis**

Edge of herpetic lesions are heaped up with swollen epithelial cells, which stain with rose bengal, whereas the central ulceration stains with fluorescein. Corneal or skin lesion scraping for multinucleated giant cells and intranuclear inclusion bodies. Viral culture.

• **Disease Severity**

Slit-lamp examination with intraocular pressure measurement. Concomitant corneal infiltrates, iritis, hypopyon, or glaucoma may occur. Bacterial superinfection must be ruled out.

• **Concept and Application**

Self-limited primary ocular herpes keratoconjunctivitis, regional lymphadenitis, vesicular blepharitis, or skin involvement. Herpes virus establishes presence in trigeminal ganglion, allowing chronic recurrent disease.

• **Management**

Skin vesicles (antibiotic ointment); eyelid margin involvement, conjunctivitis, corneal epithelial disease (topical trifluorothymidine or vidarabine); consider mechanical debridement of infected corneal epithelium; topical steroids contraindicated for corneal epithelial involvement.

C. Ophthalmic Herpes Zoster

• **H&P Keys**

Acute vesicular skin rash of fifth cranial nerve dermatome. Fever, malaise, blurred vision, eye pain, red eye. Conjunctivitis, corneal involvement (eg, pseudodendrites), uveitis, optic neuritis, retinitis, glaucoma. Postherpetic neuralgia may occur late. Involvement of tip of nose by vesicles (Hutchinson's sign) associated with corneal involvement. Immunocompromised or risk factors for AIDS?

• **Diagnosis**

Clinical diagnosis based on pattern of skin rash. Pseudodendrites stain poorly with fluorescein. Regional lymphadenopathy with associated pain occurs in primary disease.

• **Disease Severity**

Slit-lamp examination with intraocular pressure measurement. Dilated optic nerve and retinal examination. Immunodeficiency workup if less than 40 years old or immunodeficiency suspected.

• **Concept and Application**

Primary herpes zoster: Acute infection of dorsal root ganglion by chickenpox virus. Secondary eruption following ganglion involvement may be associated with immune compromise from neoplastic, inflammatory, or infectious processes.

• **Management**

Systemic acyclovir if started in first 5 to 7 days of skin rash. Antibiotic ointment to skin lesions. Consider systemic steroids and cimetidine in nonimmunocompromised, nondiabetic patients over age 60 to reduce postherpetic neuralgia.

D. Dry Eye (Keratoconjunctivitis Sicca)

• **H&P Keys**

Initial reduction of tear production leads to burning and irritation. Corneal epithelium develops scattered cellular loss called superficial keratitis; may be associated with photophobia or blepharospasm. Keratinization of the ocular surface occurs in advanced stages, often with loss of normal conjunctival fornices. Corneal ulceration, vascularization, and scarring may lead to severe visual disability. Dry eye may be an isolated phenomenon or associated with systemic diseases such as rheumatoid arthritis or lupus erythematosus (Sjögren's syndrome).

- **Diagnosis**
Reduced tear meniscus at lid margin. Fluorescein or rose bengal stains reveal superficial keratitis with scattered staining of corneal surface and premature tear drying over the corneal surface.

- **Disease Severity**
Tear production may be measured by the use of strips of blotting paper with or without topical anesthesia (Schirmer test).

- **Concept and Application**
Dryness of the eye may be associated with hypofunction of the lacrimal glands (eg, Sjögren's syndrome, familial dysautonomia, sarcoidosis, atropine), excessive evaporation of tears (eg, exposure keratopathy, dry climate, deficient blinking), mucin deficiency (eg, Stevens-Johnson syndrome, chemical burns, avitaminosis A).

- **Management**
Frequent use of artificial tears and ointments. Occlusion of the nasolacrimal punctum to reduce tear drainage or partial tarsorrhaphy to reduce tear evaporation may be tried in more severe cases.

E. Interstitial Keratitis

- **H&P Keys**
Acute: Pain, tearing, photophobia, red eye. Corneal stromal blood vessels, corneal edema, anterior uveitis. Old disease: Deep corneal scarring and haze, corneal stromal thinning, and ghost vessels. Associated with maternal venereal disease, saddle nose, frontal bossing, Hutchinson's teeth, chorioretinitis, optic atrophy (congenital syphilis); hearing deficit, tinnitus, vertigo, polyarteritis nodosa (Cogan's syndrome); hypopigmented or anesthetic skin lesions, loss of temporal eyebrow or eyelashes, thickened corneal nerves, iris nodules (leprosy); tuberculosis.

- **Diagnosis**
Slit-lamp and dilated fundus examination. Rapid plasma reagin (RPR), fluorescent treponemal antibody absorption (FTA-ABS), purified protein derivative (tuberculin) (PPD) tests with anergy panel, chest roentgenogram, sedimentation rate.

- **Disease Severity**
Slit-lamp examination for corneal edema, scarring or thinning, or uveitis.

- **Concept and Application**
Chronic nonulcerative infiltration of the deep layers of the cornea with uveal inflammation.

- **Management**
Acute corneal involvement: topical cycloplegia, topical steroids, treatment of underlying disease. Corneal transplant surgery for central corneal scarring with impaired vision.

X. DISORDERS OF THE LENS

A. Glaucoma

- **H&P Keys**

Primary Open-Angle Glaucoma. Usually asymptomatic in the early stages. Risk factors include advanced age, African ancestry, immediate family members with glaucoma, myopia (nearsightedness), diabetes mellitus, hypertension. The optic nerve may show an increased ratio of the physiologic cupping diameter to disc diameter, pallor, displacement of retinal vessels to the rim, and asymmetry compared to the contralateral eye.

Acute Angle-Closure Glaucoma. Presents with severe ocular pain, blurred vision, halos around lights, headache, nausea, and vomiting. Examination shows red eye, mid-dilated sometimes oval pupil, cloudy cornea, marked elevation of intraocular pressure, shallow anterior chamber, and closed angle by gonioscopy. Highly far-sighted patients are at greater risk. An attack may be precipitated by dim light, emotional stress, or dilating drops.

Congenital Glaucoma. Presents with light sensitivity, corneal cloudiness, and excessive tearing. Chronically there may be slow development and learning disabilities.

Secondary Glaucomas. May occur with chronic exposure to steroids (topical generally), ocular trauma, retinal vein occlusion, intraocular inflammation, intraocular tumor, diabetes mellitus, and carotid vascular disease.

- **Diagnosis**
  Intraocular pressure measurement may be performed with Schiotz' (indentation) or applanation tonometry. Individuals may present with normal intraocular pressures and have glaucoma. A patient who has elevated intraocular pressure but shows no sign of optic nerve damage or visual field loss is generally considered to be a glaucoma suspect. Visual field defects start insidiously. They are characterized by arcuate-shaped scotomas or a silent contraction of the peripheral field, sparing the central vision until late in the disease process.

- **Disease Severity**
  The severity of disease is based on the clinical appearance of the optic nerve and on the visual field. Response to treatment is evaluated with regard to relationship of lowering of intraocular pressure to stability of changes in the optic nerve appearance and visual field.

- **Concept and Application**
  Glaucoma is in general a condition in which the intraocular pressure is too elevated for the health of the optic nerve, resulting in damage and visual field loss. This is generally due to increased resistance to aqueous outflow. In primary open-angle glaucoma, there appears to be an increased resistance to aqueous outflow through the trabecular meshwork. In primary angle-closure glaucoma, the peripheral iris closes off the angle structures, preventing aqueous outflow. Neovascularization, pigmentary or inflam-

matory debris, traumatic damage, or cellular changes from chronic steroid exposure all increase resistance to aqueous outflow. Both the medical and surgical treatment of glaucoma is based on the reduction of intraocular pressure by promoting aqueous outflow or reducing aqueous production.

- **Management**

Open-Angle Glaucoma. Miotics (eg, pilocarpine) and adrenergic agonists (eg, epinephrine) reduce outflow resistance. Adrenergic agonists, β-blockers, and carbonic anhydrase inhibitors decrease aqueous production. Laser trabecular burns and surgical filtration procedures can be used to promote aqueous outflow.

Angle-Closure Glaucoma. Acutely treat with topical β-blockers, topical pilocarpine, oral carbonic anhydrase inhibitors, and osmotic agents such as oral glycerin or intravenous mannitol. A laser or surgical peripheral iridectomy must be performed for definitive treatment of the anatomic problem.

B. Cataract

- **H&P Keys**
  A cataract is a lens opacity. Complaints of painless blurred vision, glare, increasing nearsightedness, or monocular double vision. History of previous eye conditions, injury, or surgery or of concurrent diseases may suggest cause of cataract. Assessment of visual acuity with optical correction by means of Snellen letter chart or a number chart, or picture charts or ability to fixate on and follow or reach for a moving object for young children or adults with severe mental disability. Preferential viewing techniques may estimate visual acuity in infants. The lens is best examined for cataracts with a dilated pupil. The simplest way is with a hand-held direct ophthalmoscope showing dark lenticular opacities blocking the normal red reflex of the retina. The slit-lamp biomicroscope is routinely used to detect the location and density of any opacity within the lens.

- **Diagnosis**

  Potential visual acuity that might be expected with removal of the cataract may be estimated by the use of a potential acuity meter (PAM) or a laser interferometer. Both instruments are based on the ability of a patient to resolve letters or lines projected onto the retina.

  When significant lens opacification prevents direct retinal examination, B-scan ultrasonography may be used to detect severe abnormalities of the retina, such as retinal detachment or tumors.

- **Disease Severity**

  The clinical degree of cataract formation, assuming that no other eye disease is present, is judged primarily by the visual acuity. With direct ophthalmoscopy of the posterior pole through the cataract, the ocular fundus becomes increasingly more difficult to visualize as the lens opacity becomes denser. Slit-lamp biomicroscopy allows judgment of lens clarity and location of the cataract. Glare testing and contrast sensitivity testing are new methods for quantitatively estimating the functional impact a cataract has on vision.

- **Concept and Application**

  A cataract is an opacity or loss of transparency within the lens. Cataracts may be classified by their age of onset, location, and etiology (Table 13–13). The most common indication for cataract surgery is the patient's desire for improved visual function. Medical indications for cataract surgery include phacolytic glaucoma, phacomorphic glaucoma, phacotoxic uveitis, and dense cataracts that obscure the view of the fundus and interfere with the diagnosis and management of other ocular diseases such

TABLE 13–13. CLASSIFICATION OF CATARACTS

A. Age-related
1. Nuclear sclerotic
2. Posterior subcapsular
3. Cortical
4. Mature
5. Morgagnian and hypermature

B. Congenital

C. Juvenile
1. Inborn errors of metabolism
2. Chromosomal abnormalities

D. Secondary
1. Traumatic or physical damage
2. Associated with intraocular disease
   a. Chronic or recurrent uveitis
   b. Retinitis pigmentosa
   c. Retinal detachment or tumors
3. Associated with systemic disease (eg, hypoparathyroidism, Down's syndrome, diabetes mellitus)
4. Toxic
   a. Steroids
   b. Miotic agents
   c. Intraocular metals: copper or iron

as diabetic retinopathy or glaucoma. In children, cataract extraction is performed early to prevent otherwise irreversible visual impairment from amblyopia, the loss of visual maturation from visual sensory deprivation.

- **Management**

  No current medical treatment conclusively delays, prevents, or reverses the development of cataracts in adults. Pupillary dilation, increased ambient illumination, or improved spectacle correction may be temporarily helpful until cataract progression causes additional symptoms. Surgical removal of the cataract with or without artificial lens implantation is the definitive treatment.

14

Pediatrics

Charles A. Pohl, MD, and Regina Simonetti, MD

I. NEUROLOGY

A. Febrile Seizures   6 mo - 6 yr

- **H&P Keys**
  Occurs in children 6 months to 6 years of age. Signs and symptoms include generalized, tonic, atonic, tonic–clonic, or focal seizures and fever. Risk factors include positive family history develop mental delay, day care, prematurity, perinatal maternal smoking.

- **Diagnosis**
  Diagnosis of exclusion. Studies based on history and physical exam. Evaluate for source of infection or metabolic imbalance. May include lumbar puncture, blood and urine cultures, electrolytes, glucose, calcium, and complete blood count (CBC) based on clinical presentation.

- **Disease Severity**

  Simple Febrile Seizure. Generalized seizure lasting less than 15 minutes, occurring once in a 24-hour period.

  Complex Febrile Seizure. A focal seizure or a generalized seizure lasting more than 15 minutes, or more than one seizure in a 24-hour period.

- **Concept and Application**
  Genetic factors play a role, ie, an increased incidence if a first-degree relative has had a febrile seizure. Unclear etiology.

- **Management**
  ABC (airway, breathing, circulation). Lorazepam (Ativan) or diazepam (Valium) for prolonged seizures. Antipyretics. Prophylactic anticonvulsants are controversial.

B. Infantile Botulism

- **H&P Keys**
An acute neurologic disease caused by the toxin of *Clostridium botulinum*. *C. botulinum* spores can be found in soil, dust, lakes, and contaminated food products, including honey. Signs and symptoms include weakness, poor feeding, weak cry, constipation, respiratory failure, symmetric descending flaccid paralysis, loss of a gag reflex, and ptosis.

- **Diagnosis**
Stool culture for *C. botulinum* and toxin. Electrophysiologic studies.

- **Disease Severity**
Neurologic changes. Pulmonary function tests. Arterial blood gases (ABG).

- **Concept and Application**
Botulinal toxin binds to the neuromuscular junctions and inhibits exocytosis of acetylcholine, which results in flaccid paralysis.

- **Management**
Supportive care. Antitoxin (neutralizes circulating toxin before it binds to nerve endings). Must be given expediently. Parenteral penicillin. Aminoglycosides contraindicated.

C. Neural Tube Defects

- **H&P Keys**
Failure of neural tube to close in utero (normally closes by day 26). Signs and symptoms depend on the region of spinal cord involved and the extent of the lesion. Clues to diagnosis are a tuft of hair, dimple, or birthmark over the spine.

- **Diagnosis**
Prenatal ultrasonography. Maternal alpha-fetoprotein (AFP). Clinical exam. Magnetic resonance imaging (MRI).

- **Disease Severity**
Asymptomatic or disturbances of bowel, bladder, motor function. Degrees of severity include: spina bifida occulta (incomplete closure of the posterior lumbosacral spinal cord), meningocele (herniation of the meninges through the spinal canal defect without neural tissue), encephalocele (herniation of the meninges and brain substance through a skull defect), myelomeningocele (severe spinal dysraphism with herniation of the meninges and spinal cord), anencephaly (congenital absence of the cerebral hemisphere and cranial vault). More than 75% of myelomeningoceles are associated with hydrocephalus (usually related to an Arnold-Chiari malformation). Majority have normal intelligence.

- **Concept and Application**
Multifactorial. Maternal folate supplementation during pregnancy has decreased its frequency.

- **Management**
Multidisciplinary approach.

D. Malformations

1. Hydrocephalus

- **H&P Keys**
A congenital or acquired condition resulting from impaired circulation, absorption or overproduction of cerebrospinal fluid (CSF). Can cause increased intracranial pressure. Signs and symptoms include headaches, vomiting, nausea, irritability, lethargy, third and sixth cranial nerve palsies, papilledema, bulging anterior fontanelle, rapid increase in head circumference, setting-sun sign, long-tract signs, vital sign changes.

- **Diagnosis**
Clinical exam. Computerized tomographic (CT) scan. Avoid lumbar punctures (risk of herniation).

- **Disease Severity**
Evidence of herniation: Cushing's triad (bradycardia, hypertension, and irregular breathing), vomiting, change of mental status.

- **Concept and Application**

Communicating. Results from either an obstruction of CSF flow from outside the ventricular system or an overproduction of CSF. Etiologies include intraventricular hemorrhages (premature infants), postinfectious state, tumors, hemorrhagic trauma.

Noncommunicating. Results from obstruction of CSF flow within the ventricular system. Etiologies include aqueductal stenosis, Chiari malformation (low cerebellar tonsils), and Dandy-Walker malformation of the fourth ventricle.

- **Management**
  Placement of a ventriculoperitoneal (VP) shunt if needed.

2. Congenital Glaucoma

- **H&P Keys**
  Incidence of about 1 in 100 000 births; 30% are unilateral. Signs and symptoms include photophobia, tearing, blepharospasm, and clouding or enlargement of the cornea.

- **Diagnosis**
  Intraocular pressure measurements. Clinical exam.

- **Disease Severity**
  Blindness if not treated promptly.

- **Concept and Application**
  Maldevelopment of the trabecular meshwork of the eye resulting in increased intraocular pressure as a result of decreased aqueous humor outflow. Autosomal recessive. Associated with conditions such as congenital rubella, neurofibromatosis, Sturge-Weber syndrome (facial port-wine stain, seizures, central nervous system [CNS] calcifications), chromosomal abnormalities, and retinopathy of prematurity.

- **Management**
  Surgery.

3. Congenital Cataracts

- **H&P Keys**
  Unilateral or bilateral opacification of the lens. Signs and symptoms include decreased visual attentiveness, light sensitivity, decreased vision, and opacification of the lens.

- **Diagnosis**
  Ophthalmologic exam. Ocular ultrasonography. Rule out associated systemic conditions.

- **Disease Severity**
  Varies by the degree of opacification. Blindness. Amblyopia.

- **Concept and Application**
  Often idiopathic but may have an autosomal dominant inheritance pattern. May occur as part of a systemic disease including intrauterine infections (rubella, cytomegalovirus [CMV]), metabolic diseases (galactosemia), syndromes (Marfan, Alport), or be associated with chromosomal disorders (trisomies).

- **Management**
  Surgical removal of lens.

4. Congenital Deafness

- **H&P Keys**
  Conductive (abnormal sound transmission to the middle ear) or sensorineural (poorly functioning auditory nerve) hearing disorders. Signs and symptoms include delay in language skills, poor attentiveness.

- **Diagnosis**
  Clinical suspicion (especially by caretaker). Brainstem Auditory Evoked Response potentials (BAER). Audiology assessment.

- **Disease Severity**
  Depends on etiology.

- **Concept and Application**
  Genetic (dominant, recessive, or X-linked). Ototoxic drugs. Congenital infection (CMV, rubella). Prematurity (low birthweight). Associated with many syndromes (Pierre Robin, Treacher-Collins, Crouzon, Waardenburg [white forelock] and Alport [nephritis]).

- **Management**
  Early amplification. Surgical implants. Sign language. Social support.

II. RHEUMATOLOGY

A. Henoch-Schönlein Purpura

Buttock lower ext [handwritten]

- **H&P Keys**
  1-7 [handwritten]
  Small-vessel vasculitis occurring in children ages 1 to 7 years. Signs and symptoms include abdominal pain, rash, vomiting, hematemesis, and joint pain. Purpura, most commonly found on the buttocks and lower extremities, is the first sign in >50% of cases. Patients may also have fever, gastrointestinal (GI) bleeding, intussusception (3%), and hematuria.

- **Diagnosis**
  No pathognomonic laboratory tests. Normal platelet count and coagulation studies. Mild increase in erythrocyte sedimentation rate (ESR). Elevation of serum IgA and IgM in 50% of cases. Skin lesions show leukocytoclastic vasculitis.

- **Disease Severity**
  Morbidity and mortality related to the extent of GI or kidney involvement. May lead to GI hemorrhage, intussusception, or end-stage renal disease.

- **Concept and Application**
  Leukocytoclastic vasculitis often involving the synovium, GI tract, or renal glomerulus. An immune-complex disease (IgA-involved).

- **Management**
  Supportive care. Corticosteroids (if GI hemorrhage).

B. Kawasaki Disease

- **H&P Keys**
  Fever of 5 or more days associated with at least four of the following: bilateral conjunctival injection, nonsuppurative cervical lymphadenopathy, rash, mucous membrane changes (strawberry tongue, erythema of the lips or oropharynx), extremity changes (edema, erythema).

- **Diagnosis**
  Clinical presentation. Findings may include an elevated white blood cell (WBC) count with a left-shift, elevated ESR and C-reactive protein (CRP), pyuria, uveitis, hydrops of the gallbladder, thrombocytosis (second week of illness), desquamation of the hands and feet.

- **Concept and Application**
  Etiology unknown.

- **Disease Severity**
  Aneurysms of the coronary arteries and other large arteries. Electrocardiographic (ECG) changes.

- **Management**
  Intravenous gammaglobulin. Aspirin.

III. GENITOURINARY SYSTEM

A. Hypospadias

- **H&P Keys**
  Urethral meatus located proximal to its normal position at the tip of the glans (any point along the course of the anterior urethra from the perineum to the tip of the glans). Abnormal urinary stream.

- **Diagnosis**
  Clinical presentation.

- **Disease Severity**
  Dependent on the location.

- **Concept and Application**
  Failure of the urethral folds to fuse completely over the urethral groove.

- **Management**
  Surgical correction. Avoid circumcision (foreskin used in repair).

B. Posterior Urethral Valves

- **H&P Keys**
  Most common cause of anatomic bladder outlet obstruction in male children. Signs and symptoms include a poor urinary stream, dribbling, absence of voiding, ab-

dominal distention, vomiting, and failure to thrive.

- **Diagnosis**
Voiding cystourethrogram.

- **Disease Severity**
Chronic renal failure. Hydronephrosis.

- **Concept and Application**
Mucosal folds obstruct the posterior urethra.

- **Management**
Early surgical repair.

C. Prune-Belly Syndrome (Eagle-Barret Syndrome)

- **H&P Keys**
Male infant with deficiency of the abdominal wall musculature, urinary tract abnormalities, and bilateral intra-abdominal testes. Signs and symptoms include marked laxity of the abdomen with bulging of the flanks.

- **Diagnosis**
Clinical presentation. Urologic evaluation. Renal ultrasonography (dilated urinary tract).

- **Disease Severity**
Urinary tract infection. End-stage renal disease.

- **Concept and Application**
Etiology unknown.

- **Management**
Monitoring for urinary tract infections and signs of renal failure. Correction of electrolyte imbalances. Vitamin D supplementation (prevent hypocalcemia and renal osteodystrophy).

D. Vesicoureteral Reflux

- **H&P Keys**
Often asymptomatic. May develop features of urinary tract infection (fever, vomiting, flank pain, dysuria, frequency, urgency, irritability).

- **Diagnosis**
Voiding cystourethrogram.

- **Disease Severity**
Renal scarring. Pyelonephritis.

- **Concept and Application**
Abnormal backflow of urine from the bladder into the ureters or kidneys. Increased incidence of reflux in siblings.

- **Management**
Management depends on grade of reflux and the amount of renal scarring. Medical management includes treatment of the urinary tract infection and prophylactic antibiotics. Surgical correction of the anatomic defect if severe reflux or scarring.

E. Infantile Polycystic Disease

- **H&P Keys**
Signs and symptoms include enlarged palpable kidneys, oliguria, and respiratory insufficiency in the neonate. Older infants may present with hepatosplenomegaly, flank masses, renal tubular acidosis, and hypertension.

- **Diagnosis**
Renal ultrasonography.

- **Disease Severity**
Renal insufficiency. Hypertension. Portal hypertension. Hepatic fibrosis. Variable cortical atrophy.

- **Concept and Application**
Bilateral renal cystic disease. Autosomal recessive inheritance.

- **Management**
Treatment of hypertension. Management of chronic renal failure and portal hypertension.

F. Multicystic Kidney Disease

- **H&P Keys**
A unilateral, dysplastic, nonfunctioning kidney. Usually an asymptomatic abdominal mass.

- **Diagnosis**
Renal ultrasonography.

- **Management**
Kidney not routinely removed.

G. Undescended Testis

- **H&P Keys**
  Nonpalpable testis.

- **Diagnosis**
  Clinical exam. Ultrasonography (location of testis).

- **Disease Severity**
  More prone to testicular torsion, malignant degeneration, and impaired fertility.

- **Concept and Application**
  Result of mechanical hindrance, abnormal epididymal development, or endocrine dysfunction during fetal development.

- **Management**
  Hormonal therapy. Surgical orchiopexy before aged 2 years.

H. Bladder Extrophy

- **H&P Keys**
  Externalization of the bladder and epispadias.

- **Diagnosis**
  Clinical presentation.

- **Disease Severity**
  Repair depends on the capacity of the bladder.

- **Concept and Application**
  Failure of the abdominal wall to close inferior to the umbilicus with separation of the pubis symphysis. This anomaly leads to evulsion and protuberance of the posterior bladder wall.

- **Management**
  Surgery.

IV. NEONATOLOGY

A. Transient Tachypnea of the Newborn (TTN)

- **H&P Keys**
  Mild self-limited respiratory disorder seen more frequently in infants born by cesarean section. Signs and symptoms include increased respiratory rate, mild cyanosis, and retractions.

- **Diagnosis**
  Chest roentgenogram (CXR) shows prominent vascular markings with fluid in the fissures. Diagnosis of exclusion.

- **Disease Severity**
  Respiratory rate. Cyanosis. ABG. Pulse oximetry.

- **Concept and Application**
  Delayed resorption of fetal lung fluid.

- **Management**
  Supportive care. Oxygen. Parenteral fluids.

B. Respiratory Distress Syndrome

- **H&P Keys**
  Incidence inversely proportional to the newborn's gestational age and birthweight. Signs and symptoms include respiratory distress (tachypnea, grunting, nasal flaring, retractions) soon after delivery.

- **Diagnosis**
  CXR shows a fine reticular granularity of the lung fields and air bronchograms. Must differentiate from other causes of respiratory distress in newborns (sepsis, heart disease, CNS disorders, lung anomalies).

- **Disease Severity**
  ABG. Pulse oximetry. Hemoglobin. Metabolic disturbances. Cardiovascular compromise. Long-term complications include bronchopulmonary dysplasia (BPD), cor pulmonale, retinopathy of prematurity, poor growth, and persistent patent ductus arteriosus.

- **Concept and Application**
  Secondary to lung immaturity (surfactant deficiency), incomplete structural lung development, and highly compliant chest wall. Results in atelectasis, hyaline membrane formation, and pulmonary edema.

- **Management**
  Prevention of prematurity. Maternal steroid administration 48 to 72 hours prior to delivery to stimulate fetal surfactant production. Neonatal surfactant via endotracheal

tube at delivery for premature infants (surfactant serves to reduce surface tension of the alveoli). Supportive care (correction of hypoxia, acidosis, and hypercapnia).

C. Meconium Aspiration

- **H&P Keys**
  Presence of meconium in the amniotic fluid and the newborn's trachea. Signs and symptoms include retractions, increased respiratory rate, cyanosis, and hypoxia.

- **Diagnosis**
  Clinical presentation. CXR.

- **Disease Severity**
  Severe respiratory distress with increased respiratory rate, retractions, and hypoxia requiring ventilatory support. Pneumothorax. Pulmonary hypertension.

- **Concept and Application**
  Aspiration of meconium-contaminated amniotic fluid leading to airway obstruction and poor gas exchange.

- **Management**
  Suctioning the infant on the perineum. Direct visualization and suctioning of the trachea. Chest physiotherapy. Supplemental oxygen. Mechanical ventilation if needed.

D. Rh Incompatibility

- **H&P Keys**
  Infant of a gravida 2 Rh-negative mother. Signs and symptoms include pallor, respiratory distress, cardiomegaly, edema.

- **Diagnosis**
  Rh type, ABO group, Coomb test (positive), hemoglobin, blood smear (hemolysis), reticulocyte count (increased), and bilirubin (increased).

- **Disease Severity**
  Hydrops fetalis. Severe anemia leading to heart failure, ascites, pleural and pericardial effusions. Thrombocytopenia. Organ-

omegaly. Elevated bilirubin leading to kernicterus (staining of the basal ganglia).

- **Concept and Application**
  Sensitization and antibody formation in an Rh-negative mother exposed to Rh-positive fetal blood (contains D antigen). This antibody crosses the placenta causing hemolytic disease in the fetus. Rarely occurs during the first pregnancy.

- **Management**
  Supportive therapy, including volume expansion, red blood cell (RBC) transfusion, and ventilatory support if needed. Exchange transfusion. Prevention in Rh-negative mothers with the administration of $Rh_o(D)$ immune globulin (RhoGAM).

E. Neonatal Hyperbilirubinemia

- **H&P Keys**
  Signs and symptoms depend on the etiology. Ascertain a maternal history (blood type, race, illnesses during pregnancy, drug usage, family history of anemia), and an infant history (birth weight, onset of jaundice, stooling pattern, trauma, feeding pattern [breast feeding], emesis).

- **Diagnosis**
  Total and direct bilirubin (normal total levels rise to a mean of 6.5 ± 2.5 mg/dL in a full-term formula-fed infant). Hemoglobin, smear, reticulocyte count, maternal and infant blood type, direct Coomb (evidence of hemolysis, albumin level). Urine Clinitest. Culture if sepsis is suspected.

- **Disease Severity**
  Elevated bilirubin in the first 24 hours of life is pathologic. Kernicterus (bilirubin staining and necrosis of neurons in the basal ganglion) especially with hemolytic disease.

- **Concept and Application**
  Physiologic jaundice is found in 60% of newborns with maximum values reached in the second to fourth day (6 to 8 mg/dL) as a result of inefficient bilirubin conju-

gation and excretion. Jaundice due to breast feeding reaches a maximum level of 7.3 ± 3.9 mg/dL. The etiology is unknown. Elevated levels of bilirubin also occur with increased turnover of RBCs from hemolysis (ABO or Rh incompatibility), significant bruising, cephalohematomas, structural or metabolic abnormalities of RBCs, or hereditary defects of bilirubin conjugation (Crigler-Najjar syndrome, Gilbert disease).

- **Management**
Treatment of the underlying etiology. Phototherapy. Exchange transfusion.

F. Congenital Hip Dysplasia

- **H&P Keys**
A higher incidence with breech deliveries, first-born children, and oligohydramnios. Left hip more commonly involved. Twenty percent have a positive family history. Signs and symptoms include Barlow sign (posterosuperior movement of the femur over the limbus with adduction and posteriorly directed pressure), Ortolani sign (relocation of the hip with abduction, causing a dull clunk), asymmetric leg lengths, and asymmetric thigh creases. A limitation of abduction is seen in older infants.

- **Diagnosis**
Clinical exam. Hip ultrasonogram. Radiography.

- **Disease Severity**
Three degrees of hip dysplasia in order of increasing severity: subluxable, dislocatable, dislocated. Can lead to avascular necrosis and decreased range of motion.

- **Concept and Application**
Multifactorial (mechanical, hormonal, and hereditary).

- **Management**
Goal is to restore contact between the femoral head and the acetabulum. Management depends on the degree of hip dysplasia and the age at diagnosis. Harness. Closed reduction (traction). Open reduction.

V. INFECTIOUS DISEASES

A. Bronchiolitis

- **H&P Keys**
Common (60% of infants). Winter-to-spring months. Peak age under 24 months. Signs and symptoms include cough, rhinorrhea, with or without low-grade fever, scattered wheezing, with or without rales, labored breathing.

- **Diagnosis**
Clinical features (age, season, physical). Evaluation of nasopharyngeal secretions (viral culture, enzyme-linked immunosorbent assay, or immunofluorescence). CXR has nonspecific changes (hyperinflation, atelectasis, with or without interstitial infiltrates).

- **Disease Severity**
General appearance, mental status changes, labored breathing (tachypnea, nasal flaring, retractions, accessory muscle use), cyanosis, pulse oximetry, ABG if severe distress. Higher morbidity and mortality if infant has underlying pulmonary or cardiac disease, immunodeficiency disease, underlying chronic disease, history of prematurity, or is under 6 weeks old.

- **Concept and Application**
Viral infection (primary cause is respiratory syncytial virus) of lower respiratory tract. Transmission by direct contact. Respiratory mucosal injury, inflammation or edema, mucous production.

- **Management**
Supportive care. Aerosolized β_2-adrenergic agent. Oxygen (if hypoxemia). Ribavirin nebulizer (for severe respiratory distress or higher risk groups). Questionable steroid role. Prevention by hand washing.

B. Otitis Media

- **H&P Keys**
Peak age under 24 months. Winter season. Signs and symptoms include pain, fever, hearing loss, cough, and congestion as well as hyperemia, dullness, decreased mobility,

retraction or bulging (loss of landmarks) of tympanic membrane. Asymptomatic in 50% of cases.

- **Diagnosis**
Pneumatic otoscopy. Tympanometry. Audiometry.

- **Disease Severity**
Overall appearance. Degree of discomfort or hearing loss. Response to therapy. Higher morbidity if young age (<6 months), environmental setting (passive smoking, day care), genetic factors (familial, trisomy 21, Native American), immunodeficiency, congenital anomalies (cleft palate, choanal atresia).

- **Concept and Application**
Bacterial infection (usually *Streptococcus pneumoniae*, nontypable *Haemophilus influenzae*, *Moraxella catarrhalis*) of middle ear. Viral co-pathogens (40%). Often results from a dysfunctional eustachian tube.

- **Management**
First-line antibiotics include aminopenicillins and sulfonamides. Prophylactic antibiotics if recurrent episodes (≥3 bouts in 6 months, ≥4 in 12 months). Consider myringotomy tubes if persistent effusion with hearing loss, failure of prophylaxis, or high-risk groups (eg, trisomy 21, cleft palate, known sensorineural hearing loss).

C. Epiglottitis (Supraglottitis)

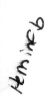

- **H&P Keys**
Ages 2 to 7 years. Winter months. Signs and symptoms include acute hyperpyrexia (39°C), hoarseness, drooling, dysphagia, anxious or toxic appearance, stridor, and respiratory distress.

- **Diagnosis**
Clinical presentation (high index of suspicion!). Lateral neck radiograph (thumb-shaped epiglottis, ballooning of hypopharynx) only if presentation not classical. Cultures of epiglottis and blood after airway secured.

- **Disease Severity**
Overall appearance. Mental status changes. Respiratory distress (tachypnea, inspiratory stridor, retractions, cyanosis). Hypoxia and hypercapnia.

- **Concept and Application**
Edema or cellulitis of epiglottis resulting in glottic narrowing. Primarily *Haemophilus influenzae* type b (>90%).

- **Management**
Early suspicion. Minimal disturbance to child. Supportive care (especially of airway). Direct visualization and culture of epiglottis in operating room followed by intubation. Emergent cricothyrotomy if complete airway obstruction. Prevention is key (*H. influenzae* type b vaccine).

D. Laryngotracheitis (Croup) parainfluenza

- **H&P Keys**
Ages 6 to 36 months. Nocturnal. Severity of disease peaks at 3 to 5 days. Signs and symptoms include barklike cough, hoarseness, upper respiratory symptoms, inspiratory stridor.

- **Diagnosis**
Clinical presentation. Steeple sign (subglottic swelling) on CXR.

- **Disease Severity**
Overall appearance. Mental status changes. Respiratory distress. Hypoxia and hypercapnia.

- **Concept and Application**
Mucosal edema and swelling of subglottis and trachea leading to hypoxia and atelectasis. Primarily caused by parainfluenza virus.

- **Management**
Supportive (especially airway). Minimal disturbance. Mist. Oxygen if hypoxemia. Racemic epinephrine or dexamethasone if severe respiratory distress.

E. Varicella (Chicken Pox)

- **H&P Keys**
Intubation period of 14 to 15 days. Winter or spring months. Contagious period is 4 to 5

days prior to exanthem and until rash scabs. Signs and symptoms include fever, malaise, vesicles with erythematous base ("tear drop on rose petal") beginning on hairline or trunk and spreading to extremities.

- **Diagnosis**
Characteristic rash. Fluorescein monoclonal antibody.

- **Disease Severity**
Worse course if under 1 year of age, teenager or adult, or visceral involvement (lungs, CNS, liver, joints, heart, kidneys).

- **Concept and Application**
Human herpes varicella-zoster virus. Respiratory (direct contact) transmission. Cutaneous tissue involvement after primary or secondary viremia.

- **Management**
Supportive (antipruritic drug). No aspirin (possibility of Reye's syndrome). Antimicrobial therapy if secondary infection (usually group A *Streptococcus*). Acyclovir if child is immunocompromised, older, or severely involved. Life-long immunity after infection. New vaccine available for prevention.

F. Pharyngitis

- **H&P Keys**
Signs and symptoms include fever, sore throat, hoarseness, cough, abdominal pain, tonsillar erythema or enlargement or exudate, petechiae of palate, anterior cervical adenopathy, "sandpaper" rash. Concomitant nasal symptoms suggest viral etiology.

- **Diagnosis**
Throat culture. Rapid streptococcus antigen test (less sensitive).

- **Disease Severity**
Clinical discomfort. Suppurative complications (cervical adenitis, otitis media, septicemia). Nonsuppurative complications (rheumatic fever, nephritis).

- **Concept and Application**
Cellulitis of pharynx and tonsils. Organisms include group A β-hemolytic streptococci,

adenovirus, influenza virus, Epstein-Barr virus.

- **Management**
Self-limiting if viral etiology. Penicillin (erythromycin if penicillin allergy) for 10 days if group A β-hemolytic streptococci.

G. Bacterial Meningitis

- **H&P Keys**
Signs and symptoms include fever, lethargy, irritability, neck stiffness or pain, headache, altered consciousness, nuchal rigidity, Kernig's sign, Brudzinski's sign.

- **Diagnosis**
Bacterial culture of CSF is gold standard. CSF cytology and biochemical parameters. Bacterial antigen test if child currently on antibiotics.

- **Disease Severity**
Mental status change. Focal or persistent neurologic deficit. Syndrome of inappropriate secretion of antidiuretic hormone (SIADH). Neonatal infection. Focal or late-onset seizures. Long-term sequelae include learning disability, hearing impairment, seizure disorders.

- **Concept and Application**
Primarily hematogenous spread to CSF. *H. influenzae* type b, *S. pneumoniae*, *Neisseria meningitidis* are usual pathogens in childhood (group B streptococcus, *Escherichia coli*, or other gram-negative enteric bacilli, *Listeria monocytogenes* in neonates).

- **Management**
Age-specific antibiotics pending cultures. Respiratory isolation. Identification and treatment of associated complications if necessary. Prevention (vaccine, treatment of carrier state). Dexamethasone (> age 2 months).

H. Congenital Infections ("Torch")

1. Congenital Toxoplasmosis

- **H&P Keys**
Characteristic features include chorioretinitis, scattered CNS calcifications, hydrocephalus, developmental delay.

- **Diagnosis**
Serology (organism isolation).

- **Concept and Application**
Intracellular protozoan parasite (*Toxoplasma gondii*).

- **Management**
Multidisciplinary approach. Pyrimethamine and/or sulfadiazine have variable effectiveness. Prevention (avoid cat litter and undercooked meat).

2. Congenital Rubella Infection (German Measles)

Blueberry muffin

- **H&P Keys**
Characteristic features include intrauterine growth retardation (IUGR), congenital cardiac defects, cataracts, deafness, thrombocytopenia, "blueberry muffin" skin lesions, hepatosplenomegaly.

- **Diagnosis**
Serology (organism isolation).

- **Concept and Application**
Multiorgan damage by the virus.

- **Management**
Multidisciplinary approach. Vaccination and prenatal screening have decreased the incidence.

3. Congenital Cytomegalovirus Infection

- **H&P Keys**
Majority of cases are asymptomatic. Characteristic features include jaundice, hepatosplenomegaly, microcephaly, chorioretinitis, deafness, periventricular CNS calcification, IUGR.

- **Diagnosis**
Organism isolation (serology).

- **Concept and Application**
Herpes virus. Multiorgan involvement. Transmission with primary or recurrent maternal infection.

- **Management**
Multidisciplinary approach. No proven antiviral treatment. Prevention by hand washing.

4. Herpes Simplex Virus

- **H&P Keys**
Incidence of HSV 1/5000 deliveries. Characteristic features include vesicular skin rash, chorioretinitis, meningoencephalitis, seizures, microcephaly.

- **Diagnosis**
Organism isolation (Tzanck test, immunofluorescent studies).

- **Concept and Application**
HSV 2 (70%). Transmission more likely during primary maternal infection.

- **Management**
Antiviral (acyclovir) therapy. Supportive.

5. Human Immunodeficiency Virus

- **H&P Keys**
One third of infants of HIV-positive mothers will develop AIDS. Presentation variable (eg, frequent infections, developmental or growth delay, lymphadenopathy, persistent thrush).

- **Diagnosis**
Serology (Western Blot not useful under age 15 months secondary to presence of maternal antibody). Immune markers. Organism isolation.

- **Concept and Application**
Human retrovirus that infects tissue cells (including helper T cells).

- **Management**
Azidothymidine (AZT). Antimicrobial therapy for infections. Poor prognosis.

6. Congenital Syphilis

- **H&P Keys**
Characteristic features include skin rash (palms and soles), hepatosplenomegaly, sniffles (blood-tinged nasal discharge), Parrot's pseudoparalysis (periostitis), saber shins, Hutchinson (peg) teeth, thrombocytopenia, anemia, jaundice, saddle nose, hepatitis.

- **Diagnosis**
Serology (rapid plasma reagin [RPR], fluorescent treponemal antibody absorption

[FTA-ABS]), darkfield examination (organism).

- **Concept and Application**
Spirochete (*Treponema pallidum*).

- **Management**
Prenatal screening. Penicillin for all infected mothers and infants with positive serology without documented adequate treatment.

I. Hemolytic Uremic Syndrome

- **H&P Keys**
Children usually between 2 months and 8 years of age. Triad of uremia, thrombocytopenia, and microangiopathic hemolytic anemia. Signs and symptoms include preceding illness (diarrhea or upper respiratory infection [URI]), irritability, bloody diarrhea, poor urinary output, pallor, petechiae, edema, hypertension.

- **Diagnosis**
CBC with platelets and smear (RBC morphology). Coombs test (negative). Electrolytes.

- **Disease Severity**
Seizures, stroke, coma, cardiac failure, metabolic imbalance (metabolic acidosis).

- **Concept and Application**
No one causative factor (viral, bacterial, drugs). Peripheral destruction of platelets. RBC hemolysis secondary to mechanical destruction by fibrin strands in small renal vessels.

- **Management**
Supportive care. Correction of fluid and electrolyte imbalance and hypertension. Dialysis and RBC transfusion if needed.

VI. GASTROENTEROLOGY

A. Cleft Lip or Palate

- **H&P Keys**
Common (1/1000 live births). Family history.

- **Diagnosis**
Clinical.

- **Disease Severity**
Feeding problems. Frequent ear infections. Speech problems. Associated with many anomalies.

- **Concept and Application**
Failure of primary (lip) and secondary (cleft) palate closure. Multifactorial inheritance (3% to 5% recurrence with an affected parent or sibling; 10% if two affected parents or siblings).

- **Management**
Multidisciplinary approach. Surgical repair.

B. Tracheoesophageal Fistula (TEF)

- **H&P Keys**
Signs and symptoms of TEF include excessive oral secretions, coughing or choking on foods, tachypnea, wheezing, rales.

- **Diagnosis**
Inability to pass nasal catheter to stomach. Surgical exploration. Barium studies rarely needed.

- **Disease Severity**
Respiratory distress. Signs and symptoms of aspiration pneumonia.

- **Concept and Application**
Failure of trachea and esophagus to separate during embryogenesis. Proximal esophageal atresia with a tracheal-to-distal esophageal fistula is most common type (85%).

- **Management**
Surgery.

C. Pyloric Stenosis   *3-4wk nonbilious*

- **H&P Keys**
Average age 3 to 4 weeks of life. First-born males. Signs and symptoms include progressive nonbilious projectile emesis, peristaltic abdominal waves in epigastrium, palpable right upper quadrant mass ("olive").

- **Diagnosis**
Clinical. Sonogram or upper GI (UGI) series ("tram-track" sign) if necessary. Hypochloremic metabolic alkalosis.

- **Disease Severity**
  Cachexia. Profound dehydration. Severe metabolic imbalance.

- **Concept and Application**
  Mechanical gastric outlet obstruction results from congenitally hypertrophied pyloric muscle.

- **Management**
  Correction of fluid and electrolyte abnormality. Surgical repair (pyloromyotomy).

D. Malrotation of the Small Intestine

- **H&P Keys**
  Bilious projectile emesis. Abdominal distention.

- **Diagnosis**
  Clinical. Barium study.

- **Disease Severity**
  Melena (secondary to intestinal ischemia). Sepsis. Signs and symptoms of peritonitis or perforation.

- **Concept and Application**
  Mechanical obstruction from either poor fixation of cecum to abdominal wall (midgut volvulus or twisting) or extrinsic bands.

- **Management**
  Surgery (15% to 20% mortality rate).

E. Intussusception

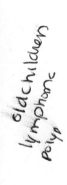
old children
lymphatic
polyp

- **H&P Keys**
  Most common cause of intestinal obstruction ages 3 to 12 months. Signs and symptoms include intermittent colicky pain, bilious emesis, mental status changes, palpable "sausage-shaped" abdominal mass, "currant jelly" stools.

- **Diagnosis**
  Clinical. Barium enema.

- **Disease Severity**
  Severe metabolic acidosis. Evidence of intestinal ischemia or infarction. Severe dehydration.

- **Concept and Application**
  Invagination or telescoping of proximal bowel into more distal bowel. Lymphatic and venous compromise. Primarily ileocolic region. Leadpoint lesion (eg, polyp, lymphoma) in older children.

- **Management**
  Gastric aspiration and fluid resuscitation. Barium enema reduction. Antibiotics if peritoneal signs. Occasionally surgical reduction.

F. Necrotizing Enterocolitis (NEC)

- **H&P Keys**
  Characteristic features of NEC include prematurity (75%), poor feeding or regurgitation, emesis, hematochezia, temperature instability, gastric retention, abdominal distention with decreased breath sounds.

- **Diagnosis**
  Clinical. Blood or reducing substances in stool. Thrombocytopenia. Prolonged prothrombin time (PT) and partial thrombin time (PTT). Pneumatosis intestinalis, bowel wall edema, biliary air, or free air in peritoneum on abdominal radiograph.

- **Disease Severity**
  Evidence of sepsis, hemorrhage, disseminated intravascular coagulation (DIC), shock, severe metabolic acidosis, mental status changes.

- **Concept and Application**
  Unknown. Presentation consistent with bowel ischemia or infarction.

- **Management**
  Bowel rest. Fluid resuscitation or parenteral nutrition. Broad-spectrum antibiotics. Surgery if failure of medical management or if complications.

G. Colonic Aganglionosis (Hirschsprung Disease)

- **H&P Keys**
  Absence of meconium stools in first week of life. Signs and symptoms include emesis, abdominal distention, minimal stool in rectal vault.

- **Diagnosis**
  Clinical. Rectal biopsy. Barium study in older children.

- **Disease Severity**
  Presentation can simulate sepsis or NEC.

- **Concept and Application**
  Absence of colonic ganglia resulting in persistent colonic contraction.

- **Management**
  Surgery.

VII. GENETICS

A. Down Syndrome (Trisomy 21)

- **H&P Keys**
  Characteristic features include epicanthal folds, upslanting palpebral fissures, transverse palmar (simian) creases, cardiac anomalies (40%) including septal defects, atlantoaxial instability (12%), duodenal atresia (4% to 7%), short stature, leukemia (1%), thyroid disease, sterility in males, early Alzheimer's disease.

- **Diagnosis**
  Clinical. Chromosome analysis (classical trisomy [95%], translocation [4%], mosaic [1%]). Prenatal screening (amniocentesis, chorionic villus sampling) in high-risk groups (advanced maternal age).

- **Management**
  Supportive. Special education. Genetic counseling. Correction of anomalies. Mortality usually result of cardiac disease. Shortened lifespan.

B. Trisomy 18

- **H&P Keys**
  Characteristic features include IUGR, micrognathia, clenched hands with overlapping fingers, congenital heart disease (ventricular septal defect [VSD], patent ductus arteriosus [PDA]), mental retardation.

- **Diagnosis**
  Clinical. Chromosome analysis.

- **Management**
  Genetic counseling. Poor prognosis. Mortality usually by age 3 months. Recurrence <1%.

C. Trisomy 13

- **H&P Keys**
  Characteristic features include cleft lip or palate (60% to 80%), microcephaly, urinary tract malformations, CNS and ocular malformations, aplasia cutis congenita, polydactyly.

- **Diagnosis**
  Clinical. Chromosome analysis.

- **Management**
  Same as for trisomy 18.

D. Gonadal Dysgenesis 45,XO (Turner Syndrome)

[handwritten: COARCT, Horseshoe kidney]

- **H&P Keys**
  Characteristic features include transient lymphedema of feet and hands at birth (80% to 90%), short stature, short webbed neck, short fourth metacarpal bone, cardiac defects (coarctation of aorta), renal anomalies (horseshoe kidney), lack of secondary sex characteristics with primary amenorrhea. Normal intelligence. Most spontaneously abort in early pregnancy.

- **Diagnosis**
  Clinical. Chromosome analysis.

- **Management**
  Correction of anomalies. Psychosocial counseling. Estrogen replacement at puberty. Consider growth hormone therapy.

E. Fragile X Syndrome

- **H&P Keys**
  Characteristic features include mental retardation (MR), hyperactivity, seizures, prominent ears, long face, macroorchidism. Common cause of MR in males (1/1000).

- **Diagnosis**
  Chromosome analysis with fragile X studies.

- **Management**
  Genetic counseling. Supportive.

VIII. PULMONOLOGY

A. Congenital Laryngeal Stridor (Laryngomalacia)

- **H&P Keys**
  Signs and symptoms include noisy "crowing" respirations (positional) and stridor.

- **Diagnosis**
  Clinical. Fluoroscopy or direct visualization.

- **Disease Severity**
  Respiratory distress (tachypnea, retractions, poor air movement).

- **Concept and Application**
  Delayed maturation of newborn larynx, resulting in increased flexibility.

- **Management**
  Self-limited.

B. Congenital Lobar Emphysema

- **H&P Keys**
  Most common congenital lung lesion. Respiratory distress in early infancy.

- **Diagnosis**
  Chest radiograph (radiolucent lobe, mediastinal shift). Mimics pneumothorax.

- **Disease Severity**
  Severe respiratory distress or cyanosis.

- **Concept and Application**
  In utero bronchial obstruction with normal alveolar histology. Usually unilateral.

- **Management**
  Surgical resection.

C. Cystic Adenomatoid Malformation

- **H&P Keys**
  Respiratory distress in infancy.

- **Diagnosis**
  Chest radiograph (mediastinal shift, multiple cystic areas). Mimics diaphragmatic hernia.

- **Concept and Application**
  Early embryonic insult with cysts and little normal lung tissue.

- **Management**
  Surgical resection. Significant mortality and morbidity.

D. Pulmonary Sequestration

- **H&P Keys**
  Fever, hemoptysis, and respiratory symptoms if intralobar. Respiratory symptoms, heart failure, or no symptoms if extralobar. Dullness to percussion. Heart murmur.

- **Diagnosis**
  CXR (mass). Further investigation includes bronchoscopy, sonogram, and aortogram.

- **Concept and Application**
  Segments of nonfunctioning embryonic lung tissue that are nourished by anomalous systemic circulation. Intralobar type occurs within normal visceral pleura. Extralobar type has separate visceral pleural covering.

- **Management**
  Surgical resection.

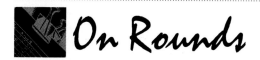

Pediatric Infections

Croup

- Ages 6–36 months, also termed "laryngo-tracheitis"
- Bark-like cough, hoarseness, inspiratory stridor, CXR positive Steeple sign (sub-glottic swelling)
- Worse at night
- Supportive treatment, mist, O_2

Epiglottitis

- Ages 2–7
- Fever, drooling, dysphagia, stridor, may have abnormal lateral neck roentgeno-gram, possible toxic appearance, anxious
- Winter most often
- Support airway, visualization in OR followed by intubation

Bronchiolitis

- Peak age under 2
- Cough, wheezing, labored breathing, non-specific CXR
- Winter to spring occurrence
- Supportive treatment

BIBLIOGRAPHY

Behrman RE, Kliegman RM, Nelson WE, et al. *Nelson Textbook of Pediatrics*. 14th ed. Philadelphia: WB Saunders Co; 1992.

Cloherty JP, Stark AR. *Manual of Neonatal Care*. 2nd ed. Boston: Little Brown & Co; 1985.

Goldberg JS. *Instant Exam Review for the USMLE Step 2*. Norwalk, CT: Appleton & Lange; 1993.

Howie VM. Otitis media. *Pediatr Rev.* 1993;14:320–23.

Oski FA, DeAngelis CD, Feigin RD, et al. *Principles and Practice of Pediatrics*. 2nd ed. Philadelphia: JB Lippincott; 1994.

Pohl CA. Practical approach to bacterial meningitis in children. *Am Fam Physician.* 1993;47:1595–1603.

Rudolph AM, Hoffman JI. *Pediatrics*. 18th ed. Norwalk, CT: Appleton & Lange; 1987.

Welliver JR, Welliver RC. Bronchiolitis. *Pediatr Rev.* 1993; 14:134–39.

15

Psychiatry

Amy Brodkey, MD

I. PSYCHOSES

A. Schizophrenia

- **H&P Keys**

History. Family history; onset most often late teens through twenties, often triggered by stressful situation; increased in lower socioeconomic groups; may have premorbid schizotypal features; symptom duration at least 6 months.

Physical and Mental Status Exam. Hallucinations, delusions, formal thought disorder, bizarre behavior; agitated, constricted, and/or inappropriate affect; social withdrawal; poor self-care; may have soft neurologic signs, motoric abnormalities.

- **Diagnosis**
  No pathognomonic signs or lab studies; rule out general medical etiology (eg, substance abuse, temporal lobe epilepsy, medications, central nervous system [CNS] infections, trauma, tumors, endocrine and metabolic disorders); psychotic affective, schizoaffective, delusional, personality disorders; obtain medical history, physical and neurologic exams, routine labs, thyroid function tests (TFTs), serology, human immunodeficiency virus (HIV), toxicology, B_{12}, folate; electroencephalogram (EEG), brain imaging indicated with first episode, unusual presentation (eg, older age, rapid onset of new symptoms, visual or olfactory hallucinations, focal neurologic signs).

- **Disease Severity**
  Worse prognosis with poor premorbid social history, early onset, insidious onset, absence of mood symptoms, neurologic abnormalities, male gender, negative symptoms (flat affect, anhedonia, poverty of speech, low motivation, social withdrawal). Course is variable, often deteriorating. Early treatment of psychosis improves prognosis. Exacerbations associated with medication

noncompliance (50% in first year), high levels of criticism and hostility in families ("expressed emotion"). Increased risk for medical illness, incarceration, victimization, poverty, suicide (10%).

• **Concept and Application**

Dopamine hypothesis: schizophrenia associated with mesolimbic and mesocortical hyperdopaminergic activity (antipsychotic efficacy function of adaptives response to dopamine receptor blockade). Negative symptoms associated with enlargement of cerebral ventricles and cortical atrophy. Functional neuroimaging demonstrates hypofrontality. Twin and adoption studies support both (polygenic) genetic and environmental contributions.

• **Management**

Acute. Hospitalization for diagnosis, stabilization, protection of self and others (may require involuntary commitment); benzodiazepines for acute agitation; neuroleptics: titrate slowly with low initial dose; require 4 to 6 weeks for full effect; observes for development of acute dystonic reactions in hours to days, pseudo-Parkinsonism in days to weeks, akathisia in weeks to months; treated with anticholinergics, eg, benztropine; dose reduction; switch to lower potency neuroleptic; akathisia also treated with benzodiazepines, β-blockers. Risperidone may cause less extrapyramidal symptoms (EPS) clozapine indicated for retractor symptoms (weekly complete blood count [CBC] to rule out agranulocylosis).

Continued Care. Continuation of neuroleptics (oral or long-acting intramuscular) reduces relapse rate; assess for development of side effects, eg, tardive dyskinesia (15% to 20% prevalence); anticholinergic effects, sexual dysfunction, weight gain; addition of lithium, anticonvulsants, benzodiazepines may benefit some; residual nonresponders (15% to 30%) may respond to clozapine; family education, social skills training, residential and day treatment, vocational rehabilitation, supportive psychotherapy.

B. Affective Psychoses: Mania and Psychotic Depression

• **H&P Keys**

History. Personal and family history of affective disorder; clinical features of mood disorders that have been present preceding psychosis; illness course generally episodic rather than continuous; alcohol abuse common.

Physical and Mental Status Exam. Mania: hyperactivity, rapid and pressured speech, flight of ideas, elated or irritable affect with lability, decreased need for sleep, distractibility, impulsivity, poor judgment, grandiose delusions, sometimes paranoia. Depression: psychomotor retardation or agitation, slowed and impoverished speech, signs of weight loss, poor self-care, guilty ruminations, somatic delusions, derogatory hallucinations, suicidal preoccupation.

• **Diagnosis**

No pathognomonic signs or studies; rule out common general medical etiologies (thyroid and adrenal dysfunction, medications, Parkinson's disease, multiple sclerosis, dementing illnesses, pancreatic and other malignancies, lupus, CNS tumors, cerebrovascular accidents [CVAs], viral illnesses); psychiatric disorders including personality disorders, substance intoxication or abuse (eg, stimulants, steroids).

• **Disease Severity**

Mania. Severe hyperactivity can lead to exhaustion, dehydration, cardiac death; impaired judgment, grandiosity, assaultiveness may result in danger to self and others; assess progression of symptoms, support system.

Depression. Increased suicide risk (15% overall) with presence of delusions; previous attempt; plan and means (especially firearm); male; concurrent substance abuse; social isolation; recent loss; family history; poor health; unemployment. Assess self-care ability, potential life-threatening medical problem.

Both. Mood-incongruent psychotic features predict poorer prognosis.

- **Concept and Application**
  See Mood Disorders below.

- **Management**

Acute. Hospitalization for diagnosis, protection of self and others, treatment (may need involuntary commitment). Acute mania: neuroleptics or benzodiazepines for initial symptom control, lithium titrated to serum levels of 1.0 to 1.5. Anticonvulsants (valproate, carbamezepine) also effective. Electroconvulsive therapy (ECT) for rapid control, pregnancy. Psychotic depression: ECT most effective and rapid; antidepressant (AD) combined with neuroleptic also effective; poor response to AD used alone.

Continued Care. See Mood Disorders below.

C. Delusional Disorder (Formerly Paranoid Disorder)

- **H&P Keys**
  Primary, often sole, manifestation is fixed, nonbizarre, systematized delusion; common types are erotomanic (one is loved by a famous other), grandiose, jealous, persecutory (most common), somatic. Average onset midlife. Psychosocial functioning variable. Migration, deafness, severe stress predispose.

- **Diagnosis**
  No pathognomonic signs or studies; rule out general medical disorders (early dementias, CNS tumor, endocrine and metabolic disorders, stimulant abuse, basal ganglia trauma); schizophrenia associated with bizarre delusions, prominent hallucinations, thought disorder, deteriorating course, younger onset; paranoid personality disorder has no true delusions.

- **Disease Severity**
  Course is variable; worsens with stress.

- **Concept and Application**
  Etiology unknown; genetically unrelated to schizophrenia or affective disorders.

- **Management**

Acute. Hospitalize for inability to control suicidal or homicidal impulses; extreme impairment, including danger associated with delusions; general medical workup.

Continued Care. Low-dose neuroleptics (pimozide); ADs for depression; supportive and psychoeducational therapies with attention to building trust.

D. Other Psychoses

1. Schizoaffective Disorder

- **H&P Keys**
  Concurrent symptoms of schizophrenia and depression or mania, with at least 2 weeks of psychotic symptoms alone.

- **Disease Severity**
  Poorer prognosis with depressive subtype, family history of schizophrenia, insidious onset, poor premorbid history, predominance of psychotic symptoms.

- **Concept and Application**
  Mood syndrome defines subtype (manic: bipolar versus depressive); depressive subtype thought to be related to schizophrenia, bipolar subtype to bipolar disorder.

- **Management**
  Rule out general medical etiology. Hospitalization as in other psychoses.

Bipolar Type. Lithium with neuroleptic; neuroleptic discontinued or reduced after stabilization; other options are carbamazepine, valproate, ECT. Li^{++} maintenance, clozapine for refractory symptoms.

Depressive Type. Neuroleptic with or without antidepressant; ECT; Li^{++} also used.

2. Schizophreniform Disorder

- **H&P Keys**
  History, signs, symptoms, and differential as in schizophrenia but duration less than 6 months.

- **Disease Severity**
  Good prognosis associated with acute onset, confusion and disorientation, full affect, good premorbid functioning.

- **Management**
  Neuroleptics for at least 6 months.

3. Brief Psychotic Disorder

- **H&P Keys**
  Acute onset psychosis with emotional turmoil and confusion often following obvious stressor, duration less than 1 month, full return to premorbid functioning. Young adult. Predisposed by personality disorder (posttraumatic stress disorder [PTSD]). Rule out schizophreniform and mood disorders, general medical etiology, factitious disorder, malingering, substance-induced.

- **Disease Severity**
  Prognostic factors as in schizophreniform disorder. Suicide risk.

- **Management**
  Hospitalization with or without neuroleptic or antianxiety agent; psychotherapy when stabilized.

4. Shared Psychotic Disorder

Patient's delusion (usually persecutory) develops in context of submissive, dependent, isolated relationship with person with established delusion. Suicide or homicide pacts. Treatment by separating patients, with or without neuroleptics.

5. Psychotic Disorder Not Otherwise Specified

Psychotic symptoms that do not meet criteria for other disorders or when enough information is unavailable. Includes postpartum psychoses, culture-bound syndromes. Former occurs 2 to 3 weeks postpartum, usually primipara, carries risk of infanticide or suicide; ensurance of safety, symptomatic treatment.

E. Psychoses Originating in Childhood

1. Autistic Disorder

- **H&P Keys**
  A pervasive developmental disorder with severe impairments in reciprocal social interaction, verbal and nonverbal communication, imaginative activity, repertoire of interests; frequent self-stimulating behaviors, rigid routines; no prominent hallucinations or delusions, no relationship to psychotic disorders. Onset by age 3, boys > girls; associated mental retardation (70%) with uneven cognitive profile; seizure disorder (25%). May have pre- or perinatal abnormalities; genetic predisposition; specific biologic etiology unknown.

- **Diagnosis**
  Neurologic exam, screening for hearing and vision, EEG, CT or MRI, heavy metals, serum ceruloplasm, phenylketonuria (PKU), karyotype, IQ testing.

- **Disease Severity**
  Better prognosis with higher IQ, language, and social skills. May be associated with neurologic or genetic medical disorders.

- **Management**
  Haloperidol for hyperactivity, Li^{++} for aggression or self-injury; fenfluramine, opiate antagonists, β-blockers also used. Special education, family support.

2. Childhood Schizophrenia

Diagnosed using adult criteria; extremely rare; average onset age 7, boys > girls; family history of psychosis, possible neonatal CNS injury; rule out autistic disorder, mood disorder, brain tumor or trauma, toxicity caused by heavy metals or poisoning, seizures, nutritional deficiencies. Monitor use of high-potency neuroleptics; family support; special schooling.

3. Psychotic Mood Disorders

In adolescence may be misdiagnosed as schizophrenia. Bipolar disorder and major depression diagnosed with same criteria used for adults; children may show irritability, somatic complaints, behavioral disturbance. Good premorbid functioning, normal IQ, prominent manic symptoms, family history of mood disorder predict bipolar diagnosis in children and adolescents, as does acute onset, psychomotor retardation, hypersomnia, psychosis, and bipolar family history in first-episode depression. Lithium with careful monitoring, supportive psychotherapy, family education.

II. MOOD DISORDERS

A. Major (Unipolar) Depression

• **H&P Keys**

Two weeks of sustained depressed mood or loss of interest and pleasure (anhedonia), and at least four of the following: weight and appetite change, insomnia or hypersomnia, fatigue, psychomotor agitation or retardation, low self-esteem or guilt, trouble concentrating, recurrent thoughts of death or suicide. Associated with social withdrawal, loss of libido, abnormal menses, constipation, diurnal mood variation, impoverished speech, somatic preoccupation (cardiac, gastrointestinal [GI], genitourinary [GU], back pain, headache), indecisiveness, obsessive rumination, tearfulness, anxiety. "Masked depression" presents with (often vague) physical complaints. Children and adolescents may have irritability, behavioral problems, somatic complaints, failure to gain weight. Elderly may present with cognitive complaints (pseudodementia). Twenty five percent identify precipitating event, often loss. Personal and family history. Females > males. Fifty percent to 60 percent recurrence rate; pattern may be seasonal. Predisposed to by chronic medical or psychiatric illness, substance abuse.

• **Diagnosis**

Clinical diagnosis. Lab tests based on neuroendocrine dysfunction (dexamethasone suppression test, thyrotropin-releasing hormone [TRH] stimulation test, sleep EEG) not specific or sensitive enough to use clinically. Rule out mood disorder caused by drugs or illness; dysthymia (chronic, less severe); personality disorder (lifelong pattern of mood instability; may be comorbid); dementia (no history of affective disorder; deficits stable; patient may try to hide deficits, rather than complain about them; insidious onset); bipolar depression (history of mania); bereavement (self-limiting, lacks morbid preoccupation with worthlessness, suicidal ideation, psychomotor retardation, marked functional impairment).

Diagnosis may be difficult in medically ill because of overlapping symptoms.

• **Disease Severity**

Same as for affective psychoses; untreated episodes last over 6 months; 60% recover, 30% partially recover, 5%–10% develop chronic course. Worse prognosis with late-life onset, concurrent personality, anxiety, substance abuse, chronic medical, or dysthymic disorder, psychosocial stress. Aggressive treatment reduces suicide risk (15%) and improves comorbid medical disorders. Each recurrence increases risk of further recurrence.

• **Concept and Application**

Decreased biogenic amine (norepinephrine, serotonin, dopamine) activity leading to neuroendocrine dysregulation; decreased serotonergic activity associated with suicide. Antidepressants increase available monoamines at nerve terminals, alter receptor sensitivity and density. Genetic component. Higher incidence and earlier age of onset in younger age groups (cohort effect) supports psychosocial contribution. Early parental loss predisposes.

• **Management**

Acute. See above for psychotic depression (20%). Hospitalization if suicide risk or incapacity warrants. Moderate to severe symptoms indication for somatic therapy. Antidepressants successful in 65% to 75%; good response predicted by vegetative signs, previous response, severe symptoms, acute onset. Titration of TCAs from low dose, monitoring blood level; allow 4 to 6 weeks at therapeutic level; monitor sedative, hypotensive, anticholinergic, and cardiotoxic effects (pretreatment ECG should be obtained); supply only one week at a time if suicide is consideration. Monoamine oxidase inhibitors (MAOIs) or serotonin receptor inhibitors (SSRIs, eg, fluoxerine) may be used preferentially to treat atypical depression (rejection-sensitivity, lethargy, mood reactivity, reverse vegetative signs); tyramine-free diet necessary with MAOIs. SSRIs have fewer side effects, less toxicity, less suicide risk for mild to moderate depression. Lithium or triiodothyronine (T_3) augmentation for nonresponders. ECT for drug nonresponders (70% to 80% respond), previous good response, rapid response, pregnancy, cardiac disease. Psychotherapy alone may be effective for mild major depression, psychotherapy plus antidepressants more effective than either treatment alone. Seasonal pattern may respond to phototherapy, exercise.

Continued Care. First episode, continuation of antidepressants for 6 to 12 months; recurrent depression indication for long-term maintenance; observation for weight gain, sexual dysfunction, dry mouth. Lithium prophylaxis also effective.

B. Dysthymia

Chronic depression of at least 2 years' duration with at least two of the following: appetite disturbance, sleep disturbance, fatigue, low self-esteem, difficulty concentrating, hopelessness; no history of major depression within first 2 years or of manic episode. May be secondary to other psychiatric or general medical illness, chronic stress. Insidious onset childhood through early adulthood; women > men; family history of depression. Rule out major depression, personality disorder (may coexist), chronic illnesses, such as uncontrolled diabetes, hypothyroidism, chronic fatigue syndrome. "10%/year develop double depression" (major depression superimposed on dysthymia), worsens prognosis of both. Treat with antidepressants, psychotherapy, exercise.

C. Bipolar Disorders

- **H&P Keys**
  (See above.) One or more manic episodes (distinct period of elated or irritable mood with at least three of the following: grandiosity, decreased need for sleep, talkativeness, racing thoughts, distractibility, hyperactivity or increased goal-directed activity, impulsivity [eg, excessive spending, gambling, promiscuity]; causing marked impairment or hospitalization) usually accompanied by one or more major depressive episodes. Bi-

ipolar depressions may have hypersomnia, severe lethargy. Manic episode may be precipitated by psychosocial stressor, sleep deprivation. Subtypes include:

Type I. History of full-blown mania and major depression.

Type II. History of hypomania (less severe manic symptoms and impairment) and major depression.

Rapid Cycling. Four or more mood episodes per year (10%).

Mixed. Full symptoms of both mania and depression intermixed or rapidly alternating.

- **Diagnosis**
  Same as for affective psychoses. Rapid cycling may be associated with thyroid abnormalities, CNS insult. Onset > age 40, look for general medical etiology.

- **Disease Severity**
  Suicide risk of 10% to 15%. Rapid cycling and mixed types have more chronic, difficult course with greater suicide risk. Women have more rapid cycling and more depressive episodes. Adolescents at high risk of relapse. Women at risk for postpartum episodes. Cycling increases with age.

- **Concept and Application**
  Strong genetic component, likely of several different mechanisms. Various data consistent with heterogeneous dysregulations of biogenic amine systems. One theory implicates kindling (repeated subthreshhold stimulation of neuron generating action potential) in temporal lobes.

- **Management**

Acute Mania. Same as for affective psychoses; >70% respond to Li^{++} serum levels 1.0 to 1.5 after 2 to 3 weeks; neuroleptics, benzodiazepines, or carbamazepine for acute control. Family history of affective disorder or Li^{++} responsiveness, euphoric mania predict good response; for rapid cycling, dysphoric mania, carbamazepine or valproic acid (obtain serum levels), possibly thyroid hormone may be added or substituted. Bipolar depression may respond to Li^{++} alone or may need additional antidepressant ECT.

Continued Care. More than 80% recurrence without prophylaxis, warranted after second episode or first with adolescents, high genetic loading, or sudden onset with suicidal or highly disruptive symptoms. Lithium levels 0.8 to 1.0; observe for nausea, diarrhea, weight gain, polyuria, tremor, cognitive dysfunction; avoid dietary Na^{++} fluctuations; monitor thyroid, renal function. Anticonvulsants for lithium nonresponders; avoid neuroleptics because of increased risk for tardive dyskinesia, depressant effects. Antidepressants may precipitate rapid cycling or mania but may be indicated for bipolar depression unresponsive to Li^{++}. Psychotherapy may increase adaptation, compliance; family support, education.

D. Cyclothymia

Chronic fluctuating mood disturbance of at least 2 years' duration with symptoms of hypomania and depression insufficient never to be diagnosed as major depression or bipolar disorder. Onset adolescence, early adulthood. Family history of affective disorder. Rule out personality disorder, substance abuse. May respond to lithium.

III. ANXIETY DISORDERS

A. Panic Disorder

• **H&P Keys**

History. Recurrent, unexpected, sudden episodes of intense fear or discomfort accompanied by autonomic hyperarousal, depersonalization, fears of dying or going crazy; often associated with agoraphobia, fear of situations where escape is difficult or help unavailable, such as outside the home alone, in a crowd, traveling, on a bridge; may be housebound. Attacks cause anticipatory anxiety, concern about implications, and/or change in behavior (eg, phobic avoidance). Increased history of separation anxiety disorder, family history of panic disorder. Onset mid-20s, women > men. Nonpsychiatric physicians usually consulted first for symptoms.

Physical and Mental Status Exam. Trembling, systolic hypertension, sweating, hyperventilation, flushing, tachycardia, palpitations, cold hands; complaints of chest pain, dyspnea, difficulty swallowing, dizziness, nausea, choking, paresthesias. Mitral valve prolapse present in 20% to 50% of cases.

• **Diagnosis**
Rule out general medical etiology: cardiac insufficiency, arrhythmias, hypoxia, hyperthyroidism, hyperparathyroidism, seizure disorders, pheochromocytoma, vestibular disease, caffeinism, hypoglycemia, carcinoid syndrome, sedative or alcohol withdrawal, stimulants. Situationally bound (Cued) panic attacks occur with phobias, obsessive–compulsive disorder (OCD), PTSD. Depression often accompanied by anxiety symptoms; look at course, predominant symptoms.

• **Disease Severity**
Chronic, intermittent course, with disability caused by phobic avoidance, substance use, depression (>50%), associated with lack of prompt diagnosis, treatment. Twenty percent attempt suicide. Excess risk of peptic ulcer disease, hypertension, cardiovascular mortality.

• **Concept and Application**
Genetic contribution, possibly compatible with single locus inheritance. Biologic models include disturbances in locus coeruleus (norepinephrine) and in γ-aminobutyric acid (GABA) neurotransmission. Benzodiazepines facilitate GABA transmission, and antidepressants down-regulate CNS β-adrenergic receptors. Substances that induce panic include carbon dioxide, lactate, isoproterenol. Onset often associated with stressful event.

• **Management**

Acute. Emergency management of panic attack via reassurance, rebreathing into paper bag, benzodiazepine. Rule out acute medical event, eg, myocardial infarction (MI), pulmonary embolism (PE), substance withdrawal, CNS insult, hypoglycemia, electrolyte abnormalities. Prompt psychiatric referral; avoidance of interminable medical workups.

Continued Care. Antidepressants first line; high-potency benzodiazepines also effective but may be difficult to discontinue. Buspirone ineffective. Taper should be attempted in 6 to 12 months; 70% eventually relapse. Cognitive-behavioral therapies effective in preventing relapses in many. Eliminate caffeine. Supportive, educational approaches.

B. Generalized Anxiety Disorder

• **H&P Keys**
More than 6 months of unrealistic, persistent anxiety and worry unrelated to another psychiatric disorder. Associated with ≥3 of following: restlessness, fatiguability, difficulty concentrating, irritability, muscle tension, sleep disturbance. Other somatic complaints common.

• **Diagnosis**
Same as for panic disorder.

• **Disease Severity**
Often seek treatment from cardiologists, etc; 25% develop panic disorder. Comorbid depression common.

• **Concept and Application**
Heterogeneous illness; possible genetic component.

• **Management**
Cognitive-behavioral therapy effective for milder cases. Medications for more severe, chronic disorder; many require prolonged or intermittent treatment. Buspirone as effective as benzodiazepines without sedation, psychomotor impairment, risk of tolerance, abuse potential, rebound; delayed onset of action, headache, nausea, dizzi-

ness. Benzodiazepines give immediate relief; abuse rare without substance abuse history.

C. Obsessive–Compulsive Disorder (OCD)

• **H&P Keys**
Recurrent intrusive thoughts, impulses, images (obsessions) and perseverative ritualistic behaviors (compulsions), that produce anxiety if resisted. Experienced as senseless product of own mind (as versus delusion). Typical obsessions involve contamination, sin, aggression, loss of control, order, doubt; common compulsions are washing, checking, counting. Onset: childhood through early adulthood; 25% have obsessions only. Comorbid depression (>50%), other anxiety disorders, Tourette's syndrome (5% to 7%), alcoholism, anorexia nervosa. Dermatologic problems due to excessive washing.

• **Diagnosis**
Clinical diagnosis; obsessive–compulsive symptoms in depression, schizophrenia accompanied by other symptoms of those disorders and respond to specific treatments. "Compulsive" behaviors such as eating, gambling give pleasure, whereas true compulsions reduce anxiety.

• **Disease Severity**
Chronic intermittent course; worse prognosis with coexisting schizotypal personality, early onset, severe depression, noncompliance with treatment.

• **Concept and Application**
Genetic contribution, also linked to Tourette's syndrome. Positron emission tomographic (PET) scans show hypermetabolism in prefrontal cortex and caudate nuclei. Psychobiologic probes suggest abnormality in serotonin system; treated with SSRIs. Autoimmunity to streptococcus linked to some childhood cases.

• **Management**
SSRIs; may need higher doses and 4 to 12 weeks for effect; typically 40% symptom re-

duction independent of depressive symptoms. Observation for nausea, agitation, insomnia (fluoxetine); weight gain, sedation, anticholinergic effects (clomipramine); sexual dysfunction (both). Rapid relapse common. Behavioral therapy based on exposure, response prevention; good long-term response in ritualizers. Combined treatment most effective. Support, education.

D. Posttraumatic Stress Disorder (PTSD)

- **H&P Keys**
Exposure to markedly stressful event causing terror and helplessness, eg, combat, rape, sexual abuse, torture, natural disaster. Symptoms from three categories: reexperiencing (eg, recollections, nightmares, play in children); emotional numbing (eg, avoidance, amnesia, restricted affect); autonomic arousal (eg, insomnia, irritability). Onset may be delayed, with initial presentation one of shock, confusion, detachment. Comorbid depression, anxiety, dissociation, substance abuse, personality problems, poor impulse control, suicide attempts.

- **Diagnosis**
Toxicology, head injury workup as indicated. Chronic PTSD may present with a variety of somatic and psychiatric symptoms; obtain trauma history routinely. PTSD symptoms following eg, divorce, bereavement diagnosed as adjustment disorder.

- **Disease Severity**
Worse prognosis in children and the elderly; with preexisting psychopathology; more severe, repetitive stressor; stressor of human design; insidious onset; poor social support; physical injury. Symptoms often persistent, worsen during periods of stress.

- **Concept and Application**
Traumatic memories may be processed differently from nontraumatic ones, making them more difficult to access and integrate in psychotherapy.

- **Management**

Acute. Early intervention important for "working through" the trauma; ventilation, immediate support, validation, encouraging assumption of control, behavioral approaches based on desensitization, group therapy all of value. Mild sedation, eg, with benzodiazepine, as indicated. Rape victims require careful documentation (including photos), thorough physical exam, speculum exam with vaginal smear; fingernail scrapings; pregnancy prevention; rule out sexually transmitted disease (STD); plan for immediate safety; legal advice.

Continued Care. Behavioral and supportive therapies, peer group therapy, family education for chronic symptoms. Antidepressants often used. Treatment of concurrent disorders.

E. Acute Stress Disorder

Symptoms of dissociation (eg, numbing detachment, derealization, depersonalization) experienced during/following extreme trauma, followed by reexperiencing, avoidance, and arousal symptoms as in PTSD. Diagnosis predicts development of PTSD. Psychotherapy aims at reducing dissociation and acknowledging trauma. If symptoms do not resolve within 4 weeks, diagnose PTSD.

F. Phobias

1. Social Phobia

Fear of scrutiny of others; may be specific (eg, eating in public, public speaking) or more generalized. Situations avoided or endured with anxiety. Onset in adolescence, chronic course, may develop depression, substance abuse. Treatment with cognitive-behavior therapy, MAOIs, high-potency benzodiazepine helpful in generalized cases; β-blockers used with specific symptoms, eg, performance anxiety.

2. Specific Phobia

Irrational, excessive fear and avoidance of object or situation (other than of panic or social situation), eg, snakes, heights, blood. Behavior therapy.

IV. ADJUSTMENT DISORDERS

- **H&P Keys**
  Pathologic, excessive emotional and behavioral responses to recognizable psychosocial stressor resulting in impaired functioning. Stressors within range of normal experience (eg, school problems, marital discord, job loss, illness). Onset within 3 months, persists no longer than 6 months unless stressor is chronic (eg, divorce). Classified by major symptom: depression, anxiety, mixed emotional features, conduct disturbance, mixed disturbance of conduct and emotions. Adolescents frequently have behavioral symptoms; adults have mood, anxiety symptoms.

- **Diagnosis**
  PTSD preceded by stressors outside range of normal experience. If one instance in typical pattern of overreaction, diagnose personality disorder. Rule out substance intoxication, abuse. Not diagnosed with uncomplicated bereavement or if meet criteria for specific mental disorder.

- **Disease Severity**
  Greater vulnerability with history of childhood parental loss, serious medical illness. Most recover fully, but 20% adults and 40% adolescents have mental disorder at 5 year follow-up. Increased risk of suicide, medical noncompliance.

- **Concept and Application**
  Vulnerability to stress may be a function of underlying constitution, developmental experiences, temperament, personality structure, as well as severity of stressor.

- **Management**
  Helping patient clarify concerns, resources, options, develop plan of action; with follow-up arranged. Stress reduction may include social support, exercise, relaxation, cognitive reframing techniques, attention to health habits, short-term therapy, peer-group support. Diagnosis and treatment of substance abuse, underlying psychopathology. Medication as indicated for short-term symptom relief.

V. PERSONALITY DISORDERS

- **H&P Keys**
  Persistent, inflexible, maladaptive patterns of thinking, feeling, and behaving causing dysfunction, subjective distress; frequent interpersonal problems, fragility under stress, depression; traits often egosyntonic. Onset late adolescence. Ten disorders (three clusters) in *Diagnostic and Statistical Manual of Mental Disorders* (DSM):

A. Odd, Eccentric

1. Paranoid: suspicious, hypervigilant; ascribes malicious intent, hidden meanings to others; hypersensitivity to criticism; nonpsychotic.
2. Schizoid: isolated, indifferent to social relationships, restricted affective expression.
3. Schizotypal: minor thought disorder (eg, ideas of reference, magical thinking), peculiar behavior, constricted affect, social anxiety.

B. Dramatic, Emotional

1. Antisocial pattern (ASP) of exploitative, socially irresponsible, destructive, impulsive behavior with no remorse; comorbid substance abuse; conduct disorder in childhood.
2. Borderline: problems with intense, unstable relationships, affect regulation, impulse control, identity; suicide gestures common.
3. Histrionic: self-absorbed, seductive, with shallow, labile affect, excess need for praise, reassurance.
4. Narcissistic: grandiose, exploitative, entitled, rageful if humiliated, lacks empathy.

C. Anxious, Fearful, Inhibited

1. Avoidant: fearful of rejection, timid, inhibited but desirous of relationships (as versus schizoid); comorbid anxiety disorders.
2. Dependent: submissive, passive, clingy; lets others make important decisions; easily hurt; preoccupied with abandonment; predisposed by chronic illness.

3. Obsessive–Compulsive: preoccupied with rules; rigid, perfectionistic, ambivalent, stingy, controlling, restricted affect; persistent, task-oriented.

• **Diagnosis**
Acute personality changes in adulthood due to Axis I or general medical disorders (eg, substance intoxication, abuse; CNS trauma, tumor, disease, eg, multiple sclerosis, lupus; mood disorders; psychosis; psychic trauma; adult attention deficit disorder; temporal lobe epilepsy); diagnose coexistent Axis I mood, anxiety, psychotic, substance use, eating, somatization disorders. Personality disorders must have long-term, persistent pattern; may need to defer diagnosis in presence of Axis I pathology.

• **Disease Severity**
Hospitalize for protection of self and others (suicide risk significant in borderlines, antisocials, schizotypals, particularly in presence of substance use); psychotic decompensation (borderline, schizotypal, schizoid, paranoid); severe Axis I pathology.

• **Concept and Application**
Personality disorders result from interaction of constitution, temperament, developmental experiences, environment; genetic contribution in antisocial, schizotypal, paranoid; childhood sexual or physical abuse in many borderlines, avoidants, antisocials; nonspecific neurologic abnormalities; decreased CNS serotonin functioning associated with impulsivity, aggression; schizotypals genetically and biologically related to schizophrenia.

• **Management**
Hospitalization as above; cognitive-behavioral, psychodynamic, group, family therapies all utilized, depending on specific disorder, resources of patient. Treatment (including medication) of comorbid Axis I disorders. Medication for predominant symptoms. Schizotypals may respond to low-dose neuroleptics; SSRIs, MAOIs, carbamazepine, low-dose neuroleptics used for borderline personality disorders. Anti-anxiety, anti-depressant medications used for anxious, fearful, inhibited disorders.

VI. SOMATOFORM DISORDERS

A. Somatization Disorder (Briquet's Syndrome)

• **H&P Keys**
Recurrent, multiple, unfeigned somatic complaints not fully explained by physical disorder, for which medical attention has been sought. Begins before age 30; half have onset before age 15, often with menstrual difficulties; rare in men. Frequent complaints, presented vaguely and dramatically, involve chronic pain in different systems; GI symptoms, eg, irritable bowel, vomiting; cardiopulmonary symptoms, eg, unexplained dyspnea, dizziness; pseudoneurologic symptoms, eg, paralysis, blindness; reproductive tract, sexual problems. High medical utilizers, treated by multiple doctors, extensive, costly evaluations; may have polysurgeries, eg, early hysterectomy. Childhood sexual abuse predisposes; at risk for concurrent spousal abuse. Comorbid alcohol, analgesic, sedative abuse; depression (80% to 90%); anxiety (25% to 45%); personality disorders common.

• **Diagnosis**
Rule out disorders that present with vague, multiple, confusing complaints, eg, multiple sclerosis, porphyria, lupus, hyperparathyroidism; physical symptoms of panic disorder occur only during attacks; conversion disorder involves pseudoneurologic symptoms without full clinical picture; in factitious disorder, person consciously controls production of symptoms.

• **Disease Severity**
Chronic course; suicide associated with substance abuse.

• **Concept and Application**
Family and adoption studies confirm that genetic and environmental factors contribute; familial association with substance abuse and antisocial personality in males. Psychologically interpreted as expression of psychologic pain, elicits care, secondary gain.

- **Management**
Regularly scheduled visits with primary care physician; tests, consultations only with evidence of illness; avoidance of opiates, benzodiazepines; treatment of depression, anxiety with antidepressants; psychiatric referral if possible.

B. Pain Disorder

- **H&P Keys**
Persistent preoccupation with pain without adequate physical findings or pathophysiologic mechanism to account for intensity or disabling psychosocial sequelae. Onset usually at ages 30 to 50 years, women > men; high utilizers of medical care, surgery; complaints may be vague, diffuse; frequent analgesic, substance abuse; comorbid depression, auxiety, insomnia; inactivity, invalidism, isolation. Resistant to psychologic interpretation.

- **Diagnosis**
Dramatic presentation of pain (cultural, personality traits) lacks related impairment; lacks plethora of symptoms of somatization disorder; psychogenic disorders with known pathophysiologic mechanisms, eg, tension headache, diagnosed as psychologic factors affecting physical condition; in malingering, symptoms intentionally produced in pursuit of obvious goal. Rule out reflex sympathetic dystrophy.

- **Disease Severity**
Addiction to prescription drugs may require hospital detoxification. Evaluate psychosocial impairment. Suicide associated with severe depression.

- **Concept and Application**
Subjective pain experience has cognitive, affective, behavioral components, which may be modified through cognitive-behavioral interventions; serotonergic, adrenergic, endorphin systems involved in pain may be modulated with antidepressants, analgesics.

- **Management**
Team approach with "gatekeeper"; cognitive-behavioral techniques (behavioral evaluation, relaxation, biofeedback, contingency management, cognitive therapy); nonsteroidal antiinflammatory agents, antidepressants for pain; family therapy, education; vocational rehab.

C. Conversion Disorder

- **H&P Keys**
Involuntary psychogenic loss or alteration of functioning suggesting a physical disorder, not limited to pain or sexual disturbance. Temporal relationship between psychologically painful stressor and onset of symptoms. Classic cases involve pseudoneurologic symptoms, eg, blindness, paralysis, seizures, difficulty swallowing because of lump in throat (globus hystericus. Antecedent physical disorder (eg, seizure disorder), exposure to persons with physical disorders, preexisting gross brain pathology predispose. More common in women, rural, lower socioeconomic strata. Comorbid somatization, depressive, panic, substance, personality dissociative disorders.

- **Diagnosis**
Diagnosis of exclusion, requiring careful neurologic exam and testing, psychiatric consultation. May have inconsistency of symptoms with known neuroanatomy and physiology, eg, glove distribution of anesthesia. Up to 30% subsequently develop neurologic or other illness that explains symptom, eg, multiple sclerosis, lupus, especially with onset >35.

- **Disease Severity**
Improvement or complete resolution associated with abrupt onset, clear precipitant, absence of general medical or psychiatric illness; recurrence predicts chronicity.

- **Management**
Reassurance, suggestion, attention to any stressful precipitant; treatment of underlying psychopathology; hypnosis or amobarbital interview may be helpful.

D. Hypochondriasis

- **H&P Keys**
Preoccupation with having serious disease despite medical reassurance to the contrary,

not of delusional intensity, duration at least 6 months. Selective attention to and misinterpretation of somatic signs and symptoms. Onset ages 20 to 40 years. History of doctor shopping, resistance to psychiatric referral. Comorbid depression, anxiety, dependence, hostility. Associated with past experience of illness in self or family member.

- **Diagnosis**
  Rule out subtle medical illness; psychotic disorder with somatic (fixed) delusions; in somatization disorder, patients preoccupied with symptoms rather than specific illness; symptoms must not be due to panic attacks or part of OCD.

- **Disease Severity**
  Usually chronic, some functional impairment frequent.

- **Management**
  As for somatization disorder; avoid repeated costly workups.

E. Body Dysmorphic Disorder

Excessive preoccupation with imagined or slight defect in appearance causing marked distress or impairment (not including anorexia nervosa). Onset adolescence, chronic course. May seek repeated cosmetic surgery. Comorbid depression, delusional disorder, social phobia, OCD. Evaluate social impairment, suicide potential. Psychotherapy, SSRI.

F. Related Disorders

1. Psychologic Factors Affecting Physical Condition (Psychosomatic Disorders)

A psychologic factor is believed to have contributed significantly to the development or exacerbation of physical symptom or illness, evidenced by temporal relationship with psychologically meaningful stressor; commonly, headaches, peptic ulcer disease, asthma, skin diseases, vomiting, obesity, low-back pain, ulcerative colitis, arrhythmias, others. Physical condition noted on Axis III. Stress manage-

ment, psychotherapy may increase adjustment, reduce medical costs.

2. Factitious Disorders (Munchausen Syndrome)

Intentional (but often compulsive) production of or feigning of physical or psychologic symptoms, presumably for psychologic reasons unknown to the patient, eg, unsatisfied dependency needs; includes reporting or intentionally producing false symptoms, eg, injection of contaminated substance, surreptitious use of medications, thermometer manipulation, self-induced bruises. Early adult onset; chronic, severe impairment; comorbid severe personality disorders, substance abuse; may have medical occupation, history of illness. Psychiatric consultation, confrontation may be helpful.

3. Malingering

Intentional production of symptoms for obvious recognizable external incentive, eg, to avoid military service, financial reward, evading prison, obtaining drugs. Discrepancy with objective findings, uncooperative.

VII. ATTENTION DEFICIT HYPERACTIVITY DISORDER (ADHD)

- **H&P Keys**
  At least 6 months of age-inappropriate degree of inattentiveness, hyperactivity, and impulsivity; manifested by difficulty following instructions, organizing and completing tasks; easy distractibility; restlessness and fidgetiness; interrupting and talking out of turn; inability to sustain play activity; accident-proneness. Onset before age 7, boys > girls. Associated with academic underachievement, low self-esteem, mood lability, low frustration tolerance, temper outbursts, academic skills disorders, soft neurologic signs, clumsiness. Older children may develop comor-

bid conduct disorder, oppositional defiant disorder. Predisposed by CNS abnormalities, eg, fetal alcohol syndrome, Tourette's disorder, chaotic environments, possibly by child abuse. Family history.

- **Diagnosis**

  Clinical diagnosis, may be assisted by careful neurologic exam, neuropsychologic testing, teachers' and parents' reports using Conner's scale; obtain EEG, TFTs, lead level, hearing assessment. Diagnose specific learning disabilities; rule out pervasive developmental disorders, mood disorder, seizure disorder, mental retardation, pathologic environment. Comorbid chronic otitis media.

- **Disease Severity**

  Poorer outcomes associated with more severe symptoms, coexisting conduct disorder, low IQ, mental disorder in parents; 50% have continued symptoms in adulthood; 25% develop antisocial personality disorder; higher rates of substance abuse, arrests, suicide attempts, accidents, comorbid psychiatric problems. Children at higher risk for abuse.

- **Concept and Application**

  Familial aggregation, also with mood, substance abuse, and personality disorders. Possible congenital and acquired CNS insults; catecholamine or dopamine abnormalities; medications increase CNS dopamine and norepinephrine levels.

- **Management**

  Seventy-five percent improve with psychostimulants, eg, methylphenidate (10 to 60 mg/d) or dextroamphetamine (5 to 40 mg/d); increase slowly; antidepressants, clonidine also used. May inhibit growth; used during school hours. Observe also for irritability, insomnia, abdominal pain, dysphoria, tics. Behavioral and environmental management by family, school. Individual, family therapy as indicated.

VIII. CONDUCT DISORDER

- **H&P Keys**

  Age-inappropriate, persistent violation of societal norms and rights of others, manifested by aggression to people and animals, property destruction, deceitfulness and theft, and serious rule violations. May lack empathy, remorse; poor frustration tolerance, irritability, recklessness, low academic achievement. Onset late childhood to early adolescence.

- **Diagnosis**

  Rule out response to immediate social context, eg, runaway episodes due to abuse, "adaptive delinquency." Obtain history from multiple sources. Evaluate suicide and violence potential, comorbid learning disorders, ADHD, mood disorders, anxiety, somatoform, substance-related disorders.

- **Disease Severity**

  Early onset, attentional problems, low intelligence, fire setting, family deviance, and large size predict worse prognosis. One third to one half develop ASP as adults; high mortality rates.

- **Concept and Application**

  Genetic, neurodevelopmental, and environmental risk factors: parental rejection/neglect; harsh and inconsistent discipline and abuse; parental ASP, substance abuse, other psychiatric disorder; poverty; evidence of genetic transmission; neurologic abnormalities, including attention deficits, seizures, perinatal insults, head injuries. Biological markers suggest autonomic underarousal, possibly associated with decreased anxiety or stimulus seeking, mediators of antisocial behavior.

- **Management**

  Pharmacologic treatment depends on comorbid neuropsychiatric diagnosis. Limit setting, containment crucial; may involve legal system, schools, parental surveillance, hospitalization, residential treatment. Individual or group therapies focus on anger management, problem solving, communication skills.

IX. EATING DISORDERS

A. Anorexia Nervosa

- **H&P Keys**

Refusal to maintain minimal normal body weight (<85%), intense fear of gaining weight, distorted body image, 3 months amenorrhea; associated features include obligate exercise, peculiar food behaviors, bulimic symptoms (see below), emaciation, hypothermia, hypotension, lanugo hair, bradycardia, edema, hair loss, hyposexuality, compulsive behaviors. Onset adolescence, 95% women, premorbid history perfectionism, anxiety, possibly sexual abuse, mid- to upper socioeconomic strata, may be precipitated by stress, dieting. Comorbid depression, personality, OCD.

- **Diagnosis**

Rule out weight loss due to major depression, AIDS, cancer, GI disorders, substance abuse; in schizophrenia, bizarre eating patterns related to psychosis; in bulimia, weight does not fall below 85%; underweight persons without anorexia recognize their low weight. May have: leukopenia, anemia, electrolyte abnormalities, signs of dehydration, decreased TFTs, elevated prepubertal hormone levels, sinus bradycardia.

- **Disease Severity**

Thirty percent have chronic course, 5% to 18% mortality; hospitalization indicated for starvation, dehydration, electrolyte imbalance, hypotension, hypothermia, suicide risk. Poorer outcome associated with longer duration of illness, older age at onset, prior psychiatric hospitalizations, poor premorbid adjustment, comorbid personality disorder.

- **Concept and Application**

Genetic component; psychologically interpreted as resistance to social or sexual demands of adolescence; cultural preoccupation with extreme slimness rare in nonindustrialized societies. biologic theories focus on hypothalamic disturbance, supported by amenorrhea preceding weight loss; reduced CNS norepinephrine activity.

- **Management**

Acute. Hospitalization as indicated; monitoring and treatment of metabolic imbalances; strict enforcement of treatment contract for weight goal with daily weights, nutritional supplements, intake-output, supervised feeding (nasogastric tube as needed), reinforcement, nutrition education. Cyproheptadine may assist weight gain. Treatment of comorbid depression with antidepressants.

Continued Care. Supportive, cognitive-behavioral, family therapies with goal of weight maintenance, normalization of eating behaviors. Residential, partial hospital treatment may prevent relapse.

B. Bulimia Nervosa

- **H&P Keys**

Recurrent binge eating (two episodes per week for 3 months) with lack of control over eating; self-induced vomiting (70% to 95%), use of laxatives or diuretics, strict dieting, vigorous exercise to prevent weight gain; overconcern with body weight. Onset in late adolescence and early adulthood, often during strict dieting; 95% women; mid- to upper socioeconomic strata; usually of normal weight; complications include dental erosion and caries, parotid enlargement, calloused fingers, electrolyte abnormalities (50%), dehydration, weakness, lethargy, GI problems, cardiac arrhythmias; rarely, esophageal tears, gastric rupture, pancreatitis, sudden death. Comorbid anorexia, depression, personality disorders, stealing, substance abuse common.

- **Diagnosis**
  Rule out seizure disorder, CNS tumor, Klüver-Bucy and Kleine-Levin syndromes; obtain ECG, electrolytes, amylase, LFTs.

- **Disease Severity**
  Chronic intermittent disorder with range of impairment; hospitalization for correction of electrolyte imbalance, suicide risk.

- **Concept and Application**
  Decreased CNS serotonin, norepinephrine activity; increased family history of mood disorders, obesity, substance abuse.

- **Management**
  Hospitalization; most treated as outpatients; SSRI helpful in reducing binging; cognitive-behavioral, individual, group therapies; nutritional counseling.

X. SUBSTANCE-RELATED DISORDERS

A. Overview

Definitions

Abuse. Recurrent maladaptive pattern of use during 12-month period despite physical hazard or legal, social, or occupational problems.

Dependence. Psychologic (craving) or physical (withdrawal syndrome, tolerance); loss of control over use; preoccupation with obtaining and using substance; continued use despite adverse social, occupational, or health consequences. Frequent denial, minimization.

Intoxication. Maladaptive behavior associated with recent ingestion.

Withdrawal. Substance-specific syndrome following cessation of regular use.

- **H&P Keys**
  Decrement in work or school performance; absenteeism; fights; family problems; injuries or accidents; acute personality change; driving under the influence, theft, prostitution; related medical and mental disorders (see below); frequent psychiatric comorbidity, particularly mood, anxiety, personality, schizophrenic, attention deficit disorders, chronic pain; may be self-medicating or symptoms may be caused by substance; defer diagnosis until patient clean 6 weeks or more. Needle tracks with IV use.

- **Diagnosis**
  History (may need to obtain from other sources) and associated physical signs; thin-layer chromatography toxicology screen specific but not sensitive, detects high-dose recent use (within 48 hours).

- **Disease Severity**
  Worse prognosis with long-term use; psychiatric comorbidity; unsupportive milieu; lack of employment, job skills; younger age of onset; may be suicidal, assaultive; dangerous withdrawal syndromes associated with alcohol, sedatives; overdoses with narcotics, stimulants, phencyclidine. High blood level without signs of intoxication indicates tolerance. Intravenous drug use may lead to AIDS, subacute bacterial endocarditis (SBE), hepatitis, thrombophlebitis, pneumonia, cellulitis; snorting cocaine, heroin may lead to nasal perforation, rhinitis, bleeding; inhaling or smoking marijuana, crack, inhalants may lead to bronchitis, asthma.

- **Concept and Application**
  Genetic component to alcohol dependence and probably others; all abused substances acutely enhance brain reward mechanisms; use reinforced by relief of withdrawal symptoms; environmental learning important.

- **Management**

  Acute. Intoxication: Observation and medical treatment for overdose, multiple substance ingestion; protection from injury. Withdrawal: symptomatic treatment; may need to detoxify (especially sedatives, alcohol, opioids) under medical supervision. Diagnosis and treatment of concurrent nonpsychiatric medical problems.

  Continued Care. Often need to confront denial; variety of approaches used to initiate and maintain abstinence, eg, inpatient, residential, and partial rehabs; individual, cognitive-behavioral and group therapies; family therapy or groups; self-help groups, eg, Alcoholics Anonymous (AA); pharmacologic treatments, eg, methadone maintenance, disulfiram (Antabuse). Relapses common, long-term treatment the rule. Diagnosis and treatment of comorbid psychiatric problems.

B. Alcohol Dependence

- **H&P Keys**

  Early: injuries, accidents, gastritis, diarrhea, absenteeism, blackouts, irritability. Later: nutritional deficiencies, hepatitis, cirrhosis, GI bleeding, pancreatitis, heart disease, hypertension, palmar erythema, acne rosacea, gynecomastia, testicular atrophy, peripheral neuropathy, GI cancers, cardiomyopathy, fetal alcohol syndrome (craniofacial abnormalities, mental retardation, behavior problems, congenital malformations), depression, anxiety, insomnia, neuropsychiatric disorders (below). Onset late teens to 30s, men > women, family history. Associated abuse of other substances. Rule out underlying bipolar, anxiety, attention deficit, antisocial disorders. Diagnosis for 20% to 40% of homeless persons. Men > women.

- **Diagnosis**

  Clinical diagnosis; screen with CAGE (attempts to Cut down; Annoyance with criticism of drinking; Guilt; morning Eyeopener; three positives give 95% certain diagnosis). Blood level of >150 mg/dL without intoxication evidence of tolerance. May have increased GGT, mean corpuscular volume (MCV), AST, ALT, uric acid, alkaline phosphatase, vertebral or rib fractures.

- **Disease Severity**

  One quarter to one third have early onset; male, antisocial, family history, poor prognosis, responds best to structured milieu treatments; two thirds to three quarters have later, gradual onset, equal sex distribution, better prognosis; women have later onset but more virulent course, family history mood disorder; complications include motor vehicle accidents, job loss, assaults, suicide, falls (rule out subdural hematoma), fires, poisonings, drownings.

- **Concept and Application**

  Multiple causes: genetic factors, cultural patterns, learning all important: High heritability in males; nondrinking sons of alcoholics have altered evoked potentials, possibly greater tolerance; certain groups, eg, Asians, have protective unpleasant responses caused by aldehyde dehydrogenase isoenzyme.

- **Management**

  Acute. Treatment of withdrawal, detoxification as below; attention to acute comorbid problems.

  Continued Care. Confrontation of denial; inpatient or outpatient programs include group, individual, family, 12-step AA, educational components; disulfiram (Antabuse), naltrexone, SSRI's used to promote abstinence in some. Anxiety, depression lasting more than 2 to 4 weeks past detoxification may require specific treatment.

C. Other Alcohol Syndromes

1. Intoxication

Maladaptive behavior, eg, disinhibition, mood lability, irritability, impaired judgment; incoordination, slurred speech, ataxia, nystagmus, flushing; may progress to blackouts, coma, death. Complicated by head injuries, motor vehicle accidents, delirium, aggressive acts, suicide. Approximate blood alcohol levels for nontolerant person:

100 to 150 mg/dL: incoordination, irritability (legal intoxication)
150 to 250 mg/dL: slurred speech, ataxia
>250 mg/dL: unconsciousness

Treat supportively; evaluate for subdural, infection, other substances.

2. Alcohol Withdrawal Syndromes

Alcohol Withdrawal. Tremulousness, nausea, vomiting, autonomic hyperactivity, malaise, headache, insomnia, irritability, transient perceptual disturbance, grand mal seizures (<3%), lasting up to 5 to 7 days postcessation.

Alcohol Withdrawal Delirium (Delirium Tremens). History of recent (2 to 3 days) cessation or reduction of heavy use in medically compromised patients with 5- to 15-year history of dependence; result of unmasking of downregulation of inhibitory GABA receptors; delirium (see below), autonomic hyperactivity, vivid auditory, visual and tactile hallucinations, paranoid delusions, agitation, tremor, fever, seizures occurring before delirium ("rum fits"); diagnosis, treatment of underlying pneumonia, GI bleed, hepatic failure, subdural hematoma, electrolyte imbalance, dehydration; obtain CBC, chemistries, vitamin B_{12}, folate, LFTs, urine analysis UA, tox screen, chest roentgenogram, ECG; possible blood cultures, lumbar puncture (LP), CT of head, EEG; frequent vital signs, observation; decrease stimulation, use seclusion, restraint as necessary; thiamine 100 mg, folate 1.0 mg, multivitamin daily; benzodiazepine, eg, chlordiazepoxide (or oxazepam with hepatic dysfunction) adjusted to control symptoms and tapered 20% to 25% daily; phenytoin with history withdrawal seizures.

Alcohol Hallucinosis. Vivid, persistent auditory or visual hallucinations within 48 hours of cessation or reduction; rarely become chronic; treatment with low-dose high-potency antipsychotic.

3. Alcoholic Encephalopathy (Wernicke's Encephalopathy)

Nystagmus, ophthalmoplegia, ataxia, confusion resulting from thiamine deficiency associated with alcoholism; early treatment with thiamine may prevent Korsakoff's syndrome. Diagnose concurrent infection, hepatic failure.

4. Alcohol-Induced Persisting Amnestic Disorder (Korsakoff's Syndrome)

Severe, persistent retrograde and anterograde amnesia, confabulation, apathy, polyneuritis resulting from thiamine deficiency, following episode of Wernicke's encephalopathy.

5. Alcohol-Induced Persisting Dementia

Dementia following prolonged, heavy ingestion; distinguished from alcohol amnestic disorder by presence of cognitive deficits other than memory; exclude other causes of dementia.

D. Drug Dependence

1. Stimulants (Amphetamine, Cocaine, "Diet Pills," Others)

Highly addictive; ingested, injected, snorted, purified to free-base form and smoked (crack); *intoxication* produces euphoria, alertness, increased energy, anxiety, talkativeness, psychomotor agitation, impaired judgment, sexual arousal, anorexia, insomnia, pupillary dilatation, hypertension, tachycardia; may progress to hyperpyrexia; nausea and vomiting; visual or tactile hallucinations ("cocaine bugs"); paranoid ideation; sudden cardiac death; treat severe agitation with benzodiazepine, tachyarrhythmia with antiarrhythmic; acidify urine. *Delirium* lasting 1 to 6 hours with olfactory or tactile hallucinations, may lead to seizures, death. Chronic use and *dependence* associated with tolerance to euphoric effects; severe social, financial, health losses including STD risk; weight loss; depression, irritability, sexual dysfunction, memory impairment, paranoia, persecutory delusions (*delusional disorder*). *Withdrawal* (crash) may be self-treated with sedatives, eg, alcohol, marijuana; associated with insomnia or hypersomnia, hunger, fatigue, dysphoria, agitation, anxiety, suicidal ideations, craving. Not physically dangerous; treat supportively, refer for drug treatment. Treat depression persisting more than 2 weeks after withdrawal.

2. Opioid Dependence (Heroin, Methadone, Meperidine, Codeine, Pentazocine, Others)

More common in urban settings, males, blacks, health care professionals, chronic pain patients. Opium smoked; heroin snorted, injected intravenously or subcutaneously ("skin popping"); speedball is heroin plus stimulant; pharmaceutic opioids ingested. *Dependence* associated with tolerance, compulsive use, weight loss, hyposexuality, amenorrhea, multiple medical problem, high mortality, criminal involvement, suicide, accidents. *Intoxication* produces euphoria, analgesia, hypoactivity, anorexia, drowsiness, constipation, nausea, vomiting, slurred speech, hypotension, bradycardia, pupillary constriction, needle tracks; CNS and respiratory depression, pulmonary edema, seizures, coma in *overdose*. Treat with IV naloxone, 0.8 mg, double dose q 15 min × 2 if no response; continue IV administration up to 3 days, support vital functions; diagnose polysubstance overdose. *Withdrawal* severely uncomfortable but not a medical emergency; flulike syndrome of rhinorrhea, myalgias, nausea, vomiting, diarrhea, lacrimation, dilated pupils, restlessness, yawning, sweating, insomnia, piloerection, anxiety, craving, tachycardia, hypertension; methadone 15 to 25 mg q 12 h until symptoms suppressed, with gradual taper according to symptoms over 10 to 14 days; clonidine also used; naltrexone used after detoxification to assist abstinence in highly motivated patient; progress to methadone maintenance or abstinence; pentazocine detoxified with pentazocine. Comorbid psychiatric disorder (ASP, depression, PTSD) in 80%.

3. Sedative-Hypnotic Dependence (Benzodiazepines, Barbiturates, Methaqualone, Others)

Young, polydrug abusers (frequently combined with alcohol, opioids, stimulants) or middle-aged women, who become iatrogenically dependent. *Dependence* produces tolerance to euphoriant and sedative effects, fatigue, psychomotor impairment, amnesia, depression, headaches, GI disturbances; *intoxication* associated with slurred speech, drowsiness, incoordination, ataxia, impaired attention and memory, disinhibition. Barbiturates have low therapeutic index, frequently used in suicide; *overdose* causes respiratory depression, coma; monitor closely, maintain airway and blood pressure. Mild *withdrawal* syndrome of anxiety, insomnia, headache, anorexia, dizziness common. Se-

vere withdrawal syndrome associated with nausea, vomiting, malaise, autonomic hyperactivity, anxiety, photophobia, tremor, hyperreflexia, hyperthermia, insomnia, delirium, seizures, death; short-acting drugs cause most severe syndrome. PO pentobarbital 200 mg, then 100 mg q 2 h (max 500 mg) until intoxication observed; substitute phenobarbital, 30 mg/each 100 mg pentobarbital; taper ≃ 10%/day, adjusting for signs of intoxication, withdrawal.

4. Cannabinoids

Intoxication produces euphoria or dysphoria, heightened sensation, time distortion, increased humorousness, impaired judgment, dry mouth, increased appetite, pupillary dilation, conjunctival injection, suspiciousness, anxiety, tachycardia, depersonalization, incoordination, rarely hallucinations, mild persecutory delusions; treatment rarely needed. Very high doses may produce prolonged (up to 6 weeks) psychosis, mild delirium, panic. Chronic use may lead to apathetic, amotivational syndrome, memory impairment, depression, anxiety, respiratory and reproductive problems; no characteristic withdrawal syndrome. Often used or mixed with other substances. Urine toxicology remains positive up to 4 weeks after cessation of heavy use.

5. Hallucinogens (LSD, Mescaline, Psilocybin, MDMA, Others)

Eaten, sucked from paper, smoked; intoxication produces wakeful hallucinosis, sympathomimetic effects, including pupillary dilation, perceptual changes, emotional intensity and lability; may be associated with anxiety, depression, paranoia, panic reactions with belief that disturbed perceptions are real ("bad trips"); treat with reassurance, ensure safe environment; benzodiazepines, antipsychotics for severe symptoms. Prolonged psychosis may develop in vulnerable patients; posthallucinogen perception disorder ("flashbacks") distressing persistent reexperiencing of hallucinations with intact reality testing low-dose benzodiazepine acutely, antipsychotic if persistent.

6. Phencyclidine (PCP, Angel Dust)

Hallucinogen, smoked with marijuana, eaten, injected, snorted; euphorogenic, commonly causes unpredictable, paranoid, agitated, assaultive behavior; accompanied by dysarthria, diaphoresis, vertical and horizontal nystagmus, hypertension, tachycardia, analgesia (may result in injury), muscle rigidity, ataxia, hyperacusis, hyperreflexia, myoclonic jerks, catatonia, seizures, respiratory depression, coma, death. Pupils are normal size, elevated CPK and SGOT. May develop chronic psychosis, mood disorder, delirium, long-term neuropsychologic damage. Ensure safety in nonstimulating environment; may need physical restraint; acidify urine to increase drug clearance, treat severe hypertension; may use benzodiazepines, haloperidol symptomatically; evaluate for medical conditions, other substance intoxication.

7. Inhalants (Volatile Glues, Solvents, Cleaners, Nitrates, Others)

Frequently abused by male adolescents; causes light-headedness, euphoria, disinhibition, dizziness, intensification of orgasm, belligerence, impaired judgment, perceptual disturbances, delusions, ataxia, confusion, disorientation, slurred speech, hyporeflexia, nystagmus; can progress to delirium, coma; chronic use can result in dementia, liver and kidney damage, bone marrow suppression, peripheral neuropathies, immunosuppression. Treat supportively.

8. Anabolic Steroid Abuse

Adolescents, athletes; may use orally, intramuscularly; associated with depression, mania, psychosis, acne, hepatic damage, infection from needle sharing, CVAs, testicular atrophy, and feminzation in males, masculinization in females.

9. Caffeine Dependence (Coffee, Tea, Cola, Chocolate, Over-the-Counter Stimulants, Cold Preps)

Restlessness, insomnia, diuresis, anxiety, excitement, GI disturbance, flushing with intake >250 mg/d (two cups brewed coffee); cardiac arrhythmia, muscle twitching, agitation, inexhaustibility with intake >1 g. Withdrawal symptoms: headache, fatigue lasting 4 to 5 days.

10. Nicotine Dependence (Tobacco Smoking, Chewing)

Strongly conditioned; assessed by number of cigarettes smoked per day, use of morning cigarette; dependence causes pulmonary, cardiac, peripheral vascular, neoplastic diseases. Withdrawal associated with craving, irritability, anxiety, difficulty concentrating, restlessness, bradycardia, increased appetite, weight gain; also GI distress, increased cough, insomnia, headache, impaired performance; treat with counseling, self-help literature, smoking cessation groups, behavioral interventions, nicotine gum or patch for moderate to severe addiction (continued smoking with nicotine treatment can cause cardiac death); highly comorbid with other psychiatric, substance use disorders; depression may develop upon withdrawal.

XI. SEXUAL DYSFUNCTIONS

- **H&P Keys**
Includes disorders of all phases of the sexual response cycle causing distress, interpersonal difficulty: *hypoactive sexual desire disorder* (deficient or absent sexual fantasies or desire); *sexual aversion disorder* (revulsion to and avoidance of sexual contact); *female sexual arousal disorder* (inability to attain or maintain adequate sexual excitement and lubrication); *male erectile disorder* (inability to attain or maintain adequate erection); *female and male orgasmic disorders* (persistent or recurrent delay or absence of orgasm following sexual excitement); *premature ejaculation* (persistent ejaculation with minimal stimulation before or shortly after penetration); *dyspareunia* (persistent genital pain with intercourse); and *vaginismus* (involuntary spasm of vaginal musculature during intercourse) classified

as sexual pain disorders. All disorders may be lifelong or acquired, generalized or situational, due to psychological or combined with general medical or substance induced factors.

- **Diagnosis**
Rule out dysfunction due to another psychiatric disturbance (eg, depression, PTSD), substance dependence, diabetes, vascular disease, neurologic disease, including MS and trauma, endocrine disorders, hepatic or other systemic disease, surgical procedures; medications, commonly including antihypertensives, anticholinergics, antihistamines, antidepressants, antipsychotics, steroids, estrogens. Spontaneous erections, morning erections, erections with masturbation rule out organic etiology of impotence. Complete gynecologic or urologic exam, measurement of nocturnal penile tumescence, pudendal nerve latency, penile blood pressure, serum glucose, LFTs, TFTs, prolactin, luteinizing hormone (LH), FSH as indicated.

- **Disease Severity**
Primary and chronic disorders more difficult to treat. Patient may have history of sexual victimization.

- **Concept and Application**
Illnesses, substance abuse, or medications that interfere with normal endocrine, neural, and vascular systems may produce sexual dysfunction. Psychological etiologies include ignorance and misinformation; unconscious guilt, anger and anxiety; performance anxiety or fear of rejection; and lack of communication between partners. Major physical and psychological stresses may inhibit sexual functioning.

- **Management**
Rule out organic etiology. Cognitive therapy, specific behavioral therapies, marital therapy, education (eg, importance of clitoral stimulation for orgasm in women), occasionally somatic treatments (eg, external vacuum device, penile prosthesis, yohimbine, bromocriptine) used for specific dysfunctions. Behavioral therapies (eg, sensate focus for erectile dysfunction, squeeze technique for premature ejaculation, directed masturbation for anorgasmia) desensitize patient and decrease performance anxiety.

XII. DELIRIUM

- **H&P Keys**
Global cognitive impairment with reduced attention; disorganized thought with rambling or incoherent speech; reduced and fluctuating level of consciousness (clear, drowsy, stupor, coma); sensory (commonly visual) misinterpretations, illusions, hallucinations; disorientation; disturbed sleep–wake cycle; psychomotor and memory disturbances; rapid onset, fluctuating course, brief duration ending in recovery, dementia, death; frequent emotional disturbance (agitated or withdrawn); fearfulness; disorders of higher cortical function; abnormal movements, eg, asterixis; autonomic hyperactivity; children, elderly, prior brain damage (eg, dementia, AIDS) increases susceptibility; prevalence 10% to 15% medical and surgical, 30% intensive care unit patients.

- **Diagnosis**
History, physical, lab studies to diagnose underlying problem; common etiologies systemic infection; metabolic disorders (hypoxia, hypoglycemia, electrolyte imbalances, hepatic or renal disease, thiamine deficiency); postoperative states; postictal states; head injury; substance intoxication, withdrawal syndromes; anticholinergic medications; toxins; hypertensive encephalopathy; focal lesions (right parietal, inferomedial occipital). Differs from psychotic psychiatric disorder with random, fluctuating symptoms; problems with attention, orientation, memory; lack of prior history. Clear sensorium in dementia. In delirium, EEG shows background slowing or low-voltage fast activity.

- **Disease Severity**
Delirium is a medical emergency, requiring rapid assessment and treatment.

- **Concept and Application**
Final common pathway for acute brain insult.

- **Management**
Diagnosis and treatment of underlying disorder (history, physical exam, electrolytes, blood urea nitrogen [BUN], creatinine, CBC, LFTs, UA, erythrocyte sedimentation rate [ESR], toxicologies, HIV, blood cultures, ECG, EEG, CT or MRI of head, LP as indicated). Monitoring vital signs, cognitive status (eg, mini-mental state exam); treatment of alcohol, sedative withdrawals as above; severe anticholinergic delirium treated with physostigmine; hydration, nutrition; reassurance; sensory environment should be individually optimized, eg, night light, soft music; restraint, protection from injury as necessary; low-dose, high-potency antipsychotic, eg, haloperidol, for agitation; careful use of benzodiazepine for insomnia or seizure risk, if no contraindication.

XIII. ABUSE SYNDROMES

A. Child Physical and Sexual Abuse

- **H&P Keys**
Risk factors include parental history of child abuse, current substance abuse, depression, impulsivity; premature, hyperactive, emotionally disturbed, physically ill, or otherwise difficult child; stepchild; current toilet training; impairment, unavailability, abuse of mother; familial isolation, stress, poverty, conflict; child's running away. History of injury inconsistent with physical findings or developmental level; inconsistent stories; multiple injuries of different ages; delay in seeking care. Suspect when see linear or geometric marks; old scars; spiral, humerus, or rib fractures; geometric or symmetric lower body burns; rup-

tured viscera; facial and head trauma; retinal hemorrhages; may see genital or anal trauma or lesions; stomach or rectal pain; urinary tract infections with sexual abuse. Signs of disturbed attachment (eg, lack of physical contact or concern, lack of separation anxiety, hypercritical attitude toward child), delayed development, disturbed play, inappropriate sexual behavior may be present.

- **Diagnosis**
Rule out unintentional trauma, bleeding diathesis, dermatologic conditions, vitamin deficiencies, osteogenesis imperfecta, self-inflicted injuries; thorough physical exam; skeletal series, serologies, bleeding screening battery, CBC, creatine kinase (CK) as indicated.

- **Disease Severity**
Deaths usually occur only after numerous episodes; psychiatric sequelae (including PTSD, depression, substance abuse, personality disorders, multiple personality disorder, sexual dysfunction, somatic complaints, repetition of abuse, suicidal or self-destructive behavior) worse with early-age onset, chronicity, severe abuse, use of force, multiple perpetrators, abuse by parental figure, lack of support.

- **Concept and Application**
Child may dissociate during abuse episode, resulting in later development of dissociative symptoms. Guilt, shame, rage, low self-esteem, self-destructive behavior, developmental delays, anxiety, withdrawal, antisocial behavior common.

- **Management**

Acute. Interview of child alone; expert may be necessary to elicit abuse history; separate interviews of parents if possible; all states mandate reporting of suspected abuse (physical, emotional, sexual, severe neglect); documentation of findings, including pictures; ensuring safety of child.

Continued Care. Treatment of child for physical, emotional sequelae; individual, group psychotherapy usually indicated; treatment for abusers ranges from support (emotional support, social services, education, Parent's Anonymous groups, hotlines, etc) through mandated therapy, removal of parent abuser or child, legal prosecution.

B. Adult Domestic Violence

- **H&P Keys**

  Risk factors include pregnancy, younger age, social isolation, child abuse in home; histories of child abuse, substance abuse, criminality in abuser; abused women not shown to have specific predisposing personality traits. History may be incompatible with injury. Trauma repetitive in most; no diagnostic injury pattern; head, face, neck, breast, abdomen frequent injury sites.

- **Diagnosis**

  Battering present in 20% of women seeking medical care; 22% to 35% of women presenting to emergency departments; 23% of prenatal patients; 25% of women who attempt suicide; 45% to 58% of mothers of abused children. Routine inquiry in privacy makes diagnosis.

- **Disease Severity**

  Increased risk of severe abuse when abused partner decides to leave; respect victim's judgment regarding her safety; high risk of marital rape; sequelae include PTSD symptoms, low self-esteem, somatic complaints, depression, anxiety, substance abuse, suicide attempts.

- **Concept and Application**

  Barriers to leaving abusive relationship include shock and denial, self-blame, feelings of helplessness, presence of children, financial dependency, lack of job skills, fear of retaliation.

- **Management**

  Treatment of injuries; evaluation of suicide risk; ensuring confidentiality and safety of victim, children; assessment of resources, continued risk (eg, threats, extent of previous injury, presence of weapon, stalking, substance abuse), acute need for social, medical, legal, psychiatric, community services (eg, battered women's shelter); careful documentation including photos; referral for marital counseling contraindicated because of risk of violence; follow-up plan essential.

C. Elder Abuse

Abuser generally relative/caretaker; victim may fear disclosure due to dependency; family system with frustration, financial, or health stress, substance abuse, history of violence; previous injuries, physical deterioration: bruising, head injury, burns, decubiti, contractures, dehydration, lacerations, diarrhea, impaction, malnutrition, urine burns, signs of neglect, sexual assault, PTSD symptoms. Interview privately; social service for assessment of living situation; mandatory reporting in most states.

XIV. BEREAVEMENT

A. Uncomplicated Bereavement

Normal reaction to death of loved one or other significant loss; acute grief characterized by intense emotional distress, somatic symptoms, dissociation, preoccupation with deceased, anger, loss of habitual patterns of conduct; mourning can include full depressive syndrome with depressed mood, sleep disturbance, anorexia, guilt, crying, difficulty concentrating, loss of interest, fatigue, anxiety most common; duration varies, up to 1 to 2 years, symptoms generally remit spontaneously, anniversary reactions common. Higher risk of general medical and psychiatric illness and mortality during mourning. Signs of pathologic grief include marked psychomotor retardation, morbid preoccupation with worthlessness and hopelessness, prolonged functional impairment, persistent suicidal preoccupation; prolonged denial; absence of grief. Encouragement of expression of feelings, reminiscences; referral to community supports; medication generally contraindicated, but autonomous depressive disorder should be treated.

B. Sudden Infant Death Syndrome

Intense, severe grief reactions frequent in parents, including guilt, anger, hostility, somatic symptoms; delayed mourning; overactivity; social isolation; psychosis; agitated depression. Associated with decline in physical health, marital difficulties, behavioral disturbance in siblings, migration. Contact with dead infant; autopsy may help; education may reduce guilt and blame; parent support groups; involvement of siblings; extended social support; counseling regarding future pregnancy recommended.

BIBLIOGRAPHY

American Psychiatric Association. *Diagnostic and Statistical Manual of Mental Disorders.* 4th ed. Washington, DC: American Psychiatric Association; 1994.

Andreasen NC, Black DW. *Introductory Textbook of Psychiatry.* 2nd ed. Washington, DC: American Psychiatric Press; 1995.

Arana GW, Hyman SE. *Handbook of Psychiatric Drug Therapy.* 3rd ed. Boston: Little Brown & Co; 1995.

Dunner DL. *Current Psychiatric Therapy.* Philadelphia: WB Saunders Co; 1993.

Kaplan HI, Sadock BJ. *Synopsis of Psychiatry.* 7th ed. Baltimore: Williams & Wilkins; 1994.

16

Pulmonary Medicine

Michael Sherman, MD, and Edward S. Schulman, MD

I. INFECTIOUS DISORDERS

A. Croup

- **H&P Keys**
  Children under 6 years old following upper respiratory illness. Barking cough, inspiratory stridor, dyspnea, hoarseness, usually worse at night.

- **Diagnosis**
  Roentgenography of upper airway (glottic and subglottic swelling).

- **Disease Severity**
  Respiratory rate, pulse oximetry, accessory muscle use, stridor, intercostal muscle retractions.

- **Concept and Application**
  Glottic and subglottic edema leading to upper airway obstruction. Multiple viral etiologies, including respiratory syncytial virus, influenza A and B, adenovirus, and rhinovirus.

- **Management**
  Supportive care. Humidification of inspired air, correction of hypoxemia, aerosol racemic epinephrine. Rarely, severe cases require intubation.

B. Acute Epiglottitis

- **H&P Keys**
  Children less than 7 years of age most common. High fever, stridor, dyspnea, hoarseness, dry cough, drooling, dysphagia, systemic toxicity, cherry-red epiglottis.

- **Diagnosis**
  Lateral neck roentgenogram (soft-tissue shadow of enlarged epiglottis), blood culture, throat culture (but see below).

- **Disease Severity**
  Roentgenographic findings, pulse oximetry, clinical distress, accessory muscle use, intercostal retractions.

- **Concept and Application**
  Edema of epiglottis obstructing upper airway. Etiologic agent usually *Haemophilus influenzae* type b.

- **Management**
  Antibiotics active against *H. influenzae* (cefuroxime, ampicillin plus clavulinic acid, others). Endotracheal intubation or tracheostomy in severe cases. Airway examination and throat culture may provoke laryngospasm and cardiopulmonary arrest!

C. Acute Bronchitis

- **H&P Keys**
  Severe, prolonged productive cough, fever, dyspnea.

- **Diagnosis**
  History and physical, sputum culture, chest roentgenogram to rule out bronchopneumonia.

- **Disease Severity**
  Respiratory rate, temperature.

- **Concept and Application**
  Infection and inflammation of large airways. Usually viral (influenza, adenovirus). May be bacterial (*Mycoplasma pneumoniae, Bordetella pertussis*).

- **Management**

Viral. Symptomatic decongestants, cough suppressants. Amantadine or rimantadine if influenza is suspected.

Mycoplasma or Bordetella. Erythromycin.

D. Acute Bronchiolitis

- **H&P Keys**
  Children under 2 years old following upper respiratory infection; tachypnea, inspiratory and expiratory wheezing, intercostal and suprasternal retractions, nasal flaring, hyperresonant chest, wheezing, inspiratory rales.

- **Diagnosis**
  Chest roentgenogram: hyperinflated lungs, peribronchial thickening; may have concurrent bronchopneumonia. Normal white blood cell (WBC) count. Inspiratory "click."

- **Disease Severity**
  Respiratory rate, intercostal retractions, pulse oximetry.

- **Concept and Application**
  Acute inflammation of small airways causing hyperinflation, obstruction, and atelectasis. Majority associated with respiratory syncytial virus.

- **Management**
  Oxygen, hydration, aerosol ribavirin for respiratory syncytial virus.

E. Pertussis

- **H&P Keys**
  Usually occurs in infants under 2 years old.

Catarrhal Stage. Lasts 1 to 2 weeks. Presents similarly to viral illness: low-grade fever, injected conjunctiva.

Paroxysmal Stage. Lasts 2 to 4 weeks. Severe, paroxysmal, short coughs with inspiratory "whoop." Thick, tenacious secretions, usually afebrile.

- **Diagnosis**
  Nasopharyngeal culture (requires special medium), elevated WBC count (mostly lymphocytes); increased polymorphonuclear neutrophils (PMNs) suggest bacterial superinfection.

- **Disease Severity**
  WBC count. Presence of bacterial superinfection.

- **Concept and Application**
  Infection of tracheobronchial tree with *Bordetella pertussis*. In severe cases, mucopurulent exudate obstructs small airways.

- **Management**
  Erythromycin in catarrhal stage (does not help in paroxysmal stage), supportive care, treatment of superinfection if present.

F. Bacterial Bronchopneumonia

1. Pneumococcal Pneumonia

- **H&P Keys**
  Acute onset of rigors, fever, productive cough of "rusty" sputum, tachypnea, respiratory distress, pleuritic chest pain, bronchial breath sounds. Dullness to percussion may indicate accompanying effusion or empyema.

- **Diagnosis**
  Chest roentgenogram (lobar infiltrate), sputum Gram's stain, sputum culture, blood culture, WBC.

- **Disease Severity**
  Pulse oximetry, arterial blood gases (ABG), tachypnea, chest roentgenogram. Multilobed

involvement, low WBC count, positive blood culture, and older age associated with worse prognosis.

- **Concept and Application**
Infection caused by *Streptococcus pneumoniae*. Most common cause of community-acquired pneumonia. Can cause otitis, meningitis, pleural effusion, empyema. Elderly, infants, asplenic, and immunocompromised patients at highest risk.

- **Management**
Penicillin G or erythromycin, chest tube drainage if empyema present. Pneumococcal vaccine for high-risk individuals after acute episode resolves. Oxygen if hypoxic. Penicillin resistance is emerging worldwide—Use vanlomycin if present.

2. Staphylococcal Pneumonia

- **H&P Keys**
Fever, dyspnea, cough with purulent sputum.

- **Diagnosis**
Chest roentgenogram (multifocal infiltrates, abscess, pneumatocele, effusions), sputum Gram's stain, sputum culture, blood culture, elevated WBC.

- **Disease Severity**
Pulse oximetry, ABG, tachypnea, chest roentgenogram. Metastatic infection (central nervous system [CNS], bone, endocarditis, sepsis).

- **Concept and Application**
Pulmonary infection caused by *Staphylococcus aureus*. Seen after influenza infection, chronic obstructive pulmonary disease (COPD), hematogenous spread from staph endocarditis (especially in intravenous drug abusers with right heart endocarditis), nosocomial infection.

- **Management**
β-Lactamase–resistant penicillin, (some strains are resistant), vancomycin. Oxygen if hypoxic.

3. *Haemophilus influenzae* Pneumonia

- **H&P Keys**
Young children, chronic lung disease, alcoholics. Fever, cough, dyspnea, purulent sputum. May present with subacute presentation over several weeks.

- **Diagnosis**
Sputum Gram's stain, sputum and blood culture, chest roentgenogram (multilobar patchy infiltrates).

- **Disease Severity**
Pulse oximetry, ABG, respiratory rate, chest roentgenogram. Empyema is rare.

- **Concept and Application**
Pulmonary infection caused by *Haemophilus influenzae*.

- **Management**
Cefuroxime, ampicillin and clavulinic acid, trimethoprim and sulfamethoxazole, chloramphenicol, others.

4. Gram-Negative Bacillary Pneumonias

- **H&P Keys**
Usually nosocomial, fever, chills, dyspnea, cough productive of purulent and sometimes bloody sputum.

- **Diagnosis**
Sputum Gram's stain, sputum and blood cultures, chest roentgenogram (lobar or multilobar, cavitary infiltrates), elevated WBC.

- **Disease Severity**
Pulse oximetry, ABG, respiratory rate, chest roentgenogram (multilobed involvement and cavitation). High mortality.

- **Concept and Application**
Aspiration of gram-negative bacilli from colonized oropharynx. *Klebsiella pneumoniae*, *Acinetobacter* and *Pseudomonas* species, Enterobacteriacae genera; common in immunocompromised and mechanically ventilated patients. *Klebsiella* common in alcoholics.

- **Management**
  Third-generation cephalosporin or semisynthetic penicillin (ticarcillin, piperacillin) plus an aminoglycoside antibiotic. Check antibiotic sensitivities (resistant strains common).

G. Atypical Pneumonias

1. Legionnaire's Disease

- **H&P Keys**
  Lethargy, headache, fever, rigors, anorexia, myalgias, nonproductive cough, nausea, vomiting, and diarrhea. Rales and rhonchi, abdominal tenderness, relative bradycardia.

- **Diagnosis**
  Chest roentgenogram (lobar, nodular, or patchy subsegmental), low sodium and phosphate, elevated WBC. Sputum culture (requires special media), serologic titers, urinary antigen.

- **Disease Severity**
  Symptoms, respiratory rate, pulse oximetry, ABG, chest roentgenogram.

- **Concept and Application**
  Infection with *Legionnella* species; transmitted through contaminated water system (not person-to-person). More common in immunocompromised, chronic disease, dialysis, alcoholics.

- **Management**
  Erythromycin, tetracycline. Addition of rifampin in severe cases; oxygen if hypoxic.

2. Mycoplasma pneumoniae

- **H&P Keys**
  Fever, chills, persistent nonproductive cough, headache, sore throat. Common in young adults.

- **Diagnosis**
  Gram's stain (many WBCs without predominant organism), chest roentgenogram (interstitial or diffuse alveolar infiltrates), cold agglutinins, serum complement fixation titers.

- **Disease Severity**
  Usually does not require hospitalization.

- **Concept and Application**
  Extrapulmonary manifestations common, including bullous myringitis, pharyngitis, meningitis, and erythema multiforme, Stevens-Johnson syndrome.

- **Management**
  Erythromycin or tetracycline.

3. *Pneumocystis carinii* Pneumonia

- **H&P Keys**
  Opportunistic infection most commonly related to HIV or other immunodeficiency states. Subacute onset fever, dyspnea, nonproductive cough, tachypnea, tachycardia, diffuse rales.

- **Diagnosis**
  Induced sputum cytology, bronchoscopic lavage or biopsy, elevated lactic dehydrogenase (LDH), HIV test, CD4 count, chest roentgenogram (diffuse interstitial or alveolar infiltrates, may be atypical or even clear).

- **Disease Severity**
  Pulse oximetry, ABG, respiratory rate, and clinical appearance.

- **Concept and Application**
  Molecular genetic data suggest organism is fungal.

- **Management**
  Trimethoprim and sulfamethoxazole (TMP/SMX) or pentamidine; oxygen and corticosteroids if hypoxic. Prophylax susceptible patients with TMP/SMX.

4. Influenza Pneumonia

- **H&P Keys**
  Abrupt onset fever, chills, headache, myalgias, and malaise. Nonproductive or productive cough, tachypnea and dyspnea follow.

- **Diagnosis**
  Sputum Gram's stain (many WBCs without organisms); chest roentgenogram (bilateral diffuse midlung and lower-lung infiltrates), viral cultures of nose and throat, acute and convalescent serum titers.

- **Disease Severity**
  Respiratory rate, clinical appearance.

- **Concept and Application**
  Viral pneumonia caused by influenza A.

- **Management**
  Amantadine or rimantadine if administered within 48 hours, otherwise symptomatic treatment. Influenza vaccine for high- and moderate-risk groups.

H. Pulmonary Tuberculosis

- **H&P Keys**
  Fever, malaise, weight loss, dyspnea, night sweats; productive cough with hemoptysis, rales in area of involvement; amphoric breath sounds may indicate cavity.

- **Diagnosis**
  Chest roentgenogram (upper-lobe cavitary disease if reactivation, lower-lobe infiltrates in primary infection, upper-lobe scarring may indicate prior inactive infection). Sputum culture, acid-fast smear; bronchoscopy if unable to get diagnosis on sputum studies. Purified protein derivative (tuberculin) (PPD) skin test.

- **Disease Severity**
  Chest roentgenogram. Extrapulmonary involvement (lymphatic, pleural, peritoneal, genitourinary, miliary, bone and joint, meningeal) may be more problematic. Drug-resistant strains more difficult to treat.

- **Concept and Application**
  Inhalation of *Mycobacterium tuberculosis* leads to primary lower-lobe infection. Localized inflammatory response usually halts infection. Reactivation disease occurs in upper lobes of lung or other areas of high oxygen content.

- **Management**

  Prophylaxis. Isoniazid for 6 to 12 months in appropriate patients with inactive infection (Table 16–1, 16–2).

TABLE 16–1. RECOMMENDATIONS FOR ISONIAZID (INH) PROPHYLAXIS

- Primary prophylaxis: Household members and close contacts of potentially infectious persons.
- Secondary prophylaxis: Newly infected persons as evidenced by a newly positive PPD.
- Patients with past tuberculosis or with a positive PPD and abnormal chest roentgenogram in whom current infection is excluded.
- Patients with a positive PPD and impaired cell-mediated immunity (steroid use, immunosuppressive therapy, AIDS, positive HIV test, hematologic malignancies, lymphoma, malnutrition, diabetes, and silicosis).
- Patients under the age of 35 with a positive PPD.

PPD, purified protein derivative (tuberculin).

Treatment. Isoniazid and rifampin for 6 months, with pyrazinamide plus either ethambutol or streptomycin for first 2 months. In cities with frequent drug resistance, therapy may be started with six drugs. Drug-resistant strains require longer treatment with additional antibiotics.

TABLE 16–2. INTERPRETATION OF TUBERCULIN SKIN TESTING

1. A reaction of more than 5 mm is classified as positive in the following groups of patients:
   A. Persons with HIV infection or suspected HIV infection with unknown HIV status.
   B. Persons with close contact to a patient with recent active, infectious tuberculosis.
   C. Persons who have chest roentgenograhpic findings consistent with old, healed tuberculosis.
2. A reaction of more than 10 mm is classified as positive in persons who have other risk factors for tuberculosis or are in high prevalence situations. These include:
   A. Foreign-born persons from countries with a high prevalence rate for tuberculosis, such as Asia, Africa, or Latin America.
   B. Intravenous drug abusers.
   C. Medically underserved low-income populations, including high-risk racial and ethnic minority populations (African Americans, Hispanics, Native Americans).
   D. Residents of long-term care facilities (nursing homes, correctional facilities, etc).
   E. Persons with medical conditions that have been reported to increase the risk of tuberculosis (silicosis, gastrectomy, jejunoileal bypass, chronic renal failure, diabetes mellitus, high-dose corticosteroid use, immunosuppressive therapy, cancer, and malnutrition).
3. Reactions greater than 15 mm are classified as positive in all other persons.

Adapted from American Thoracic Society. Diagnostic Standards and Classifications of Tuberculosis. *Am Rev Resp Dis.* 1990;142:725–35.

I. Fungal Pneumonias

3. Histoplasmosis

- **H&P Keys**
  Mostly asymptomatic, can have abrupt onset of flulike illness, with fever, chills, substernal chest pain, nonproductive cough with myalgias, arthralgias, and headache.

- **Diagnosis**
  Chest roentgenogram: Acute disease often normal, hilar adenopathy with lower-lobe alveolar infiltrates, leading to chronic calcification). Progressive form mimics tuberculosis. Diagnosis with sputum culture. Progressive disseminated histoplasmosis: blood and bone marrow culture. Serologic testing (acute and convalescent titers; poor sensitivity).

- **Disease Severity**
  Progressive and progressive disseminated more severe. Latter associated with T-cell dysfunction (AIDS).

- **Concept and Application**
  Infection with *Histoplasma capsulatum*. Inhalation of spores from soil (bat and bird droppings). Endemic areas: Ohio and Mississippi River valleys and neighboring states.

- **Management**

  Acute. None needed.

  Progressive Cavitary Disease. Itraconazole. Alternative: ketoconazole.

  Progressive Disseminated Disease. Amphotericin B.

  Chronic Suppression (for Patients with AIDS). Itraconazole.

2. Blastomycosis

- **H&P Keys**
  Abrupt fever, chills, cough with mucopurulent sputum, arthralgias, and myalgias. Signs of consolidation, erythema nodosum.

- **Diagnosis**
  KOH preparation of expectorated sputum; culture, complement fixation. Chest roentgenogram (round densities, may cavitate).

- **Disease Severity**
  Chest roentgenogram, evidence of extrapulmonary involvement.

- **Concept and Application**
  Infection with *Blastomyces dermatitidis*. Manifestations vary: asymptomatic to severe, life-threatening, disseminated illness. Midwest and South-central United States, midwestern Canada.

- **Management**

  Progressive Pulmonary, Nonsevere. Itraconazole. Alternative: ketoconazole.

  Disseminated or Severe Disease. Amphotericin B.

2. Coccidiomycosis

- **H&P Keys**
  Cough, fever, pleuritic chest pain, headache (may be indicative of meningitis); erythematous rash, "valley fever": erythema nodosum, erythema multiforme, arthralgias.

- **Diagnosis**
  Chest roentgenogram (patchy pneumonitis, hilar adenopathy, "coin lesions," cavitary lesions), KOH preparation of sputum, lung biopsy, complement fixation, skin test.

- **Disease Severity**
  Disseminated disease (meningitis, skin lesions, bone, etc). Dissemination more common in AIDS, steroids, malignant disease, African Americans, Native Americans, Mexicans.

- **Concept and Application**
  Infection with *Coccidioides immitis*. Mostly mild, self-limited, but can be life-threatening and disseminated. Southwestern United States and California valley regions, northern Mexico.

- **Management**

Nonmeningeal Disease. Fluconazole or amphotericin B. Alternative: ketoconazole, itraconazole.

Disseminated Disease or Meningitis. Fluconazole ± intrathecal miconazole, or amphotericin B; intrathecal amphotericin if fluconazole fails.

3. Cryptococcus

- **H&P Keys**

Pneumonia. Usually asymptomatic, but may have fever, malaise, chest pain, cough.

Meningitis. Subacute fever, confusion, headache. May be fulminant. Cranial nerve palsies.

- **Diagnosis**
  Cerebrospinal fluid (CSF) examination (India ink stain, latex particle agglutination), lung biopsy, chest roentgenogram (variable, large and small round lesions).

- **Disease Severity**
  Disseminated disease (CNS), presence of meningitis, chest roentgenogram.

- **Concept and Application**
  Cryptococcus neoformans, found in bird droppings and soil. Increased risk in AIDS, corticosteroid use, Hodgkin's disease, other immunocompromised states.

- **Management**
  None needed in noncompromised host with isolated pulmonary disease.

Immunocompromised Host or Disseminated Disease. Amphotericin B plus flucytosine. Alternatives: fluconazole, itraconazole.

4. Invasive Aspergillosis

- **H&P Keys**
  Immunosuppressed patient on multiple antibiotics, high fever, pleuritic chest pain, pleural friction rub.

- **Diagnosis**
  Cultures of sputum and nasal swab (suggestive, not diagnostic), lung biopsy.

- **Disease Severity**
  Chest roentgenogram (lobar, peripheral wedge-shaped infiltrates, often cavitary), pulse oximetry, ABG.

- **Concept and Application**
  Opportunistic infection with *Aspergillus fumigatus* causing pneumonia, pulmonary infarction.

- **Management**
  Amphotericin B. Prognosis poor.

5. Phycomycosis

- **H&P Keys**
  Occurs in diabetic ketoacidosis, with glucocorticosteroids, cytotoxic agents, burn victims. Rhinocerebral disease, acute pneumonia with pleuritic chest pain and hemoptysis.

- **Diagnosis**
  Chest roentgenogram (multiple wedge-shaped infiltrates), tissue biopsy.

- **Disease Severity**
  Life-threatening disease.

- **Concept and Application**
  Infection with *Mucor* (most common), also *Rhizopus* or *Absidia.*

- **Management**
  Amphotericin B and aggressive resectional surgery. Prognosis extremely poor.

II. OBSTRUCTIVE PULMONARY DISEASES

A. Pulmonary Function Tests

Obstruction. Low forced expiratory volume in one second (FEV-1), low or normal forced vital capacity (FVC), reduced FEV-1 : FVC ratio (<75%), normal total lung capacity (TLC).

Restriction. Defined by reduced TLC. Pure restriction will also have low FEV-1, FVC with normal or elevated FEV-1 : FVC ratio.

Combined Obstruction and Restriction.
Reduced FEV-1, FVC, and FEV-1 : FVC ratio
with reduced TLC.

B. Asthma

- **H&P Keys**
  Acute onset of dyspnea, wheezing, cough
  that remit spontaneously or with treatment.

- **Diagnosis**
  Pulmonary function testing (PFT) (obstructive), response to bronchodilators, response to bronchoconstricting provocational agents.

- **Disease Severity**
  PFT, use of accessory muscles, ABG, paradoxical pulse, respiratory rate, pulse oximetry, symptoms, mentation.

- **Concept and Application**
  Bronchospasm, inflammation, hyperreactivity to inhaled antigens and irritants, mucus plugging. Obstruction may improve to normal with treatment.

- **Management**

  Acute

  Bronchodilators. Inhaled β-agonist, subcutaneous epinephrine, with or without intravenous aminophylline.

  Anti-inflammatory Agents. Systemic corticosteroids.

  Chronic

  Anti-inflammatory Agents. Inhaled corticosteroids, cromolyn sodium, nedocromil sodium.

  Bronchodilator Agents. β-Agonists (inhaled, subcutaneous, oral), theophylline. Avoidance of causative agents.

C. Chronic Obstructive Pulmonary Diseases

Commonly used term with no agreed-upon definition. Term is usually applied to patients with chronic bronchitis or emphysema who have obstruction on PFTs. The obstruction may be partially reversible.

1. Chronic Bronchitis

- **H&P Keys**
  Defined as presence of chronic productive cough for *3 months in 2 successive years* without other discernible cause. Dyspnea, recurrent productive cough, "blue bloater"; cyanosis with edema, wheezes.

- **Diagnosis**
  PFTs (obstructive), history, chest roentgenogram (usually clear or hyperinflated). Sputum cultures for acute exacerbations.

- **Disease Severity**
  PFTs, pulse oximetry, ABG.

- **Concept and Application**
  In pure form, pathologic conditions in bronchi and airways, not alveoli. Tobacco smoke a causative agent. Bacterial infections may exacerbate (*Pneumococcus, Haemophilus,* others).

Simple Chronic Bronchitis. Symptoms fit criteria for chronic bronchitis but no obstruction on PFTs (therefore not truly a form of COPD).

Obstructive Chronic Bronchitis. Symptoms fit criteria for chronic bronchitis, reduced FEV-1 percent with no or partial bronchodilator response (this is a form of COPD). Obstruction caused by hypertrophic glands in airway, mucous hypersecretion.

- **Management**
  Smoking cessation, β-agonist bronchodilators, ipratropium bromide, influenza and pneumococcal vaccination, antibiotics for acute bacterial exacerbation, oxygen if hypoxic, corticosteroids if severe.

2. Emphysema

- **H&P Keys**
  Dyspnea, wheezing, cough. "Pink puffer": thin, not cyanotic, tachypnic. Diminished breath sounds, hyperinflated chest, hyperresonant to percussion.

- **Diagnosis**
  Obstructive PFTs (TLC may be increased), chest roentgenogram, history, and physi-

cal. Serum protein electrophoresis or α_1-protease inhibitor level if deficiency suspected.

- **Disease Severity**
  PFTs, ABG, exercise tolerance.

- **Concept and Application**
  Defined pathologically: enlarged respiratory air spaces beyond terminal bronchioles, with destruction of alveoli. Smoking a major risk factor; α_1-protease inhibitor deficiency a rare cause.

- **Management**
  Stopping smoking, bronchodilators, corticosteroids if severe and responsive, oxygen if hypoxic, corticosteroids may be helpful. α_1-Protease inhibitor for deficient patients.

3. Cystic Fibrosis

- **H&P Keys**
  Persistent cough, recurrent pneumonia and bronchitis, recurrent abdominal pain, meconium ileus, failure to thrive, steatorrhea, infertility, diabetes, family history. Usually diagnosed in childhood.

- **Diagnosis**
  Sweat chloride test (>60 mEq/mL before 20, >80 in adults) diagnostic. *Pseudomonas* lung infection, unexplained azospermia, and obstruction on PFTs suggests diagnosis. Chest roentgenogram (hyperinflation, enlarged pulmonary arteries, bronchiectasis, cystic areas).

- **Disease Severity**
  PFTs, pulse oximetry, ABG, chest roentgenogram.

- **Concept and Application**
  Autosomal recessive disorder; genetic defect in chloride permeability in exocrine glands; affects all exocrine secretions.

- **Management**
  Chest physiotherapy, bronchodilators, mucolytic agents, antibiotics, influenza vaccine, pancreatic enzymes (experimental: genetic replacement therapy).

4. Bronchiectasis

- **H&P Keys**
  Chronic cough, copious purulent sputum, recurrent fever, weakness, weight loss, hemoptysis, clubbing, cyanosis, edema.

- **Diagnosis**
  History, chest roentgenogram, high-resolution computerized tomographic (CT) scan, bronchography (rarely used), sputum culture.

- **Disease Severity**
  PFTs, stigmata of cor pulmonale.

- **Concept and Application**
  Abnormal dilatation of bronchi from inflammation and destruction of bronchial wall. Often associated with infection, bronchial obstruction, immotile-cilia syndrome, cystic fibrosis, allergic bronchopulmonary aspergillosis, immunoglobulin deficiency.

- **Management**
  Antibiotics for infection, chest physiotherapy, steroids for allergic bronchopulmonary aspergillosis, surgery or bronchial artery embolization for severe hemoptysis.

III. RESTRICTIVE PULMONARY DISEASES

A. Idiopathic   *Erythema nodosum*

1. Sarcoidosis

- **H&P Keys**
  May be asymptomatic. Dyspnea, cough, wheezing, hemoptysis, skin lesions (erythema nodosum, nodules, plaques), eye pain, arthralgias, cardiac arrhythmias, cranial nerve palsies. More common in African Americans, Scandinavians.

- **Diagnosis**
  Chest roentgenogram (bilateral hilar adenopathy, interstitial lung disease), tissue biopsy (noncaseating granuloma). Elevated serum calcium or angiotensin-converting enzyme suggestive.

- **Disease Severity**
  PFTs (restriction, low diffusion), chest roentgenogram, gallium scan (reflects disease activity); presence of CNS and cardiac involvement.

- **Concept and Application**
  Granulomatous disorder of unknown etiology.

- **Management**
  May be self-limited. Corticosteroids for significant pulmonary, CNS, or cardiac disease. Hydroxychloroquine sulfate (Plaquenil sulfate) or topical steroids for skin involvement.

2. Idiopathic Pulmonary Fibrosis *VIP*

- **H&P Keys**
  Insidious onset of dyspnea (may progress over many years), nonproductive cough, clubbing, fine crackles, cyanosis, stigmata of cor pulmonale, Raynaud's phenomenon.

- **Diagnosis**
  Chest roentgenogram (diffuse interstitial infiltrates), lung biopsy, PFTs (restriction, low diffusion), low positive antinuclear antibodies (ANA) titer.

- **Disease Severity**
  PFTs, ABG, exercise capacity.

- **Concept and Application**
  Pulmonary fibrosis of unknown etiology leading to hypoxia and cor pulmonale. Also called usual interstitial pneumonitis, interstitial pulmonary fibrosis, fibrosing alveolitis.

  Desquamative Interstitial Pneumonitis. Predominant alveolar component, more responsive to drugs.

- **Management**
  Corticosteroids, azathioprine, cyclophosphamide used with limited success; lung transplant only definitive therapy. Treat cor pulmonale with diuretics, oxygen.

B. Pneumoconiosis

1. Silicosis

- **H&P Keys**
  Sandblasters, miners, stoneworkers. Asymptomatic, or progressive dyspnea, cough.

- **Diagnosis**
  Exposure history, chest roentgenogram (upper lobe nodules, "eggshell calcification" of hilar nodes), PFTs (restriction), lung biopsy only if diagnosis in doubt.

- **Disease Severity**
  Chest roentgenogram and PFTs. *Progressive massive fibrosis:* coalescence of small nodules into larger conglomerate lesions.

- **Concept and Application**
  Inhalation of quartz particles damages alveolar cells and causes reactive fibrosis. Increased risk for tuberculosis.

- **Management**
  Avoidance of further exposure. No medical treatment known to be effective. Lung transplantation in severe cases.

2. Asbestosis

- **H&P Keys**
  History of asbestos exposure (mining, shipbuilding, insulation workers, construction). Asymptomatic, or progressive dyspnea, persistent cough, basilar inspiratory crackles, clubbing.

- **Diagnosis**
  Clinical diagnosis: interstitial disease with exposure history. Chest roentgenogram (lower-lobe linear infiltrates, pleural plaques and thickening); PFTs (restriction), ferruginous bodies (hemosiderin-coated asbestos fibers) in sputum, alveolar lavage fluid, or lung tissue.

- **Disease Severity**
  Chest roentgenogram, PFTs.

- **Concept and Application**
  Inhalation of asbestos fibers releases damaging enzymes and inflammatory mediators; direct damage to epithelial cells, leading to inflammation, fibrosis, and interstitial lung disease. Increased risk of lung cancer, especially in smokers.

- **Management**
  Avoidance of further exposure, stopping smoking.

Other Asbestos-related Diseases

Mesothelioma. Malignant tumor of the mesothelial cells of the pleura. Usually associated with severe chest wall pain.

Pleural Plaques. Benign, asymptomatic fibrous plaques detected on chest roentgenogram.

Pleural Thickening. Asymptomatic, detected on chest roentgenogram.

Acute Benign Pleural Effusions.

3. Coal Workers' Pneumoconiosis

- **H&P Keys**
  Coal miners, carbon manufacturers.

Simple Coal Workers' Pneumoconiosis. Asymptomatic.

Complicated Coal Workers' Pneumoconiosis (Progressive Massive Fibrosis). Dyspnea, signs of cor pulmonale, hemoptysis.

- **Diagnosis**
  Occupational exposure, chest roentgenogram (small round opacities, usually upper lobes).

- **Disease Severity**
  PFTs (usually normal in simple disease), chest roentgenogram. Progressive massive fibrosis (PMF) has enlarging, irregular nodular infiltrates, which may cavitate.

- **Concept and Application**
  Pulmonary nodules resulting from exposure to coal dust. PMF probably caused by an immunologic response. Obstructive disease usually a result of concomitant smoking. Increased risk for tuberculosis.

- **Management**
  Avoidance; surveillance for tuberculosis, stopping smoking, treatment of any underlying COPD if present.

4. Hypersensitivity Pneumonitis

- **H&P Keys**

Acute. Fever, chills, dyspnea, malaise 4 to 6 hours after exposure to antigen, lasting 18 to 24 hours.

Subacute. Insidious onset of cough, progressive dyspnea, fatigue, and weight loss, diffuse crackles.

Chronic. Insidious onset of progressive dyspnea over years.

- **Diagnosis**
  Exposure history key to diagnosis. Common antigens include: Thermophilic Actinomyces (farmer's lung: moldy hay; bagassosis: moldy sugar cane); avian secretory proteins (pigeon breeder's disease). Serum precipitins can help identify agent but are not diagnostic of disease.

- **Disease Severity**
  Chest roentgenogram (interstitial and alveolar infiltrates); PFTs (restriction, decreased diffusion).

- **Concept and Application**
  Immune-complex–mediated and cell-mediated hypersensitivity responses to inhaled antigen.

- **Management**
  Removal and avoidance of offending antigen; corticosteroids for severe attacks or if symptoms persist.

IV. PLEURAL DISEASES

A. Pleural Effusion

- **H&P Keys**
  Asymptomatic, or signs and symptoms of underlying cause. Dyspnea, pleuritic chest pain. Decreased breath sounds, dullness to percussion.

- **Diagnosis**
  Chest roentgenogram with lateral decubitus views. Pleural fluid chemistries (LDH, protein, glucose), cell count, cultures.

- **Disease Severity**
  Chest roentgenogram.

- **Concept and Application**

Transudate. Increased hydrostatic pressure or decreased systemic oncotic pressure.

Diagnosis. Pleural protein:serum protein <0.5, pleural LDH:serum LDH <0.6, pleural LDH less than two thirds of the upper limit of normal for serum LDH.

Examples. Congestive heart failure, nephrotic syndrome.

Exudate. Intrapulmonary or abdominal inflammation adjacent to pleura.

Diagnosis. Pleural:serum protein >0.5, pleural:serum LDH >0.6, pleural LDH greater than two thirds upper limit of normal for serum LDH.

Examples. Parapneumonic effusion, empyema, malignant disease, collagen vascular diseases.

- **Management**
  Treatment of underlying disease. Drainage of fluid with thoracentesis or chest tube if symptomatic or infected. Sclerosis with doxycycline or talc for recurrent effusions.

B. Pleurisy (Pleuritis)

- **H&P Keys**
  Pleuritic chest pain (sharp pain on inspiration), usually rapid onset, dyspnea, low-grade fever.

- **Diagnosis**
  Chest roentgenogram, history and physical.

- **Disease Severity**
  Usually self-limited.

- **Concept and Application**
  Inflammation of pleura.

Pleurodynia. Epidemic infection with coxsackie B or ECHO virus.

Pleuritis. Pleural inflammation, which may be due to infection, pulmonary infarction, collagen vascular disease, etc.

- **Management**
  Nonsteroidal anti-inflammatory agents.

C. Pneumothorax

- **H&P Keys**
  Chest pain, dyspnea, enlarged hemithorax, hyperresonance to percussion, absent or reduced breath sounds and fremitus on involved side, tracheal shift away from involved side.

- **Diagnosis**
  Chest roentgenogram (air in pleural space).

- **Disease Severity**
  Chest roentgenogram, pulse oximetry and ABG, pulse rate, respiratory rate, blood pressure.

- **Concept and Application**
  Communication between lung or atmosphere and pleural space.

Spontaneous Pneumothorax. Rupture of subpleural blebs or bullae; also seen with COPD and interstitial lung diseases.

Traumatic Pneumothorax. Result of direct or indirect chest trauma.

Tension Pneumothorax. Intrapleural pressure exceeds atmospheric pressure, decreases venous return, which drops cardiac output and blood pressure.

- **Management**
  Observation if stable. Chest tube if large, symptomatic, or if tension pneumothorax is present or suspected.

V. DISEASES OF PULMONARY CIRCULATION

A. Cardiogenic Pulmonary Edema (Congestive Heart Failure)

- **H&P Keys**
  Dyspnea, diapheresis, wheezing, tachycardia, cyanosis, diffuse crackles or rales, edema, cough with frothy sputum, fine and coarse crackles, S_3, displaced point of maximal impulse (PMI), peripheral edema.

- **Diagnosis**
  History and physical, chest roentgenogram (diffuse alveolar infiltrates, enlarged heart, Kerley's B lines), echocardiogram or nuclear multiple-gated arteriography (MUGA) scan, electrocardiogram (ECG) (ischemic changes),

pulmonary artery catheterization (elevated pulmonary artery and pulmonary artery occlusion pressures).

- **Disease Severity**
  ABG, clinical appearance, vital signs, pulmonary artery occlusion pressure.

- **Concept and Application**
  Increased hydrostatic pressure from left ventricular failure (ischemia, myocardial infarction [MI]) or fluid overload.

- **Management**
  Oxygen, diuresis (furosemide, low-dose dopamine), venodilators (nitroglycerin, morphine), afterload reduction agents (intrave-nous nitroglycerin, sodium nitroprusside), dobutamine. Pulmonary arterial catheter to monitor therapy may be helpful. Treatment of ischemia if present.

B. Adult Respiratory Distress Syndrome

- **H&P Keys**
  Acute onset of severe dyspnea, tachypnea, cough productive of frothy sputum, diffuse rales and rhonchi, cyanosis, signs and symptoms of underlying process (sepsis and trauma most common).

- **Diagnosis**
  Chest roentgenogram (bilateral alveolar infiltrates), ABG (hypoxemia Pao_2/Fio_2 ≤ 200), pulmonary artery catheterization (pulmonary capillary wedge pressure ≤ 18) in setting of known risk factor.

- **Disease Severity**
  Chest roentgenogram and ABG.

- **Concept and Application**
  Pulmonary edema from increased permeability across the alveolar and capillary walls. Risk factors: sepsis, diffuse pulmonary infection, trauma, aspiration, drowning, toxic inhalations, hypertransfusion, others.

- **Management**
  Treatment of underlying cause, supportive measures: mechanical ventilation, oxygen, and positive end-expiratory pressure (PEEP).

C. Newborn Respiratory Distress Syndrome (Hyaline Membrane Disease)

- **H&P Keys**
  Neonate, usually premature, with dyspnea, tachypnea, poor air movement; chest wall retractions occur shortly after birth.

- **Diagnosis**
  Chest roentgenogram (diffuse granular or ground-glass infiltrate), pulse oximetry, ABG.

- **Disease Severity**
  Clinical appearance of respiratory distress, ABG.

- **Concept and Application**
  Decreased pulmonary surfactant leading to reduced lung compliance and atelectasis.

- **Management**
  Oxygen, continuous distending airway pressure (CADP or CDP), mechanical ventilation, surfactant replacement therapy. Prevention of premature labor and use of prenatal steroid therapy to reduce incidence of disease.

D. Pulmonary Embolism

- **H&P Keys**
  Acute onset of dyspnea and pleuritic chest pain. Cough, hemoptysis, tachypnea, tachycardia; look for pleural rub, edema, or tenderness in lower extremity.

- **Diagnosis**
  ABG (acute respiratory alkalosis, usually decreased Po_2), chest roentgenogram (clear, or wedge-shaped infiltrate, effusion), ECG (sinus tach, or S1, Q3, T3 inversion pattern), ventilation perfusion lung scan (perfusion defect with normal ventilation), noninvasive or venogram studies for deep venous thrombosis (DVT) in lower extremities, pulmonary angiogram.

- **Disease Severity**
  ABG, vital signs.

- **Concept and Application**
  Venous thrombus, usually from lower extremity, embolizes to pulmonary artery. Preg-

nancy, use of birth control pills, smoking, malignant disease, obesity, immobilization (hip fracture) at highest risk for DVT.

- **Management**
Anticoagulation (heparin, then warfarin for 3 to 6 months). Thrombolytic agents for massive embolism with shock. Embolectomy in unresponsive cases. Vena caval interruption if anticoagulation is contraindicated (vena caval clip, Greenfield filter, others). Prophylaxis of high-risk patients with subcutaneous low-dose heparin, warfarin, or compression boots.

E. Pulmonary Vasculitis

- **H&P Keys**
Dyspnea; symptoms of underlying disease process.

- **Diagnosis**
Chest roentgenogram, ABG, serologic studies for systemic vasculitic processes (ANA, etc). Tissue biopsy usually required for diagnosis (open lung biopsy or biopsy of other affected organs).

- **Disease Severity**
ABG, exercise tolerance, serologic studies of underlying disease.

- **Concept and Application**
Inflammation of pulmonary blood vessels.

Leukocytoclastic Vasculitis. Neutrophilic inflammation caused by drugs, neoplasms, infection.

Granulomatous Vasculitis. Lymphocytic infiltration, eg, Wegener's granulomatosis (renal involvement), allergic granulomatosia (asthma, eosinophilia; "Churg-Strauss syndrome").

Collagen Vascular Diseases. Rheumatoid arthritis, systemic lupus erythematosis, progressive systemic sclerosis, polymyositis, dermatomyositis, mixed connective tissue disease.

- **Management**

Leukocytoclastic Vasculitis. Usually self-limited. Steroids if hypoxemia present.

Wegener's Granulomatosis. Cyclophosphamide with or without corticosteroids.

Allergic Granulomatosis, Collagen Vascular Diseases. Corticosteroids; azathioprine or cyclophosphamide in severe cases. Progressive systemic sclerosis usually does not respond.

F. Vasculitis: Goodpasture's Syndrome

- **H&P Keys**
Hemoptysis, hematuria, fever, dyspnea. Pulmonary involvement associated with smoking.

- **Diagnosis**
Antiglomerular basement membrane antibodies, renal biopsy (linear immunofluorescence pattern).

- **Disease Severity**
Amount of hemoptysis, chest roentgenogram, blood urea nitrogen (BUN), creatinine, ABG.

- **Concept and Application**
Circulating glomerular basement membrane antibodies damage glomerular and alveolar basement membranes.

- **Management**
Corticosteroids plus cyclophosphamide or azothioprine; plasmapheresis.

G. Cor Pulmonale

Defined as right-ventricular failure secondary to pulmonary disease.

- **H&P Keys**
Breathlessness, hepatic discomfort, symptoms of underlying disease. Right-ventricular heave, loud split S_2, peripheral edema, ascites.

- **Diagnosis**
Chest roentgenogram (large pulmonary artery, right-ventricle hypertrophy [RVH]); ECG (RVH, pulmonale), echocardiogram (RVH, elevated pulmonary artery pressures), PFTs (reflect underlying disease).

- **Disease Severity**
  ABG, cardiac catheterization (direct measurement of pulmonary artery pressures), symptoms, and exercise tolerance.

- **Concept and Application**
  Hypoxic vasoconstriction leads to pulmonary hypertension and hypertrophy of right ventricle. Occurs in severe primary pulmonary diseases, including COPD, sleep apnea.

- **Management**
  Oxygen, diuretics. Treatment of underlying disease.

VI. PULMONARY NEOPLASTIC DISEASES

A. Bronchogenic Carcinoma

- **H&P Keys**
  Smoking, asbestosis produce highest risk. Asymptomatic or cough, hemoptysis, dyspnea, chest pain, fever, weight loss, hoarseness, focal wheezing or decreased breath sounds, adenopathy.

- **Diagnosis**
  Chest roentgenogram (coin lesion or mass, adenopathy), CT scan, bronchoscopic or percutaneous needle biopsy or cytologic aspiration.

- **Disease Severity**
  Severity depends on stage, cell type, and patient's general condition.

- **Concept and Application**

  Adenocarcinoma. Usually peripheral; gland-like structure on path.

  Squamous Cell. Usually central, often cavitates, best prognosis.

  Oat Cell (Small Cell). Usually central, high metastatic potential.

  Alveolar Cell. Subtype of adeno, originates in terminal bronchioles or alveoli, peripheral.

Large Cell. Poorly differentiated, tends to be peripheral, rapid-growing with high metastatic potential.

- **Management**

  Non-small Cell. Staging, surgery if resectable. Radiation for palliation.

  Small Cell. Chemotherapy. Rarely resectable (usually metastatic when discovered).

  All. May metastasize to other lung, mediastinum, brain, adrenal glands, other organs. Watch for superior vena cava syndrome, hypercalcemia.

B. Carcinoid Tumors

- **H&P Keys**
  Asymptomatic or wheezing, cough, hemoptysis, obstruction. Carcinoid syndrome (episodic flushing, bronchospasm, and diarrhea) is rare.

- **Diagnosis**
  Chest roentgenogram (clear, mass, or obstructive pneumonia). Lung biopsy, urine 5-hydroxyindoleacetic acid.

- **Disease Severity**
  Metastatic workup.

- **Concept and Application**
  Tumors are slow-growing with low metastatic potential. Classified as "neurosecretory," but cellular origin is now unclear.

- **Management**
  Surgical resection. Chemotherapy or radiation for recurrent or metastatic disease.

C. Metastatic Malignant Tumors

- **H&P Keys**
  Often asymptomatic, or cough, hemoptysis, wheezing, dyspnea, pain, symptoms of obstructive pneumonia. Signs and symptoms of primary malignant disease.

- **Diagnosis**
  Chest roentgenogram (single or multiple masses or nodules, pleural effusion, hilar or mediastinal adenopathy), biopsy of pulmonary lesion or primary lesion.

- **Disease Severity**
  Metastatic workup.

- **Concept and Application**
  Metastatic tumor cells enter via hematogenous or lymphatic route. Colon, breast, lymphoma, testicular, kidney, thyroid, melanoma, others.

- **Management**
  Surgical excision for single metastases if possible. Otherwise, systemic therapy determined by primary tumor cell type and site.

VII. ILL-DEFINED SYMPTOM COMPLEX

A. Cough

- **H&P Keys**
  Smoking history, sputum characteristics (color, viscosity), postnasal drip, throat clearing, reflux symptoms, wheezing, occupational history, medication history help pinpoint cause.

- **Diagnosis**
  History and physical, PFTs, bronchoprovocation challenge tests, chest roentgenogram, sputum culture, trial of medication. Common causes of cough:

  Asthma. Wheezing may not be present. Diagnose by history, bronchoprovocation challenge.

  COPD. Diagnose by history and physical, trial of decongestants.

  Gastroesophageal Reflux. Worse at night and recumbent.

  Others. Recurrent aspiration, lung carcinoma, congestive heart failure, medications (β-blockers, angiotensin converting enzyme [ACE] inhibitors), bronchiectasis, others.

- **Disease Severity**
  Cough intensity and number.

- **Concept and Application**
  Nonspecific symptom caused by (1) direct stimulation of cough receptors (foreign body, tumor), (2) increased sensitivity of cough receptors (asthma), (3) inadequate glottic closure (aspiration, reflux), or (4) altered mucus quantity or quality (chronic bronchitis, bronchiectasis).

- **Management**
  Treatment of underlying disorder. Therapeutic trial of bronchodilators, ant-acids, H_2 blockers, decongestants may be diagnostic. Guaifenesin, dextromethorphan, or codeine may alleviate symptoms.

B. Dyspnea

- **H&P Keys**
  Shortness of breath, chest tightness, air hunger, signs and symptoms of underlying disease.

- **Diagnosis**
  History and physical examination, PFTs, exercise testing, ECG, chest roentgenogram. Differential diagnosis of dyspnea includes pulmonary diseases, congestive heart failure (CHF), neuromuscular disease, anemia, hyperventilation disorders (eg, metabolic acidosis, psychogenic).

- **Disease Severity**
  Exercise tolerance, symptom scores. Usually dyspnea correlates with degree of pulmonary dysfunction.

- **Concept and Application**
  Sensation of increased respiratory effort.

- **Management**
  Specific treatment of underlying disease (bronchodilators for COPD, diuretics for CHF, etc). General supportive measures include oxygen for hypoxia, nutritional and psychologic support, pulmonary rehabilitation.

C. Chest Pain

- **H&P Keys**
  Quality of pain, location, and relationship to breathing keys to diagnosis. Signs and symptoms of underlying disease.

- **Diagnosis**

Breathing-Associated Pain. Pleuritis, lung infection, pulmonary embolism, pneumothorax, musculoskeletal pain, pericarditis.

Pain Not Associated with Breathing. Pulmonary hypertension, airway, or mediastinal inflammation, cardiac ischemia, dissecting aortic aneurysm, esophagitis, costochondritis.

- **Disease Severity**
Symptoms, exercise test, chest roentgenogram, PFTs, ECG.

- **Concept and Application**
Sensation of pain resulting from tissue injury or inflammation.

- **Management**
Diagnostic workup to identify source of pain, then specific therapy of underlying disease. Analgesics, therapeutic trial of antacids, nitrates, nonsteroidal antiinflammatory drugs when diagnostic workup is unrevealing.

D. Hemoptysis

- **H&P Keys**
Cough productive of bloody or blood-tinged sputum.

- **Diagnosis**
Differential diagnosis (common causes).

  - *Tracheobronchial disorders:* Acute or chronic bronchitis, bronchogenic carcinoma, bronchiectasis, cystic fibrosis, trauma, telangiectasia.
  - *Cardiovascular disorders:* Pulmonary infarction, mitral stenosis, CHF, atrioventricular malformation, aneurysm, others.
  - *Hematologic disorders:* Anticoagulation, thrombocytopenia, hemophilia, disseminated intravascular coagulation.
  - *Parenchymal lung disorders:* Bacterial pneumonia, tuberculosis, paragonimiasis, contusion.
  - *Vasculitic disorders:* Systemic lupus erythematosus, Goodpasture's syndrome, Wegener's granulomatosis.

- **Disease Severity**
Massive hemoptysis: >600 mL blood/48 h.

- **Concept and Application**
Damage to pulmonary parenchyma, tracheobronchial tree, or pulmonary vasculature; defects in coagulation, increased hydrostatic pressure. Mechanism depends on underlying etiology.

- **Management**
Diagnostic workup (chest roentgenogram, complete blood count [CBC], platelet count, prothrombin time [PT], partial thrombin time [PTT], sputum culture, cytology, acid-fast bacilli [AFB] smear, cytology), quantitate hemoptysis, bronchoscopy. Treatment of coagulation abnormalities and CHF if present, cough suppressant (codeine), antibiotic if infection present. Surgical excision of bleeding segment or angiographic embolization if persists.

E. Wheezing and Stridor

- **H&P Keys**
Audible, continuous, musical adventitial sound. Location and timing to respiratory cycle a help in diagnosis.

- **Diagnosis**
PFT, flow volume loop, bronchoprovocation challenge, chest roentgenogram, soft-tissue neck films, bronchoscopy.

Stridor. Inspiratory "wheeze" heard best over trachea and upper airway (eg, epiglottiditis, croup, tracheal stenosis, angioedema, laryngeal ("psychogenic") asthma.

Focal Inspiratory and Expiratory Wheeze. Bronchogenic tumor, foreign body.

Diffuse Expiratory Wheeze. Asthma, COPD, CHF.

- **Disease Severity**
Clinical symptoms, PFT.

- **Concept and Application**
Sound caused by vibrations of airway narrowed by bronchospasm, inflammation, mass, or edema.

- **Management**
Treatment of underlying disease, bronchodilators, oxygen if hypoxic.

F. Solitary Pulmonary Nodule (Coin Lesion)

- **H&P Keys**
Asymptomatic, or cough and hemoptysis. Smoking history, occupational exposures, previous malignant disease help in diagnosis.

- **Diagnosis**
Chest roentgenogram (single round lesion <6 cm), old chest roentgenogram, CT scan, bronchoscopic or transthoracic needle biopsy or aspirate, open biopsy.

- **Disease Severity**
Lung biopsy.

- **Concept and Application**
Round mass may be benign or malignant tumor, tuberculoma, granuloma, artifact, cyst, resolving pneumonia, others.

- **Management**
Old films key: if present more than 2 years, probably benign. Follow periodic chest roentgenography. If unavailable or new lesion, CT scan and biopsy mass. Unless a firm benign diagnosis can be made, surgical excision required. Laminated or solid calcification suggests benign granuloma.

G. Sleep Apnea Syndrome

- **H&P Keys**
Daytime sleepiness, restlessness, unrefreshed sleep, morning headaches, neuropsychiatric changes, signs and symptoms of cor pulmonale. Hypothyroidism, use of sedatives, ethanol should be ruled out.

- **Diagnosis**
Physical examination (obesity, narrowed pharyngeal opening); polysomnography.

- **Disease Severity**
Polysomnography, degree of nocturnal oxygen desaturation.

- **Concept and Application**

Central Sleep Apnea. Defective central drive causing transient apneic periods.

Obstructive Sleep Apnea. Occlusion of oropharyngeal upper airway during sleep.

- **Management**

Central Sleep Apnea. Oxygen, respiratory stimulants (acetazolamide), noninvasive mechanical ventilation (BiPAP).

Obstructive Sleep Apnea. Nasal continuous positive airway pressure (CPAP), tracheostomy, weight reduction, avoidance of sedatives and alcohol.

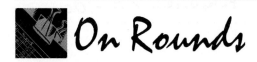

Bacterial and Other Pneumonia

Pneumococcal Pneumonia

- Acute onset of rigors, fever, and "rusty sputum"
- Lobar infiltrate on CXR
- Caused by Streptococcus pneumonia
- Is the most common cause of community acquired pneumonia

Staphlococcal Pneumonia

- Fever, cough, and purulent sputum
- Multifocal infiltrates, abscess, and effusions on CXR
- Caused by *Staphlococcus aureus*

Haemophilus Influenzae Pneumonia

- Fever, cough and, purulent sputum
- Found in young children, alcoholics, COPD patients
- Multilobar patchy infiltrates on CXR

Mycoplasma Pneumonia

- Fever, chills, sore throat, nonproductive cough, and headache
- Common in young adults
- Interstitial or diffuse alveolar infiltrate on CXR

Pneumocystis Carini Pneumonia

- Opportunistic infection, often HIV related
- Fever, dyspnea, tachypnea, tachycardia, rales, nonproductive cough
- CXR may be clear or demonstrate diffuse infiltrates

BIBLIOGRAPHY

American Thoracic Society. Diagnostic standards and classifications of tuberculosis. *Am Rev Resp Dis*. 1990;142:725–35.

Fishman AP, ed. *Pulmonary Diseases and Disorders*. 2nd ed. New York, McGraw-Hill Book Co; 1988.

Hodgkin JE, ed. *Clinics in Chest Medicine: Chronic Obstructive Pulmonary Disease*. Philadelphia: WB Saunders Co; 1990.

Light RW. *Pleural Diseases*. 2nd ed. Philadelphia: JB Lippincott Co; 1990.

Murray JF, Nadel JA, eds. *Textbook of Respiratory Medicine*. 2nd ed. Philadelphia: WB Saunders Co; 1994.

National Asthma Education Program Expert Panel Report. *Guidelines for the Diagnosis and Management of Asthma*. Publication No. 91-3042. Bethesda, MD: National Institutes of Health; 1991.

Azotemia = ↑BUN/creat
anuria: <100cc/day
Oliguria: <400cc/day
Polyuria: >3L/day.

BUN/creat Ratio >20:1 Prerenal.

17

Disease of the Renal and Urologic Systems

S. Bruce Malkowicz, MD

Hyaline cast - pre or post renal failure
Eosinophils (Hansel's stain) = interstitial nephritis
RBC cast = Glomerulonephritis

I. INFECTIOUS DISEASES AND INFLAMMATORY CONDITIONS

A. Urinary Tract Infection

- **H&P Keys**

  Dysuria, urgency, frequency, nocturia, suprapubic pain, back or flank pain, tenesmus, voiding of small volumes of urine, urethral discomfort.

- **Diagnosis**

  Urinalysis: pyuria, white blood count/high-power field, bacteriuria, hematuria. Urine culture, dip-slide method. Cystoscopy, voiding cystourethroscopy, intravenous (IV) urography in chronic cases.

- **Disease Severity**
  Gross hematuria, pain, ascending infection, fever and chills, initial or persistent or recurrent infection, pregnancy status, renal function.

- **Concept and Application**
  Male-female difference because of anatomy; bacterial-mucosal adherence principal reason for recurrent infection. Urinary stasis, *Escherichia coli* is principal pathogen. Fecal flora are primary source during in-dwelling or short-term catheterization. Asymptomatic bacteriuria in pregnant females (3% to 15%).

- **Management**
  Uncomplicated: TMP-SMZ for 5 to 7 days, also nitrofurantoin monohydrate macrocrystals 100 mg twice a day BID for 7 to 10 days. Three-day regimens effective. Persistent/recurrent infection: chronic or prophylactic use of antibiotics. Timed voiding, urodynamics, and imaging for complicated cases. Rule out nonbacterial causes such as TB, chlamydia, and yeast.

B. Painful Bladder and Urethral Syndromes

- **H&P Keys**
  Urinary urgency and frequency or dysuria, absence of documented chronic urinary tract infection (UTI), negative neurologic findings, absence of carcinoma.

- **Diagnosis**
  Cystoscopy: hydrodistention, urodynamics, bladder biopsy. Diagnosis of exclusion.

- **Disease Severity**
  Degree of *urinary* frequency, level of pain, and bladder capacity and deterioration of quality of life.

- **Concept and Application**
  Etiology undefined; grouping of syndromes rather than specific disease. Theories of mast-cell activity and glycosaminoglycan layer defects. Epithelial permeability.

- **Management**
  Hydrodistention, anticholinergics, dimethylsulfoxide intravesical instillation, therapies for chronic pain.

C. Prostatitis

- **H&P Keys**
  Slow or sudden onset, perineal discomfort, voiding dysfunction, prostate tenderness on digital rectal exam. UTI.

- **Diagnosis**
  Urine culture and sensitivity, extraprostatic secretion culture, urinalysis (pyuria).

- **Disease Severity**
  Fever or rigors, urinary retention, constant or intermittent discomfort, degree of voiding dysfunction.

- **Concept and Application**
  Distinguish true bacterial prostatitis (acute and chronic) from nonbacterial (inflammatory states, chlamydia) and prostadynia. Acute bacterial prostatitis responds dramatically to antibiotics. Fifty percent empiric response to antibiotics in other conditions. Prostatodynia in pelvic floor or sphincter spasm.

- **Management**
  Acute bacterial infection requires culture-appropriate antibiotics. Chronic bacterial or nonbacterial infection requires ciprofloxacin and ofloxacin or tetracyclines for 4- to 6-week course. Warm soaks and nonsteroidal anti-inflammatory drugs (NSAIDs). Chronic pain evaluation for prostatodynia.

D. Epididymitis

- **H&P Keys**
  Pain, tenderness, discomfort distinct from testis parenchyma. Normal testis, palpable epididymal discomfort. Slow or sudden onset. No trauma, sexual activity, voiding symptoms, genitourinary (GU) instrumentation.

- **Diagnosis**
  Pyuria; culture and sensitivity are usually negative. Scrotal ultrasound or Doppler good flow state, inflammation of epididymis.

- **Disease Severity**
  Fever or rigors, testis and epididymis are indistinguishable, scrotal induration, incapacitation.

- **Concept and Application**
Rule out torsion or tumor in young men (Prehn's sign is unreliable). Bacterial infection in older men with voiding dysfunction; chlamydia in younger men. Irritative urine reflux in acute or chronic states. Most respond to antibiotics in 3 to 6 weeks.

- **Management**
Warm soaks, elevation, intermediate course of antibiotics (ciprofloxacin or tetracyclines), NSAIDs.

E. Urethritis

- **H&P Keys**
Purulent or mucoid discharge. Dysuria and frequency during urination. History of sexual activity.

- **Diagnosis**
Gonococci (GC) culture in Thayer-Martin media, gram stain (−) diplococci, or specific chlamydia culture.

- **Disease Severity**
Ranges from painless discharge to severe voiding symptoms, epididymal and testicular involvement, systemic illness.

- **Concept and Application**
Generally gonococcal and nongonococcal (*Chlamydia trachomatis, Ureaplasma urealyticum, Trichomonas*) complications of urethral stricture or Reiter's syndrome.

- **Management**
Gonococcal infection: ceftriaxone, 250 mg intramuscularly (IM); procaine-penicillin, oral probenecid; ofloxacin, 400 mg oral, one dose. Nongonococcal infection: tetracycline 500 mg 4 times/day QID; doxycycline, 100 mg BID for 7 to 10 days, or ofloxacin, 300 mg BID for 7 to 10 days. Metronidazole for *Trichomonas*. Acyclovir for herpes.

F. Orchitis

- **H&P Keys**
Rapid or slow onset, fever and malaise, absence of trauma. Scrotal contents can be normal, inflamed, or distorted (torsion). Sexual or voiding dysfunction. Child or adolescent versus adult.

- **Diagnosis**
Pyuria, scrotal ultrasound, urine culture.

- **Disease Severity**
Scrotal induration, fistula, abscess on ultrasound, rule out torsion-hyperemic blood flow and systemic infection.

- **Concept and Application**
Rule out torsion in young men; bacterial infection in older men and sexually transmitted disease (STD) in younger men. Mumps orchitis in children and adolescents. Chronic orchalgia can be present without infection.

- **Management**
Four to six weeks of ciprofloxicin-ofloxacin or doxycycline. NSAIDs, warm soaks, and elevation.

G. Gonorrhea

- **H&P Keys**
Sexual exposure; thick, creamy urethral discharge; urethritis. May involve epididymis.

- **Diagnosis**
Gram-stain gram-negative diplococcus. GC culture in Thayer-Martin media.

- **Disease Severity**
Severity of pain and discharge; associated epididymitis or orchitis.

- **Concept and Application**
Beta-lactamase plasmid-penicillin resistance. Pili contribute to virulence. Different infection rate per exposure (male 20%, female 90%). Coexisting chlamydial infection.

- **Management**
Ceftriaxone, 250 mg IM, and doxycycline, 100 mg BID for 7 days. Penicillin, 4.8 million units IM with 1 g probenecid.

H. Syphilis

- **H&P Keys**
Sexual activity. Painless genital ulcer, lack of vesicles. Negative travel history.

- **Diagnosis**
  Rapid plasma reagin and fluorescent treponemal antibody-absorption test for syphilis, patient's history.

- **Disease Severity**
  Primary, secondary, or tertiary disease; systemic symptoms, neurosyphilis; cardiovascular changes.

- **Concept and Application**
  Treponema pallidum or spirochete family of bacteria. Three stages of disease with different systemic findings.

- **Management**
  Benzathine, 2.4 million units IM, one dose. Erythromycin base 2 g/day for 2 weeks. Tertiary stage: procaine-penicillin, 600 000 units per day for 2 weeks.

I. Chlamydia

- **H&P Keys**
  Sexual activity, younger age group, clear or mucoid discharge.

- **Diagnosis**
  No routine culture; tissue culture 8 to 10 days, fluorescent antibody stains, history.

- **Disease Severity**
  Pain, spread to testis or prostate.

- **Concept and Application**
  Obligate intracellular parasite. Cannot produce adenosine triphosphate. Antibiotics effective. Neonatal infection is serious—conjunctivitis or pneumonitis. Think of mycoplasma and ureaplasma in differential diagnosis.

- **Management**
  Doxycycline, tetracycline, quinolones.

J. Herpes

- **H&P Keys**
  Genital ulcer, painful vesicles, multiple lesions.

- **Diagnosis**
  Tzanck test with Wright's or Giemsa's stain and cell culture.

- **Disease Severity**
  Pain, coalesced vesicles, persistence or recurrence of infection.

- **Concept and Application**
  Double-strand DNA virus. Subclinical infections, systemic complications—aseptic meningitis, fever, urinary retention in women, and, in rare cases, hepatitis or pneumonia.

- **Management**
  Oral acyclovir, 200 mg 5 times/day for 10 days. Topical application for pain relief.

K. Human Immunodeficiency Virus (HIV/AIDS)

- **H&P Keys**
  Night sweats, fever, adenopathy, weight loss, opportunistic infections.

- **Diagnosis**
  HIV antibody test. Western blotting.

- **Disease Severity**
  HIV positivity versus systemic disease.

- **Concept and Application**
  RNA virus, AZT therapy. Lymphocyte counts.

- **Management**
  Per current therapy. Evaluation of GU symptoms as per uninfected patients. Minimize invasive procedures in immunocompromised patients.

II. BENIGN CONDITIONS OF THE GENITOURINARY TRACT

A. Cryptorchidism

- **H&P Keys**
  Immature birth, absence of testis on scrotal exam. If hypospadias is present, consider sex ambiguity.

- **Diagnosis**
  Physical exam. In adults, consider CT scan.

- **Disease Severity**
  Retractile testis; inguinal canal versus intra-abdominal, unilateral, or bilateral.

- **Concept and Application**
Mal-descent of testes hormonally controlled. Gubernaculum provides path of descent with or without mechanical assistance. Rule out retractile, ectopic, or absent testis (blind-ending vas deferens at exploration).

- **Management**
Surgical correction at 6 to 12 months of age. Hormonal manipulation.

B. Testicular Torsion

- **H&P Keys**
Common scrotal swelling in children. Acute severe onset. Possible nausea and vomiting, abdominal pain.

- **Diagnosis**
Negative urinalysis, distorted or rotated gonad, Doppler ultrasound, nuclear flow scan.

- **Disease Severity**
Degree of pain and scrotal swelling. Duration of less than or more than 5 hours. Absence of contralateral testis.

- **Concept and Application**
Twisting of spermatic cord with mechanical ischemia. Congenital tunica vaginalis attachment is irregular; thus favors twisting (bell-clapper deformity). Contralateral side at risk.

- **Management**
Surgical correction in 5 hours. Bilateral orchiopexy with permanent suture.

C. Intersex

- **H&P Keys**
Salt loss, salt retention. Phallic enlargement. Precocious pubic hair, early masculinization, early epiphyseal closure (congenital adrenal hyperplasia [CAH]). Sparse axillary pubic hair (testicular feminization). Penile scrotal hypospadias and bilateral cryptorchidism. Groin mass (gonad).

- **Diagnosis**
Buccal smear, karyotype. Metabolic studies for congenital adrenal hyperplasia. Genitography, ultrasound gonadal histology.

- **Disease Severity**
Degree of underdevelopment or ambiguity of genitalia. Neonatal versus pubertial diagnosis. Reproductive and gender role dysfunction.

- **Concept and Application**
Four major groups:

1. Female pseudohermaphrodites, normal ovaries, 46XX, virilization (CAH).
2. Male pseudohermaphrodites, normal testis, 46XY, failure to masculinize (testicular feminization), androgen insensitivity (receptor block, other 5-α-reductase deficiency.
3. True hemaphrodites, testicular and ovarian tissue. Appearance and karyotype variable.
4. Dysgenetic gonads, replaced by fibrous stroma, mosaicism with XY,XX (Turner's syndrome) and XO lines.

- **Management**
Variable. Treatment depends on specific syndrome and time of recognition. Gender reassignment usually male to female. Support in assigned role (testicular feminization).

D. Infertility

- **H&P Keys**
Failure to conceive after 1 year of unprotected intercourse. Asymetric or undescended testicles. Testicular mass. Varicocele. Secondary sexual characteristics. Drug and chemical exposure. Stress.

- **Diagnosis**
Semen analysis (>20 million/cc, 1.5–5 cc volume). Urinalysis, semen fructose (obstruction/dysfunction of seminal vesicles). Luteinizing hormone (LH), follicle stimulating hormone (FSH), and testosterone level. Sperm function tests.

- **Disease Severity**
Mild disorders of semen parameters (motility or morphology) to azoospermia (total absence of sperm).

- **Concept and Application**
  Need to distinguish treatable (blockage, varicocele) from untreatable (gonadal failure, FSH three times normal) conditions.

- **Management**
  Varicocele repair. Repair of anatomic blockage. Clomiphene citrate administration (idiopathic infertility). Assisted reproductive techniques. Adoption.

E. Hydrocele and Varicocele

- **H&P Keys**

  Hydrocele. Painless scrotal mass; fluid accumulation in tunical layer of testis; symmetrical swelling, occasionally bilateral; transillumination.

  Varicocele. Spermatic venous varices; "bag of worms" palpation; commonly occurs on left side; occasionally, painful or heavy sensation.

- **Diagnosis**
  Physical exam, urinalysis, scrotal ultrasound. Check tumor marker in young men if diagnosis is questionable.

- **Disease Severity**

  Hydrocele. Cosmetic deformity.

  Varicocele. Deformity, pain, testicular atrophy, infertility problems.

- **Concept and Application**

  Hydroceles. Benign; membranes actively secrete serumlike fluid. Reaccumulation with simple drainage.

  Varicoceles. Gonadal venous valve insufficiency; occasionally subclinical on right side. Unclear mechanisms for effect on fertility in some men. Most men with varicoceles do not have fertility problems. Sperm parameters improve after procedure in two thirds of infertile men.

- **Management**

  Hydrocele. Drainage with sclerotherapy or surgical correction (5% to 15% recurrence).

  Varicocele. Venous ligation or embolization.

F. Benign Urethral Stricture

- **H&P Keys**
  Prior history of STD or urinary instrumentation, decreased force of stream, meatal stenosis.

- **Diagnosis**
  Physical exam, urinalysis, retrograde urethrogram, cystoscopy.

- **Disease Severity**
  Blood urea nitrogen (BUN) and creatinine, degree of voiding dysfunction, dysuria.

- **Concept and Application**
  Usually occurs at meatus, fossa navicularis (glans–shaft border), or bulbar urethra; bulbar is site for most STD infections. Ischemia from instrumentation or catheterization while on cardiopulmonary bypass.

- **Management**
  Dilatation, optical internal urethrotomy, plastic staged repair. Biopsy irregular stricture to rule out neoplasia.

G. Peyronie's Disease

- **H&P Keys**
  Painless, firm, nonindurated area on penile shaft.

- **Diagnosis**
  Physical exam. Color-flow Doppler ultrasound.

- **Disease Severity**
  Firm area, degree of pain with erection, deformity of erection, impotence.

- **Concept and Application**
  Idiopathic fibrosis of tunic of corpora cavernosa. Asymmetric thickening leads to erectile thickening and pain. Natural history is unclear. Ten percent are associated with Dupuytren's contracture.

- **Management**
  Observation, oral antioxidants, surgical excision and graft repair.

H. Erectile Impotence

- **H&P Keys**
  Neurological disease, diabetes, peripheral vascular disease, medications, radical pelvic surgery, Peyronie's plaque, psychological factors.

- **Diagnosis**
  History and physical exam, color-flow Doppler ultrasound, nocturnal penile tumescence studies, hormone profile (testosterone), LH, FSH, prolactin.

- **Disease Severity**
  Occasional or permanent inability to attain erection sufficient for vaginal penetration.

- **Concept and Application**
  Vascular, muscular, or neurologic etiology is the site of primary dysfunction; psychogenic issues much less common.

- **Management**
  Oral yohimbine (modestly effective). Intracavernosal injection (prostaglandin E_1 or papaverine-regitine); vacuum suction device; penile prosthesis.

I. Hypospadias

- **H&P Keys**
  Ectopic position of urethral meatus on ventral shaft of penis. Lack of ventral foreskin. Check for undescended testicles.

- **Diagnosis**
  Physical examination.

- **Disease Severity**
  Glandular position to more proximal location on shaft (penile or scrotal). Associated anomalies.

- **Concept and Application**
  Occurs at the rate of one in 300 live male births. Failure of mesothelial folds to close in the midline. Epispadias (dorsal urethral opening) is extremely rare. Associated with midline closure defects.

- **Management**
  Surgical correction.

J. Vesicoureteral Reflux

- **H&P Keys**
  Associated family history. Occurs in 50% of infant UTIs and 30% of childhood UTIs; recurrent UTIs in infancy and childhood.

- **Diagnosis**
  Ultrasound, IV urography, renal nuclear scan.

- **Disease Severity**
  Grades 1–5, international classification.

- **Concept and Application**
  Ectopic ureteral bud leading to lateral placement of ureter in bladder. Decreased flap-valve mechanism. May improve with maturity. High-pressure voiding states also can overwhelm normal anatomy. Goal is to preserve upper tracts. Avoid renal scarring and hypertension.

- **Management**
  Prophylactic antibiotics: trimethoprim-sulfamethoxazole, nitrofurantoin. Initial medical management of grades 1–3; grade 4, medical or surgical; grade 5, surgery. Cohen reimplant. Breakthrough infection, noncompliance, reflux persistent at puberty are indications for surgery.

K. Urolithiasis

- **H&P Keys**
  Prior history of stone, geography, metabolic disorders, flank or groin tenderness.

- **Diagnosis**
  Urinalysis, IV urogram, ultrasound.

- **Disease Severity**
  Stone burden on imaging studies; degree of urinary obstruction or renal impairment; pain, nausea, vomiting.

- **Concept and Application**
  Most stones are "idiopathic" calcium oxalate. Struvite stones are associated with infections (proteus) and uric acid; cysteine is less common.

- **Management**
  Small calculi: hydration, pain control, spontaneous passage. Upper tract: extracorporal

uric acid; cysteine —
need HCO_3 (keep pH > 7.5)

shockwave lithotripsy; lower tract: ureteroscopic extraction or lithotripsy.

L. Neurogenic Bladder

- **H&P Keys**
Neurologic exam, palpable bladder, rectal exam. Rule out stricture disease.

- **Diagnosis**
Urodynamics: pressure-flow, cystometrogram, electromyography, uroflowmetry, cystoscopy.

- **Disease Severity**
Voiding dysfunction versus complete retention, total incontinence, chronic urinary tract infection, deterioration of renal function.

- **Concept and Application**
Several classification schemes: (1) failure to empty versus failure to store is most functional scheme, (a) emptying failure resulting from decompensated detrusor mechanical obstruction or overactive sphincters (smooth and striated), (b) failure to store because of overactive detrusor or incompetent sphincters, and (2) motor versus sensory. Classification of uninhibited versus autonomous is used least often.

- **Management**
Failure to empty (detrusor): clean intermittent catheterization; bethanechol is ineffective. Failure to empty (mechanical): cystoscopy to rule out stricture or enlarged prostate. Failure to empty (sphincter dyssynergia): alpha-blockage, bladder neck incision, sphincterotomy. Failure to store (detrusor): anticholinergics, surgical bladder augmentation. Failure to store (sphincter incompetence): bladder sling surgery, collagen injections, artificial sphincter placement. (NOTE: Diabetes can induce a sensory neurogenic bladder. Initial good motor function can be maintained with *timed* voiding. Chronic overdistention creates dilated myopathy with motor decompensation as well. Treatment involves intermittent catheterization.

M. Stress-Related Urinary Incontinence

- **H&P Keys**
Childbirth, pelvic surgery (total abdominal hysterectomy), loss of urine with cough or movement.

- **Diagnosis**
Incontinence cystogram, urodynamics, cystoscopy.

- **Disease Severity**
Occasional leakage to gravity incontinence.

- **Concept and Application**
Forms of failure to store: type 1, hypermobility of urethra and mild leakage; type 2, descensus of bladder and cystocele; type 3, nonfunctional bladder neck.

- **Management**
Initial management is conservative: pelvic floor strengthening exercises, possible biofeedback training, use of alpha-agonists to tighten bladder neck (phenylpropanolamine, 50 mg daily). Then consider bladder neck suspension. Type 3 is treated with collagen injections or bladder sling surgery.

N. Enuresis

- **H&P Keys**
Lack of neurologic history, structural disorder that precludes normal toilet training, polyuria.

- **Diagnosis**
Urinalysis and culture and sensitivity. Radiography if infection is present, wetting is diurnal and present beyond age 12 years.

- **Disease Severity**
Frequency and persistence into adolescence.

- **Concept and Application**
Persistence of immature reflex pattern of bladder emptying.

- **Management**
Reassure patient about spontaneous resolution. Restrict fluids in evening. Administer imipramine to maximum dose of 2.5 mg/kg

at bedtime; 1-deamino-8-D-arginine vaso-pressin, 10 to 40 μc intranasally.

O. Ureteropelvic Junction Obstruction

- **H&P Keys**
Flank pain or abdominal pain or mass.

- **Diagnosis**
Renal ultrasound, cystoscopy as indicated, retrograde pyelogram.

- **Disease Severity**
Renal function, preserved renal parenchyma. Can occur with or without dilation of collecting system.

- **Concept and Application**
A dynamic segment of ureter, patent but functionally obstructive. Can occur at ureteral vesical junction (megaureter). Severe prostatism, neurogenic bladder, or ureteral reflux can cause general hydronephrosis.

- **Management**
Surgical correction, open or endoscopic, of ureteropelvic junction, Megaureter: observation or surgery. Treat prostatism or reflux according to recommendations.

P. Urologic Trauma

- **H&P Keys**
Cardiovascular stability, hematuria, pelvic stability, prostate location on rectal exam. Penile and scrotal ecchymosis, blood at urethral meatus, blunt or penetrating trauma.

- **Diagnosis**
Urinalysis, CT scan, IV urogram, retrograde urethrogram, cystogram. Ultrasound for oliguria.

- **Disease Severity**
Mild contusions treated with observation. Renal fracture involving collecting system, ureteral disruption, intra- versus extraperitoneal bladder extravasation. Penile or testicular fracture.

- **Concept and Application**
Much renal trauma can be managed conservatively; ureteral injuries usually iatrogenic

(ureteroscopy or gynecologic); urethral disruption and pelvic hematoma mitigate against immediate repair. Diagnosis of genital injury is aided by ultrasound.

- **Management**
Renal (stable): observation and bed rest, serial imaging; renal (unstable) surgery or angiography. Ureteral (minor): diversion of urine with stent; ureteral (major): early or immediate repair; (major, delayed diagnosis): urine diversion with later repair. Bladder (intraperitoneal): catheter drainage; bladder (extraperitoneal): open repair. Urethra (suprapubic): drainage and later repair in most cases. Penile-testicular: debridement and repair.

III. NEOPLASIAS OF THE GENITOURINARY TRACT

A. Benign Prostatic Hyperplasia

- **H&P Keys**
Hesitancy, decreased force of stream, postvoid dribbling, nocturia, urgency, frequency. Enlarged prostate. Rule out palpable bladder.

- **Diagnosis**
Uroflowmetry, postvoid residual urine, urinalysis, pressure-flow urodynamics if indicated, cystoscopy if indicated, serum prostate-specific antigen (PSA).

- **Disease Severity**
American Urological Association symptom score of 0 to 35. UTIs, renal deterioration, urinary retention.

- **Concept and Application**
Testosterone and aging are principal factors in enlargement. Static component is enlarged gland; dynamic component is smooth muscle-tone in prostate, prostate capsule, and bladder neck.

- **Management**
Expectant management. Reduce bulk with finasteride, 5 mg/day for life. Transurethral resection of prostate (transurethral pros-

tatectomy [TURP]). Laser prostatotomy. Decrease tone via incision of prostate (transurethral incision of prostate) or α-blockers (eg, Terazosin 1–10 mg at bedtime.

B. Prostate Cancer

- **H&P Keys**
  Digital rectal exam and serum PSA. Ultrasound is not part of routine exam. Hematuria and obstruction symptoms are less specific.

- **Diagnosis**
  Needle biopsy of prostate. Staging: Bone scan. Endorectal coil magnetic resonance imaging (eMRI) investigational. Computed tomography (CT) scan and MRI of body are not useful.

- **Disease Severity**
  Tumor grade and stage (Jewett-Whitmore, A-D, TMN system). (A/T1) local, PSA, or incidental biopsy, nonpalpable disease; (B/T2) palpable organ, confined disease; (C/T3) extracapsular disease; (D/T4, N^+, M^+) lymph node or distant metastasis.

- **Concept and Application**
  41,500 cancer-related deaths per year. Etiology is unknown. Adenocarcinoma. Disparity in racial incidence: high in African American men, low in native Asians. PSA plus digital rectal exam detects more cancer than either test alone. True value of screening awaits long-term follow-up. Androgen-sensitive and androgen-resistant tumor.

- **Management**
  Prostate cancer is a progressive disease. Slow rate of progression suggests that active observation is an option in patients with local disease and expected lifespan of less than 10 years. *Local disease:* Radical prostatectomy or radiation therapy. *Extracapsular disease:* Radiation therapy. *Advanced disease:* Androgen ablation (orchiectomy, LH-releasing hormone agonists with or without antiandrogen). Brachytherapy and cryosurgery for local disease is investigational. Palliative therapy for hormone-refractory disease.

C. Bladder Carcinoma

- **H&P Keys**
  Gross or microscopic hematuria. Irritative voiding symptoms. Occasionally, pelvic pain. Exposure to tobacco, cyclophosphamide, analine dyes.

- **Diagnosis**
  IV urogram, cystoscopy, barbitage cytology. Transurethral resection biopsy of bladder lesion.

- **Disease Severity**
  Key determinant is presence or absence of muscle invasion by the tumor. Degree of hematuria does not correlate with tumor stage. TNM staging system. Patients with gross nodal and distant disease do poorly.

- **Concept and Application**
  Cancer-related deaths per year, 10 000. Two thirds of tumors are superficial and treated by resection; two thirds of these will recur, and 10% to 20% progress to muscle-invasive disease. Associated carcinoma in situ is a bad prognostic feature regarding recurrence and progression. Tumor grade is strong indicator of recurrence.

- **Management**
  Superficial: Resect initial tumor and observe, on standard schedule (see below), multiple tumors or recurrence. Treat with intravesical chemotherapy or bacillus Calmette-Guérin vaccine (BCG); best response with BCG. Decreases papillary recurrence, decreases recurrence and progression in carcinoma in situ. *Cysto schedule:* Every 3 months for 1 year, every 6 months for 1 year, yearly thereafter. Recurrence resets schedule. *Muscle invasive:* Best result with radical cystectomy and urinary tract reconstruction (ileal conduit or continent neobladder). Transurethral resection, radiation therapy, and chemotherapy used separately or in combination in some instances. Advanced disease treated with combination of methotrexate, vinblastine, Adriamycin, and cisplatin (MVAC), with 40% to 50% response and 15% sustained complete remission. Alternatives are being sought.

D. Renal Cell Carcinoma

- **H&P Keys**
Classically called "internists tumor" because it was found after workup for general weight loss, fatigue, and so on. Now, it is usually discovered as incidental mass on an imaging study. Classic hematuria, flank pain, and mass are present in only 11% of patients.

- **Diagnosis**
Mass on IV urogram, ultrasound, CT, or MRI. Angiography rarely performed now. CT criteria: Mass with slight increase in Hounsfield units after contrast: Paraneoplastic effect of hypercalcemia and elevated liver function tests (LFTs) (Stauffers syndrome) does not indicate metastases. Anemia is more common than erythrocytosis.

- **Disease Severity**
Robeson or TNM tumor stage. Weight loss, fatigue, and large-mass organ-confined disease easily treated with surgery. Metastatic disease responds poorly to therapy.

- **Concept and Application**
Annual mortality rate is 12 000. Arises from proximal tubule. Exposure to tobacco increases the relative risk twofold. Surgical disease; not responsive to irradiation, chemotherapy.

- **Management**
Radical nephrectomy. *Advanced disease:* Interleukin-2 or vinblastine, or research protocol. Vinblastine is best single agent. Progesterones are used for palliation and have few side effects. Some positive results with biological response modifiers.

E. Wilms' Tumor

- **H&P Keys**
Pediatric tumor. Noticed as flank mass on exam. Hematuria.

- **Diagnosis**
History and physical exam, CT scan or ultrasound, IV urogram.

- **Disease Severity**
Clinical staging, performance status.

- **Concept and Application**
Arises from metanephric blastema tissue. Occurs in young children (peak age 3 years); rarely presents in adolescents and adults.

- **Management**
Radical nephrectomy for localized or regional disease and chemotherapy (actinomycin and vincristine). Radiation therapy for advanced disease.

F. Testicular Carcinoma

- **H&P Keys**
Painless testis mass, testis rupture after mild trauma. Advanced disease includes gynecomastia, shortness of breath, adenopathy, abdominal mass.

- **Diagnosis**
Scrotal ultrasound, tumor markers (beta human chorionic gonadotropin and alpha fetoprotein [AFP]). Diagnosis by radical orchiectomy (inguinal incision).

- **Disease Severity**
Marker level, retroperitoneal CT scan, organ confined versus subdiaphragmatic lymph nodes versus pulmonary/visceral disease.

- **Concept and Application**
Annual mortality rate, 350. Major distinction: seminoma versus nonseminomatous lesion (eg, embryonal, teratoma, choriocarcinoma). Nonseminoma: any elevated AFP and more than twice the normal β-human chorionic gonadotropin (β-HCG). Tumors sensitive to platinum-based chemotherapy.

- **Management**
Radical orchiectomy. Staging. Seminoma (local): 2500 cGy of radiation; seminoma (node positive): chemotherapy. Nonseminoma (local): retroperitoneal lymph node dissection (RPLND); nonseminoma (advanced, 6 positive nodes or >2.5 cm): Chemotherapy followed by salvage RPLND. Bleomycin, etopiside, and cisplatin (BEP).

G. Penile, Urethral, and Scrotal Carcinoma

- **H&P Keys**
  If patient is not circumcised, check under foreskin and look for bloody urethral stricture and scrotal mass. Check for inguinal adenopathy.

- **Diagnosis**
  Physical exam and biopsy.

- **Disease Severity**
  Degree of penile shaft destruction, adenopathy, weight loss.

- **Concept and Application**
  Rare cancer in developed world; usually squamous in origin. Adenopathy may be secondary to infection.

- **Management**
  Treat local lesion. Treat adenopathy with 6 weeks of the antibiotic doxycycline. Sample pelvic nodes. Treat by inguinal lymphadenectomy only if regional disease. Bleomycin base chemotherapy in advanced disease.

IV. RENAL DISORDERS

A. Pyelonephritis

- **H&P Keys**
  History of UTIs, voiding dysfunction, flank pain, fever, malaise. Differentiate acute from chronic pyelonephritis.

- **Diagnosis**
  Urine culture, urinalysis (pyuria, white blood cell casts), renal ultrasound to rule out obstruction by stone or other cause.

- **Disease Severity**
  Discomfort to frank sepsis. Acute infection versus chronic deterioration (renal scarring, insufficiency, proteinuria, hypertension).

- **Concept and Application**
  Ascending urinary tract infection can cause significant initial damage in pediatric population (usually associated with reflux).

Infection and obstruction enhance renal damage. Can be associated with stone disease. Usually standard pathogens.

- **Management**
  Rule out obstruction and calculus. Treat with culture-appropriate antibiotics. Monitor renal function in chronic patients.

B. Acute Renal Failure

[handwritten margin note: Prerenal ↓perfusion; Postrenal—obstruct; Parenchymal— ATN ischem, nephrot toxn]

- **H&P Keys**
  Increased creatinine and BUN, edema, hypertension, toxicity exposure, rhabdomyolysis, hemolysis.

- **Diagnosis**
  Urine diagnostic indexes, renal failure index, electrolyte measurements, possible renal biopsy.

- **Disease Severity**
  Acute progression versus rapid progression; oliguric versus nonoliguric. Rate of improvement and associated pathology.

- **Concept and Application**
  Prerenal, 55%; intrinsic, 40%; and postrenal causes, 5%. Conversion of oliguric to nonoliguric state improves management and may improve outcome. Prerenal conditions include congestive heart failure (CHF), hypovolemia, plasma protein deficiency. Hepatorenal syndrome probably reflects renal response to prerenal circulatory environment. Intrinsic disease caused by restricted blood flow to glomeruli, decreased basement membrane permeability, tubular plugging, disrupted tubules. Intrinsic disease; also acute glomerular nephritis and allergic interstitial nephritis. Acute anuria suggests urologic origin. Also consider solitary kidney. Acute tubular necrosis. Mortality can range between 25% and 70%.

- **Management**
  Assess clinical and laboratory parameters.

Prerenal. Restore adequate circulating plasma volume. Correct nonrenal pathology.

Renal. Convert to nonoliguric state, remove toxins, dialyze as needed. Urologic evaluation (ultrasound, cystoscopy, retrograde stent placement) as needed.

C. Chronic Renal Failure

- **H&P Keys**
  Diabetes, hypertension, pericarditis, glomerulopathy, obstructive uropathy, edema, anemia, puritis, osteodystrophy (osteitis fibrosa).

- **Diagnosis**
  Shrunken kidneys on imaging, uremia, creatinine clearance, edema, hyperkalemia normochromic, normocytic anemia.

- **Disease Severity**
  Creatinine clearance, edema, electrolyte derangement, neurologic complications of uremia.

- **Concept and Application**
  Multiple causes, majority of cases involve hypertension, diabetes mellitus, and glomerulonephritis. Early reduction of glomerular filtration (GFR) (30% to 50%) compensated. Azotemia between 20% and 35% GFR and overt renal failure below 20% of normal.

- **Management**
  Initial dietary restriction of protein, control hypertension, correct electrolyte imbalances, dialysis and transplantation.

D. Tubulointerstitial Disease

- **H&P Keys**
  Toxin exposure (analgesics, heavy metal), immune disorders, neoplasia, vascular disease, family history of renal disorders.

- **Diagnosis**
  Electrolyte irregularities, eosinophilia, impaired creatine clearance, renal biopsy.

- **Disease Severity**
  Acute or chronic, tubular defects versus marked GFR deterioration.

- **Concept and Application**
  Pathology is morphologically in tubules and interstitium, not glomerulus. *Acute disease:* inflammation, tubule necrosis, edema. *Chronic forms:* Fibrosis is common. Condition has many causes. Look for dysfunction

in tubular transport. Proteinuria usually not severe. Eventual GFR dysfunction.

- **Management**
  Remove offending agent and compensate tubular defect. Treat primary disease.

E. Renal Transplant Rejection

- **H&P Keys**
  Oliguria, azotemia, graft tenderness, fever, proteinuria.

- **Diagnosis**
  Ultrasound to rule out obstruction, urine output, proteinuria, renal scan, renal biopsy.

- **Disease Severity**
  Mild azotemia, frank renal failure, rapidity of onset and progression.

- **Concept and Application**
  Immunologic reaction, cellular and humoral. Hyperacute, acute accelerated, acute, and chronic rejection.

- **Management**
  Hyperacute and acute accelerated: Rare, nephrectomy. *Acute:* Immunosuppression—methylpreniselone, antilymphocyte globulin. *Chronic:* Rule out obstruction, no treatment, kidney-sparing diet.

F. Nephrotic Syndrome

- **H&P Keys**
  Edema.

- **Diagnosis**
  Urinalysis, proteinuria, 24-hr collection, hypoalbuminemia, renal biopsy.

- **Disease Severity**
  Rapid versus chronic course. Degree of proteinuria/renal insufficiency.

- **Concept and Application**
  Albuminuria, hypoalbuminemia, hyperlipidemia, and edema. Minimal change disease, mesangial proliferative IgA glomerulonephritis (Berger's disease), focal and segmental glomerulosclerosis, membranous Berger's disease.

• **Management**
Treatment with combination of steroids, cytotoxic drugs, cyclosporine.

G. Glomerulonephritis

• **H&P Keys**
Infectious disease, primary renal disease, multisystem disease. Abrupt azotemia, oliguria, edema, hypertension.

• **Diagnosis**
Serum electrolytes, proteinuria, urinalysis for hematuria, red-cell casts.

• **Disease Severity**
Degree of edema, renal insufficiency, acute versus rapidly progressing disease.

• **Concept and Application**
Glomerular damage, capillary wall damage (anionic charge/pore size), vascular changes resulting from vessel damage and surrounding inflammation.

• **Management**
Acute supportive disease: Diuresis, bedrest, antihypertension drugs as needed. *Rapidly progressing disease:* Glucocorticoid pulse treatment, cytotoxic agents, plasma exchange. Long-term preservation of renal function is poor.

H. Diabetic Nephropathy

• **H&P Keys**
History of diabetes, diabetic stigmata, edema, hypertension.

• **Diagnosis**
BUN and creatinine, creatinine clearance, oliguria.

• **Disease Severity**
Degree and duration of diabetes, level of renal impairment.

• **Concept and Application**
Microangiopathy of renal system and glomeruli (Kimmelstiel-Wilson lesions), nodular deposits in glomeruli.

• **Management**
Early: Compensate for electrolyte-fluid derangement. *Later:* Dialysis or transplantation.

I. Renal Osteodystrophy

• **H&P Keys**
Renal insufficiency, growth retardation, rickets. Bone pain or proximal muscle weakness in adults.

• **Diagnosis**
Calcium and phosphorus levels. Parathyroid activity. Plain film findings.

• **Disease Severity**
Renal dwarfism versus growth retardation or maturation, degree of orthopedic disability in adults. Extent of calcium imbalance, pathologic calcification.

• **Concept and Application**
Impaired vitamin D metabolism, parathyroid hormone overproduction. Dialysis accelerates bone pathology secondary to aluminum deposition. Osteitis fibrosa cystica, renal rickets, osteosclerosis.

• **Management**
Early treatment to reduce morbidity. Reduce dietary phosphate with calcium carbonate as phosphate binder, balanced dialysate. Keep PO_4 at 4.5 mg/dL and Ca at 10 mg/dL.

J. Papillary Necrosis

• **H&P Keys**
Hematuria and flank pain, patient may be asymptomatic, disease often associated with severe infection and other conditions.

• **Diagnosis**
Urinalysis, culture, filling defect on urogram; ring shadow may be present.

• **Disease Severity**
Asymptomatic or flank pain infection, obstructive uropathy with papillary sloughing.

• **Concept and Application**
Infection or microangiopathy of renal pyramids. Associated with diabetes, alcoholism, sickle cell anemia.

• **Management**
Asymptomatic finding: Treat primary disease. Endpoint of hematuria evaluation, or mechanical removal of obstruction.

K. Renovascular Hypertension

- **H&P Keys**
  Hypertension, rapid onset, poorly controlled, epigastric bruit.

- **Diagnosis**
  Renal vein renin sampling (ratio greater than 1.5); angiography (classic, digital, MRI); occasionally, IV urogram (not a screening test).

- **Disease Severity**
  Pharmacologic control, severity of stenosis on imaging.

- **Concept and Application**
  Usually secondary to atherosclerotic vascular disease; several forms of fibromuscular hyperplasia.

- **Management**
  Medical, angioplasty, surgical repair.

L. Preeclampsia

- **H&P Keys**
  Pregnancy related, edema, proteinuria, and hypertension after 24th week of pregnancy.

- **Diagnosis**
  Blood pressure 140/90, proteinuria, 30 mm Hg systolic or 15 mm Hg diastolic relative to earlier pregnancy readings.

- **Disease Severity**
  Progression to eclampsia; need for intervention beyond bedrest.

- **Concept and Application**
  Etiology unknown. Glomerular capillary endotheliosis is major pathologic alteration.

- **Management**
  Bedrest, antihypertensives (hydralizine), delivery. Magnesium sulfate 4–6 g, then 1–2 g per hour.

M. Eclampsia

- **H&P Keys**
  Preeclampsia and seizures.

- **Diagnosis**
  Preeclampsia and seizure evaluation.

- **Disease Severity**
  Proteinuria, level of hypertension and degree of seizure activity.

- **Concept and Application**
  Etiology unknown.

- **Management**
  Control blood pressure and seizures.

N. Polycystic Kidney Disease

- **H&P Keys**
  Flank mass, renal insufficiency, family history.

- **Diagnosis**
  Azotemia, uremia, CT scan, proteinuria.

- **Disease Severity**
  Age of onset, infection, hypertension, rate of renal deterioration, abdominal distension.

- **Concept and Application**
  Ten percent of end-stage renal failure. Cortical and medullary cysts. Hepatic cysts, cerebral aneurysms. Presents in third and fourth decade. Hypertension in 75%. Autosomal dominant disease (usually adult, wide range and penetrance). Two genes identified. Autosomal recessive, infancy or childhood (renal failure or portal fibrosis) medullary ductal ectasia.

- **Management**
  Hypertension control, antibiotics, dialysis, transplantation.

O. Nephrosclerosis

- **H&P Keys**
  Mild, moderate, or malignant hypertension; neurologic signs; papilledema.

- **Diagnosis**
  Urinalysis, proteinuria, renal imaging (size).

- **Disease Severity**
  Mild sclerosis with mild-to-moderate physiologic changes (slight azotemia, exaggerated natriuresis with fluid challenge versus malignant hypertension, neurologic symptoms.

- **Concept and Application**
  Mild-to-moderate secondary changes of essential hypertension, vascular atherosclerotic changes (afferent arterioles). Severe disease with fibrinoid necrosis and hyperplastic arteriolitis.

• **Management**
Control hypertension (acute and chronic).

P. Lupus Nephritis

• **H&P Keys**
Associated history of systemic lupus erythematosus (SLE) and physical exam, edema.

• **Diagnosis**
Urinalysis, azotemia, low C_3 and C_4 concentrations. Positive double-stranded DNA antibody, proteinuria, nephrotic syndrome, renal biopsy.

• **Disease Severity**
Asymptomatic, clinical SLE, mild-to-severe renal status.

• **Concept and Application**
Renal involvement in 35% to 90% of SLE patients, deposition of circulating immunocomplexes, autoantibody activity.

• **Management**
Steroids, azothiaprine, cyclophosphamide.

V. ELECTROLYTE AND ACID/BASE DISORDERS

A. Hyponatremia

• **H&P Keys**
Nausea, confusion, lethargy, coma, seizures, decreased deep-tendon reflexes.

• **Diagnosis**
Serum sodium under 130 mg/dL.

• **Disease Severity**
Abnormal laboratory value to severe clinical derangement.

• **Concept and Application**
Free-water retention, exogenous free water, TURP or water intoxication, syndrome of inappropriate secretion of antidiuretic hormone (SIADH), renal and cardiac decompensation.

• **Management**
Restrict free water, replace salt.

B. Hypernatremia

• **H&P Keys**
Dehydration, hyperpnea, oliguria, thirst, hypotension.

• **Diagnosis**
Serum sodium greater than 145 mg/dL.

• **Disease Severity**
Laboratory finding to severe clinical derangement.

• **Concept and Application**
Impaired thirst mechanism, excessive water loss, solute and free-water loss (diabetic ketoacidosis).

• **Management**
Slow replacement of free water to avoid cerebral edema.

C. Hypokalemia

• **H&P Keys**
Dysrhythmia, rhabdomyolysis, muscle weakness or cramps.

• **Diagnosis**
Serum potassium under 3.5 mg/dL. Changes in electrocardiogram (ECG): wide decrease in T wave, U wave, atrioventricular block.

• **Disease Severity**
Laboratory finding to severe clinical derangement.

• **Concept and Application**
Inappropriate gastrointestinal (GI) or GU loss, cellular sequestration, decreased intake. Because of body stores, small decrease in serum value can indicate significant total-body depletion.

• **Management**
Oral replacement for chronic loss (diuretic use). IV replacement is not advised except in monitored situation (keep below 20 mEq/hr).

D. Hyperkalemia

• **H&P Keys**
Renal insufficiency, diarrhea, weakness.

- **Diagnosis**
Laboratory findings, ECG: widened QRS waves and peaked T waves.

- **Disease Severity**
Laboratory value or severe clinical derangement.

- **Concept and Application**
Reduced renal excretion of potassium; adrenal insufficiency, excessive intake; hyperchloremic acidosis.

- **Management**
Limit exogenous potassium, correct underlying acidosis, exchange resin, insulin/D50 glucose, dialysis.

E. Volume Depletion

- **H&P Keys**
Decreased skin turgor, orthostasis, thirst, coma, sunken eyes.

- **Diagnosis**
Serum electrolytes, increased sodium, BUN, osmolality increased.

- **Disease Severity**
Laboratory derangement to severe clinical compromise.

- **Concept and Application**
Third spacing, insufficient replacement of free water, excessive loss of free water.

- **Management**
Slow replacement of free water. Replace sodium as needed.

F. Volume Excess

- **H&P Keys**
Renal insufficiency, CHF, pathologic free-water consumption (water intoxication), syndrome of inappropriate antidiuretic hormone secretion (SIADH), nausea, seizures, weakness, coma.

- **Diagnosis**
Serum electrolytes, clinical scenario.

- **Disease Severity**
Mild electrolyte disturbance to severe clinical derangement.

- **Concept and Application**
Excessive exogenous free water or poor elimination of free water.

- **Management**
Restrict fluids.

G. Metabolic Alkalosis

- **H&P Keys**
GI loss, renal loss, H^+ translocation (hypokalemia), $NaHCO_3$ administration.

- **Diagnosis**
Elevation of arterial pH, increase in plasma HCO_3, compensatory hypoventilation (up P_{CO_2}).

- **Disease Severity**
Compensated disturbance or severe metabolic derangement.

- **Concept and Application**
Generally a loss of H^+, retention of bicarbonate, or contraction alkalosis.

- **Management**
Correct primary cause. Compensate electrolyte abnormality.

H. Respiratory Alkalosis

- **H&P Keys**
Hypoxemia, CHF, pulmonary disease, severe anemia, gram-negative sepsis, hepatic failure.

- **Diagnosis**
Elevated arterial pH, hypocapnea, plasma HCO_3 decreased.

- **Disease Severity**
Mild compensated disorder or severe metabolic derangement.

- **Concept and Application**
Hyperventilation caused by hypoxemia or central stimulation of respiration. Primary respiratory disease and mechanical ventilation also a cause.

- **Management**
Correct underlying medical defect. Rebreathing (increase P_{CO_2}).

I. Metabolic Acidosis

- **H&P Keys**
Low arterial pH, reduced plasma HCO_3 concentration, compensatory hyperventilation.

- **Diagnosis**
Electrolytes, blood gas, associated metabolic disorders.

- **Disease Severity**
Mild electrolyte disturbance to severe metabolic derangement.

- **Concept and Application**
Generally characterized as anion gap (ingestions, ketoacidosis, lactic acidosis, renal failure, rhabdomyolysis), and hyperchloremic (normal anion gap) renal dysfunction, GI loss of HCO_3, renal loss of HCO_3, ingestion.

- **Management**
Correct primary etiology. Replace HCO_3 with accompanying additional cation load (Na^+).

J. Respiratory Acidosis

- **H&P Keys**
Medications, acute cardiac arrest, obesity, upper-airway obstruction, chest-wall pathology, adult respiratory distress syndrome, and chronic obstructive pulmonary disease.

- **Diagnosis**
Blood gas and electrolytes. Elevated serum HCO_3, reduced arterial pH. Elevated P_{CO_2}.

- **Disease Severity**
Mild disorder to severe decompensation.

- **Concept and Application**
Inability to excrete respiratory CO_2, multiple mechanical and structural disorders.

- **Management**
Correct primary ventilatory defect.

K. Hypomagnesemia

- **H&P Keys**
Alcoholism, malnutrition, diuretics, diabetic ketoacidosis, lethargy, delirium, irritability of central nervous system.

- **Diagnosis**
Low serum magnesium (less than 1.1 mEq/dL); electrocardiogram (ECG), prolonged QT waves; hypokalemia; hypocalcemia.

- **Disease Severity**
Electrolyte abnormality to severe neurologic decompensation.

- **Concept and Application**
Metabolism similar to calcium; generally difficult to deplete body stores.

- **Management**
IV or IM exogenous replacement.

L. Hypercalcemia

- **H&P Keys**
Carcinoma, hyperparathyroidism or hyperthyrosis, dartoid, milk alkali syndrome.

- **Diagnosis**
Serum-free calcium over 2.9 mEq. ECG, short QT and long PR waves.

- **Disease Severity**
Abnormal electrolytes to tetany and cardiac arrest.

- **Concept and Application**
Inappropriate calcium storage mobilization, hormonal etiology, neoplasia. Excretion linked to sodium and state of hydration.

- **Management**
Saline infusion, furosemide, diuresis, calcitonin, mithramycin, sodium etironate.

M. Hypocalcemia

- **H&P Keys**
Renal failure, hypoparathyroidism, vitamin D deficiency, malabsorption, Chvostek's sign, Trousseau's sign, perioral parasthesias, muscle cramps.

- **Diagnosis**
Serum calcium (free Ca less than 2.2 mEq).

- **Disease Severity**
Electrolyte finding to tetany, neurologic, cardiovascular complications.

- **Concept and Application**
Secondary to parathyroid surgery, poor absorption, inability to access bone stores.

- **Management**
Correct underlying defect. Administer exogenous calcium and vitamin D.

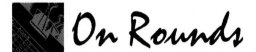

Urologic Disorders

Prostate Cancer

- Diagnosis by digital rectal exam and PSA followed by needle biopsy, bone scan
- Staging: Jewett-Whitmore A–D.
  - A = Local, nonpalpable
  - B = Palpable, confined
  - C = Extracapsular
  - D = Lymph node or distant mets
- Treatment if local includes radical prostatectomy or radiation
- Treatment if extracapsular is radiation
- Treatment for advanced disease includes androgen ablation (orchiectomy, LH-releasing hormone agonists)

Wilms' Tumor

- Pediatric tumor (peak age 3), flank mass, hematuria

Bladder Cancer

- Risk factors include exposure to tobacco, cyclophosphamide and analine dyes

Hydrocele

- Painless scrotal mass, transillumination, fluid in tunical layer of testes, a cosmetic problem

Varicocele

- Spermatic venous varicies, "bag of worms" feel, pain, infertility

Testicular Torsion

- Scrotal swelling in children, acute severe onset, nausea, abdominal pain

BIBLIOGRAPHY

Aaronson IA. Sexual differentiation and Intersexuality. In: *Clinical Pediatric Urology.* 3rd ed. Kelalis PP, King LR, Belman AB, eds. Philadelphia: WB Saunders; 1992: 977–1014.

Catalona WJ. Urothelial tumors of the urinary tract. In: *Campbell's Urology.* 6th ed. Walsh PC, Retik AB, Stamey TA, Vaughan ED, eds. Philadelphia: WB Saunders; 1992: 1094–1158.

Fowler JE Jr. *Urinary Tract Infection and Inflammation.* Chicago: Year Book Medical Publishers; 1989.

Hanks GE, Myers, CE, Sardino PT. In: *Cancer of the Prostate, Cancer Principles and Practice of Oncology.* 4th ed. DeVita, VT Jr., Hellman, S, Rosenberg SA, eds. Philadelphia: JB Lippincott Co.; 1993:1073–1113.

Hodge EE, Flechner SM, Novick AC. Renal Transplantation. In: *Adult and Pediatric Urology.* 3rd ed. Gillenwater JY, Grayhack, JT, Howards SS, Duckett JW, eds. St. Louis: Mosby; 1996:999–1068.

Krieger JN. Urethritis: Etiology, Diagnosis, Treatment and Complications. In: *Adult and Pediatric Urology.* 3rd ed. Gillenwater JY, Grayhack, JT, Howards SS, Duckett JW, eds. St. Louis: Mosby; 1996:1879–1916.

Malkowicz SB. Clinical aspects of renal Tumors. *Sem Roentgen.* 1995;30:102–115.

McAninch JW. Injuries to the genitourinary tract. In: *General Urology.* Tanagho EA, McAninch JW, eds. Norwalk, CT: Appleton & Lange; 1988:302–18.

Partin AW, Oesterling JE. The clinical usefulness of prostate specific antigen: Update 1994. *J Urology.* 1994;152:1358–68.

Richie JP. Neoplasms of the testis. In: *Campbell's Urology.* 6th ed. Walsh PC, Retik AB, Stamey JA, Vaughan ED, eds. Philadelphia: WB Saunders; 1992:1222–63.

Wein AJ. Neuromuscular dysfunction of the lower urinary tract. In: *Campbell's Urology.* 6th ed. Walsh PC, Retik AB, Stamey TA, Vaughan ED, eds. Philadelphia: WB Saunders; 1992:573–642.

18

Surgical Principles

David P. Coll, MD, and Morris D. Kerstein, MD

I. DISORDERS OF THE SKIN AND SUBCUTANEOUS TISSUE

A. Cellulitis

- **H&P Keys**
  Skin trauma; pain; fever; tender, erythematous, or edematous skin; ulcer; surgical wound; skin puncture; red or tender streaks; indistinct advancing edge; history of venous or lymphatic insufficiency.

- **Diagnosis**
  Physical examination, blood culture, biopsy ulcers.

- **Disease Severity**
  Malaise, fever, lymphangitis, bullae. Sepsis/bacteremia.

- **Concept and Application**
  Injury to skin, bacterial invasion of skin and subcutaneous tissue (*Streptococci, Staphylococci,* anaerobes) spread by way of lymphatics.

- **Management**
  Warm packs, rest, elevation of limb, intravenous antibiotics, local wound care.

B. Lipoma

- **H&P Keys**
  Swelling, rarely painful; soft fluctuant lobulated mass, subcutaneous in position.

- **Diagnosis**
  Physical examination.

- **Disease Severity**
  Hard mass, calcification.

- **Concept and Application**
  Benign tumor of mature fat cells.

- **Management**
  Observation, surgical excision.

C. Hemangioma

- **H&P Keys**
  Red, raised, or blue lesion; painless.

- **Diagnosis**
  Physical examination.

- **Disease Severity**
  Rate of growth, degree of disfigurement, ulceration, infection, cardiac failure.

- **Concept and Application**
  True neoplasm or malformation of normal vascular structures.

- **Management**
  Observation, corticosteroids, injection sclerotherapy, partial or complete surgical excision.

D. Neurofibroma   *Consider VonRecklinghausen*

- **H&P Keys**
  Mass, peripheral nerve dysfunction, occlusive pain, sensory deficit, muscular weakness (motor or sensory). If multiple must consider von Recklinghausen disease.

- **Diagnosis**
  Physical examination, nerve conduction studies, electromyography, magnetic resonance imaging (MRI) scan.

- **Disease Severity**
Motor or sensory deficit, multiple lesions, recurrent lesions, malignant degeneration, involvement within craniospinal axis, diffuse growth.

- **Concept and Application**
Neoplastic activity in nerve sheath, part of von Recklinghausen disease complex.

- **Management**
Observation, surgical excision.

E. Sebaceous Cyst

- **H&P Keys**
Asymptomatic swelling, spherical mass with punctum.

- **Diagnosis**
Physical examination.

- **Disease Severity**
Size of lesion, presence of infection, ulceration.

- **Concept and Application**
Thin layer of epidermal cell lining, contains keratinous debris.

- **Management**
Surgical excision, incision and drainage if infected.

F. Basal Cell Carcinoma

- **H&P Keys**
Lesion on face or other sun-exposed areas; bleeding; pearly nodule; central ulceration; rolled, raised, or beaded edge. Seen most commonly in elderly population, most common skin cancer.

- **Diagnosis**
Physical examination, biopsy.

- **Disease Severity**
Size and site of lesion, destruction of adjacent tissue, intracranial extension, massive ulceration.

- **Concept and Application**
Ultraviolet light exposure, fair-skinned persons.

- **Management**
Curettage and electrodesiccation, surgical excision, radiation, topical chemotherapy, close follow-up.

G. Squamous Cell Carcinoma

- **H&P Keys**
Erythematous plaque or nodule, ulceration with raised edges, chronic ulcer, lymphadenopathy. Second most common form of skin cancer.

- **Diagnosis**
Physical examination. Biopsy.

- **Disease Severity**
Burn-scar carcinoma (Marjolin's ulcer), fixed to surrounding structures, ulceration, lymphadenopathy (regional), histologic differentiation.

- **Concept and Application**
Invasive neoplasms devised from keratinocytes, ultraviolet exposure, irradiation, chronic irritation, chronic granulomas, burn scar, chronic sinus.

- **Management**
Radiotherapy, surgical excision, block dissection of lymph nodes.

H. Melanoma

- **H&P Keys**
Increase in size or change in color of mole, or any pigmented nevus, bleeding, itching, pain, lymphadenopathy, family history, hepatomegaly. Presence of dysplastic nevus, presence of congenital nevus.

- **Diagnosis**
Physical examination, punch biopsy, lymphoscintigraphy.

- **Disease Severity**
Mole or moles on trunk, especiallly if congenital or dysplastic, thickness of tumor, Breslow's classification, ulceration, melanosis, satellitosis, lymphadenopathy, subungual lesions, pattern of growth, multiple nevi, location of the lesion.

- **Concept and Application**
Ultraviolet exposure, genetic predisposition, presence of dysplastic nevi, malignant tumor of melanocytes.

- **Management**
Wide surgical excision, therapeutic nodal dissection, regional hyperthermic limb perfusion, chemotherapy, immunotherapy.

I. Sarcoma

Arsenic   neurofibramatos
vinylchloride
HIV

- **H&P Keys**
Painless discrete mass in limb, abdominal mass, hepatomegaly. Patient often gives an antecedant history of trauma.

- **Diagnosis**
MRI scan, computed tomography (CT) scan of abdomen and pelvis, needle biopsy, incisional biopsy, chest roentgenogram, CT scan of chest. Positron-emission tomography (PET) scan.

- **Disease Severity**
Tumor size, depth, and site; histological grade, presence of metastatic disease, recurrence of tumor.

- **Concept and Application**
Invasive neoplasm derived from mesodermal connective tissue. Radiation exposure, oncogenic viruses. Arsenic, vinyl chloride, HIV, neurofibromatosis.

- **Management**
En bloc surgical resection, radiotherapy, chemotherapy, hyperthermic limb perfusion.

J. Decubitus Ulcer

- **H&P Keys**
Blanching erythema, shallow or extensive dermal defects, contractures, fever, cellulitis. Immobilized patient.

- **Diagnosis**
Physical examination, roentgenogram of ulcer (to rule out osteomyelitis).

- **Disease Severity**
Depth and size of defect, osteomyelitis, nutrition, albumin, associated cardiopulmonary disease.

- **Concept and Application**
Ischemia from prolonged pressure, immobilization, incontinence of urine or feces, malnutrition, inadequate nursing care. Inadequate antipressure bed or mattress.

- **Management**

Prevention. Keep dry, turn patient frequently, use air or foam mattress, improve nutrition.

Definitive. Drainage of infected spaces, antibiotics, debridement, musculocutaneous flap closure.

K. Venous Ulceration

- **H&P Keys**
Ulceration in leg, commonly over medial malleolus, varicose veins, history of deep-vein thrombosis, saphenofemoral incompetence, perforator incompetence, brawny skin in distal one third of leg, scars from healed ulcers, hyperpigmentation, icthyosis, dependent edema, fever, cellulitis.

- **Diagnosis**
Doppler venous flow mapping, venogram. Impedance plethysmography (IPG) or photoplethysmography (PPG) study.

- **Disease Severity**
Cellulitis, subfascial perforators, obesity, cardiac failure, anemia, malnutrition.

- **Concept and Application**
High venous pressure, pericapillary fibrin deposition, hypoxia, loss of subcutaneous fat, frank ulceration of skin.

- **Management**

Conservative. Elevation, compressive dressing, antibiotics, debridement.

Surgical. Ligation of perforators, skin graft.

L. Arterial Ulcer

- **H&P Keys**
Intermittent claudication, pain at rest, cold feet, ulcer, pale or cold skin, gangrenous toes, absent pulses. Punched-out appearance of ulcer, extremely painful.

- **Diagnosis**
Ankle/brachial index, Doppler arterial flow mapping, arteriography, magnetic resonance angiography.

- **Disease Severity**
Pain at rest, established gangrene, infection, diabetes mellitus, previous amputation,

cerebrovascular accident, myocardial infarction or angina. Previous vascular surgery.

- **Concept and Application**
  Skini schemia resulting from atherosclerotic peripheral vascular disease.

- **Management**
  Antibiotics, angiography, anigoplasty, arterial bypass surgery, debridement, skin graft.

II. DISEASES OF THE ENDOCRINE SYSTEM

A. Thyroid Neoplasm

- **H&P Keys**
  Neck mass, dysphagia, dysphemia, respiratory difficulty, hoarseness, hard or fixed mass, vocal cord paralysis, bony pain, lymphadenopathy. Female patient, childhood neck irradiation.

- **Diagnosis**
  Thyroid function tests, fine-needle aspiration, thyroid suppression trial, cytology, ultrasound scan, radioisotope scan. CT scan, MRI.

- **Disease Severity**
  Symptoms of local invasion, metastatic disease, age, sex, size of tumor, histology, lymphadenopathy, cellular differentiation.

- **Concept and Application**
  Genetic predisposition, neck radiation, pre-existing goiter.

- **Management**
  Lobectomy, total thyroidectomy, cervical lymph node dissection, thyroxine, radioiodine, radiation, chemotherapy.

B. Hyperparathyroidism

- **H&P Keys**
  Lethargy, confusion, depression, constipation, anorexia, muscle weakness, renal failure, hypertension.

- **Diagnosis**
  Hypercalcemia, elevated parathyroid hormone (PTH), hypophosphatemia, ultrasonography (US), CT, MRI, thallium-technetium scan, sestomebe scan.

- **Disease Severity**
  Renal failure; primary, secondary, tertiary disease.

- **Concept and Application**
  Excess PTH production, from parathyroid adenoma, parathyroid hyperplasia, very rarely parathyroid carcinoma.

- **Management**
  Adenoma resection. 3½ gland excision, consider multiple endocrine neoplasia (MEN) evaluation

C. Cushing Disease/ Cushing Syndrome

- **H&P Keys**
  Alteration in appearance, "mooning" of face, truncal obesity, acne, hirsutism, buffalo hump, bruising, weakness of shoulders or thighs, purple striae, back pain, impotence or amenorrhea, hypertension, diabetes.

- **Diagnosis**
  Plasma cortisol/adrenocorticotropic hormone (ACTH) levels, 24-hour urine cortisol, dexamethasone suppression test, metyrapone test, cortisol releasing hormone test, isotope-scanning, CT scan of abdomen, angiography, venous sampling.

- **Disease Severity**
  Hypertension, stroke, diabetes mellitus, muscle wasting, duration of disease.

- **Concept and Application**
  Excess cortisol production, pituitary adenoma producing ACTH, adrenal adenoma or carcinoma, ACTH-secreting tumors.

- **Management**

  Medical. Ketoconazole, metyrapone, aminoglutethimide.

  Surgical. Pituitary ablation, adrenalectomy, postoperative corticosteroid therapy, removal of source of ectopic ACTH.

D. Pheochromocytoma   VmA

- **H&P Keys**

  Episodic headache, sweating, blurred vision, weight loss, flushing, anxiety, hypertension, palpitations, tachycardia.

- **Diagnosis**

  Twenty-four-hour urine vanillylmandelic acid, serum catecholamine, glucagon stimulation test, phentolamine suppression test, CT scan of abdomen, metaiodobenzylguanidine (MIBG) isotope scanning, venous sampling.

- **Disease Severity**

  Myocardial infarction, arrhythmias, renal failure, pregnancy, stroke.

- **Concept and Application**

  Tumors of adrenal medulla and chromaffin tissue, associated MEN II; excess catecholamine production.

- **Management**

  Medical. Alpha-adrenergic blockade (phenoxybenzamine), beta-blocker agents, sedatives. Blood pressure control paramount.

  Surgical. Hemodynamic monitoring, adrenalectomy, fluid therapy, nitroprusside and propranolol.

III. DISORDERS OF THE KIDNEY AND URINARY TRACT

A. Testicular Tumors

- **H&P Keys**

  Asymptomatic painless swelling (85%), associated hydrocele (5%).

- **Diagnosis**

  Physical examination, ultrasound surgical exploration via inguinal approach.

- **Concept and Application**

  Staging: CT scan, chest tomograms, cavagrams, lymphangiogram tumor markers for beta human chorionic gonadotropin (hCG), and alpha fetoprotein. Seminomatous versus nonseminomatous.

- **Management**

  Remove tumor via inguinal approach. For seminoma, radiation to retroperitoneum. For nonseminoma germ-cell tumor, retroperitoneal lymphadenectomy, adjuvant chemotherapy.

B. Carcinoma of the Bladder

- **H&P Keys**

  Hematuria, pyuria, mass, tobacco, β-napthylamine and paraaminodiphenyl exposure.

- **Diagnosis**

  Excretory urography, ultrasound for extent of local disease, cystoscopy, CT scan for nodal metastatic disease. *Urinary cytology:* MRI to detect local and nodal lesions, chest roentgenogram, bone scan, cell-surface antigen.

- **Concept and Application**

  Staging of cell type (transitional, squamous, ademomatous), grade, and depth of invasion.

- **Management**

  Carcinoma in situ. Chemotherapy (controversial), intravesicular fulgaration.

  Superficial. Intravesical chemotherapy, local immunotherapy, cystectomy. Intravesicular fulgaration, recurrence common.

  Invasive. Intensive local therapy, partial cystectomy, radiotherapy. Radical cystectomy is treatment of choice, chemotherapy.

C. Prostate Cancer

- **H&P Keys**

  Often asymptomatic; average age, 73 years. Rectal examination. Most common malignant tumor in men, incidence 10% over age 65.

- **Diagnosis**

  Confirmation by needle biopsy, staging by rectal examination. Transrectal ultrasound, CT scan, MRI. *Metastatic disease:* Chest roentgenogram, intravenous pyelogram (IVP), bone scan, CT scan. Acid phosphatase is elevated in 80% of patients with metastatic disease, prostatic-specific antigen.)

- **Concept and Application**
Adenocarcinoma (95%). Exposure to cadmium, genetic and hormonal factors. At diagnosis, 40% of tumors have metastasized; in 40% of patients, tumor extends beyond capsule.

- **Management**
Stage A and Stage B (disease confined to prostate): Treat with radical prostatectomy or interstitial/external radiaiton, impotence seen in 50%, incontinence 10%–30%. *Stage C* (disease outside capsule): Treat with radiaiton. *Metastatic carcinoma:* Castration and estrogen administration, chemotherapy. LHRH, Flutamide.

D. Renal Cell Carcinoma

- **H&P Keys**
Flank mass, pain, gross hematuria (40% of patients with classic triad), hypertension, fever, anemia, erythrocytosis.

- **Diagnosis**
Excretory urography with nephrotomograms, ultrasound with needle biopsy, CT scan, renal angiogram.

- **Concept and Application**
Staging via TNM system; cavagram, bone scan, MRI; tumor markers: renin and erythropoietin. Tumor has characteristic of spontaneous remission.

- **Management**
Stage related: Stages I and II radical nephrectomy; Stage III radical nephrectomy with lymphadenectomy possible adjuvant immuno/chemotherapy; Stage IV still radical nephrectomy; if lung or brain metastatic disease is isolated surgical excision is optimal; immuno/chemotherapy. Diffuse metastatic disease or locally invasive disease (Stage IV) immunotherapy, chemotherapy.

E. Renal Calculi

- **H&P Keys**
Pain (upper back to testicle or vulva) secondary to dilation of urinary tract, hematuria, nausea, vomiting, urinary frequency or urgency, no comfortable position, decreased bowel sounds.

- **Diagnosis**
Urinalysis: hematuria, crystals in urine; ultrasound to define hydronephrosis or acoustic shadow. CT scan not helpful except to differentiate a possible soft-tissue lesion (cyst versus solid).

- **Disease Severity**
Hydration, allopurinol (uric acid stones).

- **Concept and Application**
Infection related to calculi (structure), urea-splitting bacteria (eg, proteus); uric acid calculi 5% to10% of all stones, radiolucent, cystine calculi: decreased reabsorption of dibasic amino acids. Autosomal recessive. Cacium stones (three times more in men than women), calcium metabolism, hyperparathyroidism. Composition: Calcium oxalate and phosphate, calcium oxalate, struvite, uric acid, cystine.

- **Management**
Shock wave lithotripsy, transurethral extraction if less than 4 mm (90% chance of success) to 6 mm (50% chance of success), nephrostomy (percutaneous), open. Half may pass spontaneously, analgesics imperative.

F. Benign Prostatic Hypertrophy

- **H&P Keys**
Frequency, nocturia, hematuria, dribbling, decreased force of stream (retention), difficulty initiating stream, nodules or firm areas within the gland. Degree of obstruction relates to gland's size.

- **Diagnosis**
Urinalysis, endoscopy, biopsy, cystometry.

- **Concept and Application**
Obstruction of outflow in the aging male, stromal and epotheal hyperplasia.

- **Management**

Medical. Proscar to shrink gland. Balloon dilatation.

Surgical. TURP or open prostatectomy relates to size.

IV. TRAUMA

A. Cranial Injury

- **H&P Keys**

  Loss of consciousness, amnesia, headache, lethargy, irritability, memory loss, seizures, ingestion of alcohol or other drug, speech disorder, weakness of extremities, scalp laceration or hematoma, hemotympanum, rhinorrhea, otorrhea, periorbital or mastoid ecchymosis.

- **Diagnosis**

  Neurologic examination, CT scan of the head, cervical spine roentgenogram.

- **Disease Severity**

  Age, Glasgow coma scale, amnesia longer than 24 hours, focal neurologic deficits, hypoxia, assessment of injuries, hypertension, bradycardia, decerebrate rigidity, Cheyne-Stokes respiration, loss of gag or cough reflex.

- **Concept and Application**

  Sudden movement of brain relative to skull, inflammation of white matter, punctate hemorrhage in white and gray matter, cerebral laceration, diffuse axonal injury, intracranial hemorrhage, raised intracranial pressure.

- **Management**

  Secure airway; correct hypoxia; restore blood pressure; hyperventilate; administer hyperosonistic agents, antibiotics, anticonvulsant prophylaxis; suture scalp laceration; perform craniotomy; intraventricular bolt to monitor intracranial pressure, hypothermia, phenobarbitol coma.

B. Abdominal Injury

- **H&P Keys**

  Abdominal pain; abdominal distention, tenderness, guarding, or rigidity; tachycardia, hypotension, tachypnea, narrowed pulse pressure, cool extremities; associated injuries.

- **Diagnosis**

  Physical examination (repeated), serum amylase, urinalysis, chest roentgenogram while erect, abdominal roentgenogram while supine, CT scan of abdomen or pelvis, diagnostic peritoneal lavage, selective arteriography; abdominal ultrasound.

- **Disease Severity**

  Hypotension, response to therapy, peritonitis, associated injuries, evisceration, positive blood on nasogastric aspirate or rectal exam, positive DPL.

- **Concept and Application**

  Blunt or penetrating missile injury to abdomen or lower chest.

- **Management**

  Secure airway; use fluid resuscitation, observation, blood transfusion, exploratory laparotomy; address injury to all intra-abdominal organs.

Spleen. Splenorrhaphy, splenectomy. Can manage conservatively if blood pressure and hematocrit stable with serial CT scans.

Liver. Pringle maneuver, direct ligation of bleeding vessels, hepatic lobectomy, insertion of atriocaval shunt, drainage, packing and second look laparotomy. Optimal management is nonoperative with red cell replacement and serial CT scans.

Biliary Tract. Cholecystectomy, T-tube in common bile duct, choledochojejunostomy.

Pancreas. Drainage, Whipple procedure; debridement of devitalized pancrease, ligation of main duct if visualized, internal drainage; can also manage expectently with serial CT scans in stable patient.

Gastrointestinal (GI) Tract. Primary repair, drainage, exteriorization of injury less common.

Kidney. Observation, partial or total nephrectomy, serial imaging.

V. POSTOPERATIVE INFECTIONS

A. Wound Infections

- **H&P Keys**
Fever, wound pain, malaise, anorexia, tachycardia, local redness, tenderness, swelling, hemoserous/purulent discharge, postop day 3–5 most commonly.

- **Diagnosis**
Physical examination, wound culture.

- **Disease Severity**
Fever, mentation, abscess formation, wound dehiscence, evisceration, general debility, nutritional status, systemic or local infectious problem.

- **Concept and Application**
Contamination of wound at surgery, postoperative formation of hematoma or seroma, wound-tissue ischemia, classification of surgical wound.

- **Management**
Minimize risk factors, evacuate pus, administer antibiotics, provide local wound care.

B. Urinary Tract Infections

- **H&P Keys**
Dysuria, frequency of micturition, suprapubic or flank pain and tenderness, fever.

- **Diagnosis**
Urinalysis, urine Gram stain and culture, blood cultures.

- **Disease Severity**
High fever, mentation. Response to therapy.

- **Concept and Application**
Contamination of urinary tract, urinary retention, urinary tract instrumentation.

- **Management**
Maintain adequate hydration and catheter hygiene, remove catheter if unnecessary, administer antibiotics.

C. Pneumonia and Atelectasis

- **H&P Keys**
Fever, dyspnea, productive cough, green or yellow sputum, tachycardia, tachypnea, cyanosis, decreased breath sounds, bronchial breathing.

- **Diagnosis**
Physical examination, arterial blood gases (ABG), sputum culture, chest roentgenogram, complete blood count.

- **Disease Severity**
Cyanosis, tracheal deviation, dyspnea at rest, mentation, ABG, gastric response to therapy.

- **Concept and Application**
Obstruction of tracheobronchial airway, abnormality of surfactants, loss of lung volume, secondary bacterial infection. Increased work of breathing. Pain induced decreased lung volumes.

- **Management**
Deep breathing or coughing exercises, ambulation, bronchodilator therapy, physical therapy for chest, intermittent positive-pressure breathing, antibiotics, bronchoscopy, nasotracheal sectioning, pain control is mandatory.

VI. DISEASES OF THE CIRCULATORY SYSTEM

A. Carotid Artery Disease

- **H&P Keys**

Definitions. Transient ischemic attacks (TIA): Brief paresis or numbness of an arm or leg contralateral to the affected carotid territory—by convention, less than 24 hours. Resolving ischemic neurologic deficits (RIND): A neurologic deficit of the contralateral carotid territory that lasts longer than 24 hours but is resolved within 7 days of the event. Amaurosis Fugax (AF): Transient episode of monocular blindness or partial blindness that usually lasts no more than 10 minutes. Stroke: A complete neurologic deficit that does not resolve.

Symptoms and Signs of Cerebral Vascular Disease. Many patients have significant disease without exhibiting any symptoms. Symptomatic patients experience transient ischemic attacks, temporary monocular blindness, or resolving neurologic deficit. Patients with unstable neurologic deficits may experience crescendo transient ischemic attacks, stroke in evolution, or waxing and waning neurologic deficits. Patients with complete stroke have experienced a stroke but continue to be at risk for further stroke and neurologic damage.

Vertebral-basilar artery symptoms are another form of cerebrovascular disease. These symptoms result from TIA's or hypoperfusion to the cerebellum and brain stem and consist of vertigo, drop attacks, dizziness, and clumsiness.

Signs of disease include the auscultation of carotid bruit, presence of Hollenhorst plaques. Significant disease can exist without signs, including occlusions of the internal carotid artery, high-grade stenosis, and ulceration without stenosis.

- **Diagnosis**

Noninvasive Testing. Duplex ultrasound for initial investigation. Duplex scanning is 95% accurate and 90% sensitive compared to arteriography.

Arteriography. The gold standard for analyzing cerebral vascular disease. Not obtained unless operative intervention is contemplated.

- **Disease Severity**
  Controversy surrounds the treatment of cerebral vascular disease. In symptomatic disease, patients experience the symptoms of cerebral vascular disease and have a stenosis of 70% or more of the internal carotid arteries. These patients have been shown by prospective randomized trials to benefit from carotid endarterectomy. In asymptomatic disease, similar trials have shown that patients with 60% or greater degree of stenosis benefit from prophylactic carotid endarterectomy.

- **Concept and Application**
  A majority of symptomatic disease is caused by atherosclerosis. Ulceration of atherosclerotic plaque results in the release of microemboli (usually platelets) that lodge downstream. This embolization results in interruption of the blood supply to the cerebral parenchyma resulting in ischemia and infarct.

- **Management**
  Medical therapy is indicated for patients with stenosis less than 60% whether symptomatic or asymptomatic (acetylsalicylic acid, persantine, ticlopidine). Prospective randomized trials show that surgery is beneficial for symptomatic patients with stenosis of 70% or more. With the recent report of surgical efficacy in the asymptomatic 60% stenotic lesion, most agree now that all patients (symptomatic or not) should be considered for endarterectomy if the degree of stenosis is 60% or greater. Generally accepted combined morbidity and mortality is approximately 2%–4%.

B. Renovascular Disease

- **H&P Keys**
  Two to 7% of patients with hypertension will have a renovascular disease. In over three quarters of these renal artery lesions are secondary to atherosclerosis. The second most common etiology is fibrodysplasia (bilaterally in 90% of males). Irritability, headache, and depression; family history of hypertension; early onset; marked acceleration of the degree of hypertension, resistance to control with antihypertensive drugs, rapid deterioration of renal function, persistent elevation of the diastolic blood pressure, upper abdominal bruit are all signs of renovascular hypertension. Progressive deterioration of renal function with start of angiotensin-converting enzyme (ACE) inhibitor is a tell-tale sign.

- **Diagnosis**

Renal Vein Renins. Ratio of renin from the involved kidney compared to the uninvolved kidney is greater than 1.5. Duplex evaluation, renal systemic renin index (RSRI) 70.48 implies significant disease.

Renal Arteriography. For deteriorating renal function of persistent diastolic hypertension above 110 mm Hg.

- **Disease Severity**

  Surgery is successful in 90% of patients with fibromuscular dysplasia. Improvement or cure in 60% of patients with atherosclerotic disease. Factors suggesting potential renal salvage include urographic visualization of the kidney, renal length of 9 cm or more, retrograde filling of the distal arterial tree, lateralizing renal vein renins, intraoperative biopsy to determine functional glomeruli.

- **Concept and Application**

  Unilateral renal artery stenosis leads to release of renin. Increased renin causes an increase of angiotensin I and subsequently of angiotensin II with vasoconstriction and sodium retention.

- **Management**

  Medical. Attempt to control hypertension with ACE inhibitors and other antihypertensive drugs especially β-blockers. Percutaneous arterial dilatation (with or without stenting) is most successful for fibromuscular dysplasia. Good results in short, isolated atherosclerotic lesions that do not involve the renal artery ostium.

  Surgical. Revascularization if medical therapy fails. Focal atherosclerotic lesions treated most successfully. Aortorenal bypass or, in special circumstances, hepatorenal, splenorenal, or ilial renal bypass. Endarterectomy may also be employed for atherosclerotic lesions and can sometimes be employed through the aorta at the time of aortic reconstruction.

C. Arterial Occlusive Disease

- **H&P Keys**

  Definitions. *Claudication* is a deep ache (most commonly in the calf) that is secondary to muscle ischemia during exercise. This pain progresses to the point where ambulation must stop to resolve the pain. *Rest pain* is a burning pain usually confined to the forefoot and is indicative of severe disease. *Tissue loss* is necrosis of tissue secondary to inadequate blood flow.

  Risk Factors. Smoking, hypertension, diabetes, hyperlipidemia, history of myocardial infarction or stroke, family history of atherosclerotic cardiovascular disease, claudication of the calves, thighs, or buttocks. Distal aortic occlusion (Leriche's syndrome) is characterized by claudication of the hip, thigh, and buttock muscles; atrophy of the leg; impotence, and diminished or absent femoral pulses.

  Physical Examination. Diminished or absent pulses distal to the point of stenosis. Bruits, pallor on elevation, rubor with dependency temperature change, loss of hair, paresthesia, and rest pain.

- **Diagnosis**

  Noninvasive vascular tests include the following: Pulse volume recordings, segmental pressure measurements, segmental Doppler and arterial duplex.

  Ankle-Brachial Index (ABI). Normal, 1.0. A value of less than .75 would be indicative of disease. Rest pain is associated with a value of .4 or lower, and tissue loss is associated with a value of .2 or lower.

  Imaging Studies. Arteriography defines the site and amount of arterial obstruction and delineates proximal and distal arterial anatomy. Reserved for preoperative patients or in special instances of diagnostic difficulty. Complications include hematoma, arteriovenous fistula, false aneurysm, distal embolization of clot, or atheromatous plaque. Digital subtraction arteriography (DSA) uses computer subtraction to enhance images. Poor spatial resolution when compared with arteriography. Requires less contrast media. Magnetic resonance angiography provides arterial anatomy without the risk of contrast agents and may be of greater accuracy in assessing the distal tibial vessels.

- **Disease Severity**

  Claudication, rest pain, and tissue loss are the stages of disease progression. Tissue loss includes both wet and dry gangrene.

- **Concept and Application**
Atherosclerotic narrowing (stenosis). Capillary dilatation and ischemia produce a purple rubor that is characteristic of ischemic vasodilatation associated with disease progression.

- **Management**

Medical. Reduction of risk factors, improvement of collateral circulation, avoidance of foot trauma. Antiplatelet and vasodilatory agents.

Surgical. For incapacitating claudication or limb salvage. Aortoiliac or aortofemoral reconstruction for aortoiliac occlusive disease. Patency is 80% at 5 years. Operative mortality is 5%. For patients with poor cardiovascular or pulmonary reserve, an extra-anatomic bypass, a femorofemoral, iliofemoral, or axilobifemoral bypass can be used. Iliac angioplasty with or without stenting is also employed for disease at this level with good results.

Femoropopliteal Occlusive Disease. Femoropopliteal reconstruction is indicated in claudication and absolutely indicated in patients with rest pain and tissue loss. The optimal graft is autogenous greater saphenous vein. When a saphenous vein does not exist, alternatives such as polytetrafluoroethylene (PTFE) or composites of PTFE and short segments of autologous arm or lesser saphenous vein are used. Femorodistal reconstruction to the tibial, peroneal, or pedal arteries is indicated only for limb salvage. Saphenous vein is the best material. Infrainguinal angioplasty and stenting also are treatment options, but at this level they are inferior to surgical reconstruction.

D. Aneurysms of the Thoracic Aorta

- **H&P Keys**
Compression pressure and chest pain are main symptoms; hoarseness and superior vena caval syndrome, cough and dyspnea from tracheobronchial obstruction. Hemoptysis is indicative of erosion into the trachea and main-stem bronchus.

- **Diagnosis**
Plain roentgenogram of specific location; involvement of surrounding structure requires angiography. CT scan and MRI can be helpful. Echocardiography and cardiac catheterization may be diagnostic. Transesophageal echo has become a standard imaging technique in this disease state.

- **Disease Severity**
Ascending aortic: Excellent results—mortality less than 10%. *Transverse aortic:* Reimplantation of brachycephalic vessels. Mortality rate, 10% to 15%; neurologic complications, 10%. *Descending aortic:* Mortality, 10%; paraplegia, 5% to 30%.

- **Concept and Application**
Etiology: atherosclerosis, cystic medial degeneration, myxomatous degeneration, dissection, infection, trauma, and post-stenotic dilatation. Syphilitic aortitis is unusual. Incidence of aneurysm increases with age. Atherosclerosis occludes vasa vasorum, producing medial necrosis and subsequent aneurysm formation.

- **Management**
Rupture is the most common cause of death. Aneurysms over 6 cm should be resected even if asymptomatic. Documented enlargement is indication for surgery.

Ascending Aortic. Replacement with dacron graft. Simultaneous replacement of aortic valve, if necessary. Frozen homograft can be used in mycotic aneurysms.

Transverse Aortic. Reconstruction with dacron graft. Deep hypothermic circulatory arrest on cardiopulmonary bypass.

Descending Aortic. Replacement with dacron graft. Partial bypass used in attempt to lower complications of paralysis and organ failure.

E. Dissecting Aortic Aneurysms

- **H&P Keys**

  Onset of pain is sudden and severe. The tearing substernal pain may radiate to the back or into the abdomen and extremities. Patients may present with neurologic deficit as well as dyspnea, pulmonary edema, nausea, and vomiting. The patient may be normotensive or hypotensive. Three times more frequent in males. Acute dissection most frequent between the ages of 45 and 70 years. Hypertensive history in 80% to 90% of patients. The patient may be in shock. Pulmonary edema and a murmur of aortic insufficiency may be noted. Comparative blood pressure readings different in extremities. Pulses in extremities may be diminished. Differential diagnosis: myocardial infarction, cerebrovascular accident, pulmonary embolism, acute aortic thrombosis, and acute surgical abdomen.

- **Diagnosis**

  Chest roentgenogram may show a dilated aorta, widened mediastinum, pulmonary edema, or mass effect with or without pleural effusion. Electrocardiogram may show left axis deviation, left ventricular hypertrophy, ischemic changes, dysrhythmias. Aortogram is diagnostic test of choice. Usually reveals splitting of contrast column, distortion of column, or aortic insufficiency. CT, MRI, and transesophageal echocardiogram also used in diagnostic workup.

- **Disease Severity**

  Dissections classified as ascending or descending. Ascending dissections involve the entire aorta in 90% of the cases. Descending dissections involve the aorta distal to the left subclavian artery. May be managed medically or require immediate surgical intervention. Mortality rate is 10% for both methods of management.

- **Concept and Application**

  Underlying defect is destruction of elastic fibers of medial layer. Necrosis of medial layer can be caused by hypertension, atherosclerosis, coarctation, endocrine factors, Marfan's syndrome, trauma, and pregnancy-induced hypertension. Hemodynamic forces, longitudinal shear stress of blood passing through the aorta, together with medical necrosis lead to the development of an intimal tear. A hematoma forms within the torn aorta and dissects distally as well as proximally. This disection plane is within the media.

- **Management**

  Ascending Dissections. Should be managed surgically on diagnosis. Majority (90%) involve the entire aorta. Approach through median sternotomy with cardiopulmonary bypass. Repair the ascending dissection first. The distal extension can be repaired later. The most important thing is to repair the initiation point of the dissection.

  Descending Dissections. Medical management with nitroprusside. Propranolol and methyldopa administered after stabilization. One third of patients will require surgery for enlargement of their aneurysm. Immediate surgery indicated for failure to control hypertension, expansion of the aneurysm, or signs of rupture into the pleural space; development of a neurologic deficit; or compromise of visceral or lower-extremity arteries.

F. Abdominal Aortic Aneurysmal Disease

- **H&P Keys**

  Most patients are asymptomatic; some may be aware of a pulsatile abdominal mass. Sudden onset of severe abdominal pain radiating to the back and associated with hypotension indicative of ruptured aneurysm. On physical examination, palpable mass in the supraumbilical area. In obese patients or patients with tortuous aortas, physical examination may be unremarkable. Abdominal bruit may be present.

- **Diagnosis**

  Plain roentgenograms to detect calcification of the aneurysmal wall, if present. CT scan to assess size of aneurysm as well as extent above and below the renal and iliac vessels. Ultrasound to assess size of aneurysm. Aortography preoperatively to determine suprarenal involvement, suspected renovascular disease, compromised renal function, visceral arterial involvement, possible distal occlusive or aneurysmal disease. Not valuable to assess aneurysm size.

- **Disease Severity**

  Risk of rupture increases with increasing dilatation of abdominal aorta. The majority of aneurysms will continue to enlarge and may rupture if untreated. Rate of expansion is correlated with diastolic blood pressure, initial diameter of aneurysm, and degree of obstructive pulmonary disease. Twenty percent of aneurysms 6 cm or less will rupture compared with 40% of aneurysms larger than 6 cm. Recommend repair of all aneurysms 5 cm or greater in diameter. Coexistent coronary and carotid atherosclerotic disease common.

- **Concept and Application**

  Aneurysmal dilatation secondary to atherosclerotic changes. Inability to withstand increased wall tension secondary to damage of elastic fibers of media. Hereditary deficiency of collagen cross-linking and abnormal copper metabolism.

- **Management**

  Aortic replacement with grafts constructed of polytetrafluoroethylene or dacron indicated when aneurysmal dilatation of 5 cm. Complications include renal failure, myocardial infarction, stroke, graft infection, limb loss, bowel ischemia, impotence. Paraplegia is rare.

G. Thoracic Outlet Syndrome

- **H&P Keys**

  History should establish previous clavicle or rib trauma or fracture, exercise or occupation, poor posture. Must rule out cervical disk disease and carpal tunnel syndrome. Symptoms of thoracic outlet syndrome dependent on compression of brachial plexus, axillary or subclavian artery or vein. Neurologic symptoms include weakness, paresthesia, pain, and numbness, usually in the fingers and hands in an ulnar distribution. Late manifestations include motor weakness, atrophy, and sensory loss. Symptoms of arterial compression include ischemic pain, numbness, fatigue, paresthesia, coldness, and weakness in the hand or arm. Symptoms are intensified by exercise. Embolization, or thrombosis, of the artery may occur. Venous symptoms of compression are edema of extremities, pain, and cyanosis. Patients also may complain of heaviness and tightness in upper extremities.

  Physical examination should focus on neural, arterial, and venous signs. Must rule out weakness, atrophy, and neural deficits, usually in distribution of the ulnar nerve. Arterial signs include absent or weak brachial and radial pulses, delayed capillary refill, distal gangrene. Venous signs include distention of veins of chest, arm, or hand; edema; cyanosis.

- **Diagnosis**

  Adson maneuver: While palpating pulse, patient inhales deeply and turns head to examined side with neck extended. Positive if bruit heard or pulse is lost. Costoclavicular compression maneuver, hyperabduction maneuver, elevated-arm stress test. Diagnostic studies include the following: Plain roentgenograms may demonstrate cervical ribs, ab-normal first ribs, prominent transverse processes, abnormalities of the clavicle. Plethysmography may demonstrate arte-rial component by showing obstruction to arterial flow. Phlebograms may demonstrate compression or obstruction of the axillary or subclavian veins. Arteriograms may show partial or complete arterial occlusion. Should be performed while performing diagnostic maneuvers outlined. Also may demonstrate poststenotic dilatation or embolization. Electromyography may detect compression of peripheral nerves, conduction delay. Somatosensory evoked potentials may provide objective evidence of nerve dysfunction. Duplex can also be employed to evaluate arterial and venous anatomy.

- **Disease Severity**

  Three basic types of thoracic outlet syndrome (TOS): Neurogenic TOS makes up 95% of cases, venous TOS 2%, arterial TOS 1%.

- **Concept and Application**
Compression areas include the interscalene triangle, the scalenus anticus space between the first rib and clavicle, the costocoracoid fascia, the pectoralis minor tendon. In addition, compression may be associated with anatomic variants, including cervical ribs, long transverse process of C7, scalene muscle fiber variants with degenerative changes and increased intramusclar fibrosis.

- **Management**
Four to six months of intensive physical therapy if no evidence of vascular occlusion, distal embolization, or poststenotic aneurysm. Surgical treatment consists of resection of the first rib, anterior scalenectomy, middle scalenectomy; removal of a cervical rib if one is present. Improvement noted in 60% to 75%, no change in symptoms in 10% to 15%, and a worsening of symptoms in 5% to 10%.

H. Infrainguinal Aneurysmal Disease

- **H&P Keys**
Femoral and popliteal aneurysms are often asymptomatic. They may present as a groin or popliteal mass. Ischemia of foot and toes may be the presenting symptoms in some cases. Fifty percent of popliteal and 74% of femoral arterial aneurysms are bilateral. Thirty percent of patients with popliteal aneurysms have abdominal aortic aneurysms, and 85% of patients with femoral aneurysms have other associated aneurysms.

- **Diagnosis**
Ultrasound is noninvasive method of diagnosis and delineates size of the aneurysm. Angiography is indicated in all patients in whom surgical correction is considered. Because of the high incidence of coexistent aortic, iliac, and femoral aneurysms, workup must include a close assessment of the entire arterial tree.

- **Disease Severity**
Immediate treatment indicated when acute thrombosis causes ischemia. Early surgery indicated for recurrent embolization.

Asymptomatic aneurysms should always be repaired

- **Concept and Application**
Etiology is atherosclerosis, previous surgery, trauma (either blunt or penetrating); infection, especially associated with femoral aneurysm from intravenous (IV) drug abuse; and associated with femoral catheterization or angiography.

- **Management**

Femoral Artery Aneurysm. Excision and replacement. Preferable to use autologous artery or vein, but prosthetic material can be used.

Popliteal Artery Aneurysm. Proximal and distal ligation of native popliteal artery, with bypass using autogenous saphenous vein.

I. Arterial Embolism/Thrombosis

- **H&P Keys**
Acute occlusion, pulselessness, pallor, paresthesia, pain, and paralysis. Irreversible limb loss may occur within 6 hours. No previous history of claudication and no physical findings of vascular disease. Normal pulses in the unaffected extremity.

- **Diagnosis**
Clinical assessment includes echocardiography because cardiac system is most common source of emboli. Noninvasive vascular evaluation includes the ankle-brachial index (ABI). Arteriogram employed if diagnosis is in question or time permits.

- **Disease Severity**
Usually secondary to cardiac source. Therapy initiated (ie, atrial fibrillation, myocardial infarction, congestive heart failure). Severity clearly depends on the number and degree of medical comorbidities.

- **Concept and Application**
Primary source of acute occlusion is cardiac source. Embolic occlusion is more common than thrombotic occlusion. Thrombotic occlusion is caused by chronic degenerative atherosclerotic disease. Compromise of oxygenation leads to anaerobic metabolism

acidosis, membrane destabilization, and cellular edema and death.

- **Management**
Embolectomy (by balloon catheter or completion angiogram). Thrombolytic agents (urokinase, streptokinase) are used when thrombus has progressed into small vessels. Four-compartment fasciotomy is recommended with delayed surgery or excessive swelling. Maintenance of urine output and alkalinization recommended to prevent renal injury, antioxidants, and mannitol employed.

J. Hemangioma

- **H&P Keys**
Most common and rapidly growing tumor in infants. Incidence during first year, with majority appearing in second to fourth week of life. Three forms are (1) superficial, (2) combined superficial and deep, and (3) deep. Noninvoluting hemangiomas are present at birth and do not grow by rapid expansion. Do not undergo involution and grow in proportion to the child into adulthood. Port wine stains are the most common type of noninvoluting hemangioma.

- **Diagnosis**
Clinical assessment and physical exam.

- **Disease Severity**
Include strawberry nevus and capillary hemangiomas. Appear in the first 2 to 3 weeks of life, and grow rapidly for the first 4 to 6 months. Rapid growth ceases after sixth month, and involution process takes place. Disappear by age 5 to 7 years. Minimal surgery is indicated. Noninvoluting hemangiomas are usually an esthetic problem.

- **Concept and Application**
Involuting hemangiomas are composed of endothelial cells during the rapid growth phase. Fibrous stroma during the involution phase. The port wine stains are composed of thin-walled capillaries with mature endothelial cells and large venous sinuses. Cavernous hemangiomas are composed of large, dilated, packed vascular sinuses lined by mature endothelium.

- **Management**
Treatment of hemangiomas is governed by their size and growth. Involuting hemangiomas should be followed, not treated surgically. Treatment of port wine stains yields poor results.

K. Deep Venous Thrombosis

- **H&P Keys**
Patient can either be asymptomatic or exhibit the classic findings of calf swelling and tenderness, elevated temperature, and a positive Homans sign (leg pain on dorsiflexion of the foot). Phlegmasia cerulea dolens is complete iliofemoral venous occlusion, with massive swelling, pain, and cyanosis of the leg, which may progress to venous gangrene. A swollen tender extremity, tenderness of the calf, and differences in circumferential measurements are commonly seen. Symptoms are unilateral, patient often gives a history of previous DVT or superficial thrombophlebitis.

- **Diagnosis**
Clinical findings on examination are incorrect in approximately 50% of the cases. False-negative ultrasound results can occur with partially occluding thrombi. Doppler ultrasound is accurate in 80% to 85% of time. B-mode duplex ultrasound and Doppler color-flow analysis can be used to assess for thrombosis. Sensitivity and specificity for above-the-knee thrombi is 90% to 100%. Most errors with this method occur with below-the-knee thrombi, where sensitivity is only 75%. Duplex scan has become the standard test for diagnosis in most institutions. Venograms are still employed and accepted as the gold standard.

- **Concept and Application**
Thrombosis is related to three factors: endothelial abnormalities, blood flow stasis, and hypercoagulability (Virchow's triad). Platelet aggregation and procoagulants compromise the venous lumen and result in a hypercoagulable state.

- **Management**
Prevention is the best management. Attempts to overcome venous stasis include

leg exercise, leg elevation, elastic stockings, pneumatic stockings, and early ambulation. Patients with deep venous thrombosis should be confined to bed until the pain and swelling begin to resolve. Bed rest will reduce the edema associated with the condition. After this period, the patient can undergo gradual ambulation with limited sitting or standing and use of elastic stockings. Drug therapy consists of intravenous heparin to prevent propagation of the thrombus and to prevent pulmonary embolus. The partial thromboplastin time should be extended to 1.5 times the normal value. Heparin should be continued for 3 to 5 days until warfarin therapy (which is initiated once diagnosis is established) is therapeutic. Warfarin therapy is continued for 3 to 6 months. Surgical therapy includes vena cava interruption to prevent embolism of thrombus to the lungs. Surgery is indicated when anticoagulation is contraindicated or when patient has pulmonary embolism on adequate anticoagulation, multiple small emboli creating chronic pulmonary insufficiency, septic emboli refractory to treatment, or has undergone a pulmonary embolectomy. Thrombolytic therapy is also employed in cases of iliofemoral DVT to abate the late sequelae of venous thrombosis, namely valvular incompetence, and the development of chronic venous insufficiency.

L. Varicose Veins

- **H&P Keys**
  It is estimated that 10% to 20% of the population has some difficulty with varicose veins. Patients may have no symptoms or may complain of aching, swelling, heaviness, cramps, itching, and disfigurement. Symptoms increase with prolonged standing. Varicose veins secondary to chronic venous insufficiency are associated with more severe symptoms. Ankle ulcers are common with this form of varicosity. Dry, scaling skin; edema and brawny induration; and, occasionally, hemorrhage may be noted. Physical examination shows dilated, tortuous, subcutaneous veins of the thigh and leg (often involving the greater and lesser saphenous systems). Pitting edema of the ankles and legs as well as brawny discoloration of the medial lower leg is noted.

- **Diagnosis**
  Valvular competence of the deep, superficial, and perforating veins between the deep and the superficial systems must be determined. The Brodie-Trendelenburg test should be used to determine competence of valves in the greater saphenous vein and perforating veins.

- **Concept and Application**
  Fundamental abnormality is sequential incompetence of the valve. Incompetent valves create a higher pressure at the next lower valve and result in localized dilation. A second theory assumes an inherent weakness in the wall of the vein, producing dilatation despite normal venous pressures. Secondary varicosities result following obstruction of deep veins. Recanalization of the veins leaves the valves incompetent, especially in the superficial system, which has little surrounding support. The result is increasing venous pressure transmitted from the deep to the superficial system and venous dilatation.

- **Management**
  Nonoperative management consists of improving venous return and reducing venous pressure by elevation and graduated elastic stockings. Surgical therapy is indicated for severe symptoms, large varicosities, attacks of superficial phlebitis, hemorrhage from a ruptured varix, or ulceration from venous stasis or for cosmetic reasons. Sclerotherapy is used for small "spider" varicosities.

M. Superficial Thrombophlebitis

- **H&P Keys**
  History of intravenous catheters or drug abuse. Lower extremity thrombophlebitis is associated with varicose veins, thromboangiitis obliterans, or bacterial infection. Abdominal cancer may be expressed as recurrent or migratory superficial thrombophlebitis (Trousseau's sign). Other symptoms include erythema, pain, induration,

heat, tenderness along the course of a superficial vein, fever, and leukocytosis.

- **Diagnosis**
  History and physical examination.

- **Disease Severity**
  Disease is limited, with a short and uncomplicated time course. Recurrent superficial phlebitis is an indication for venous stripping.

- **Concept and Application**
  Introduction of bacteria with either IV catheters or IV drug abuse. Local infection and inflammatory response result in thrombosis. There is a significant inflammatory response in thrombosis alone. The introduction of bacteria aggravates this response.

- **Management**
  Condition is symptomatic in most cases and includes analgesia, nonsteroidal antiinflammatory agents, local heat, and elastic compression bandages. If inflammation of saphenous vein involves the saphenofemoral junction, pulmonary embolism may result. Ligation of the greater saphenous vein is indicated in these cases. In cases of suppuration, surgical excision of involved vein is indicated.

VII. DISEASES OF THE GASTROINTESTINAL TRACT

A. Zenker's Diverticulum

- **H&P Keys**
  Dysphagia, noisy sound in the throat, regurgitation of undigested food, spasm, coughing, mass on the left side of the neck, foul mouth odor.

- **Diagnosis**
  Barium esophagogram.

- **Disease Severity**
  Pulmonary complications, poor nutrition, weight loss, size of pouch, presence of carcinoma, is rare. This is the most common esophageal diverticulum.

- **Concept and Application**
  Acquired false mucosal pouch (caused by pressure) at Killian's dehiscence. Incoordination of the oricopharygeal muscle at its junction with the thyropharyngeus causing a posterior pharyngeal mucosal herniation.

- **Management**
  Adequate pulmonary care, diverticulectomy, cricopharyngeal myotomy.

B. Midesophageal Traction Diverticulum

- **H&P Keys**
  Often associated with mediastinal granulomatous disease. Most commonly assymptomatic and incidentally discovered.

- **Diagnosis**
  Barium esophagram.

- **Disease Severity**
  Only dependent on associated symptoms.

- **Concept and Application**
  Mediastinal adenopathy from TB or histoplasmosis adheres to the esophagus, "dragging" a section of esophagus toward the mediastinum and creating a diverticulum.

- **Management**
  Only in symptomatic patients is excision indicated. This is a true diverticulum.

C. Achalasia

- **H&P Keys**
  Dysphagia, effortless regurgitation of undigested food, weight loss, dyspnea.

- **Diagnosis**
  Barium esophagogram, panendoscopy, esophagomanometry.

- **Disease Severity**
  Aspiration, pneumonia, carcinoma, old age, recurrent dysphagia.

- **Concept and Application**
  Absent esophageal peristalsis and dilatation, incomplete relaxation of lower esophageal sphincter, hypertensive lower esophageal sphincter, decreased ganglion cells in Auerbach plexus. Risk of carcinoma is increased.

• **Management**

Medical. Calcium channel blockers, esophageal dilatation.

Surgical. Distal esophagocardiomyotomy and antireflux procedure.

D. Esophageal Varices

• **H&P Keys**
Asymptomatic, hematemesis, melena, signs of liver failure, patient with history of alcohol abuse.

• **Diagnosis**
Barium esophagogram and panendoscopy.

• **Disease Severity**
Recurrent bleeding. Child's classification, ascites, encephalopathy, nutritional status, degree of coagulopathy.

• **Concept and Application**
Significant elevation of portal pressures. Majority of patients have cirrhosis or had extrahepatic portal obstruction in childhood.

• **Management**
If bleeding is acute, fluid resuscitation vasopressin, somatostatin, sclerotherapy, balloon tamponade, endoscopic banding. Portosystemic shunt most commonly employed in an urgent or elective status to relieve portal hypertension.

E. Cancer of the Stomach

• **H&P Keys**
Anorexia, epigastric pain, weight loss, dysphagia, vomiting, hematemesis, epigastric mass, ascites, hepatomegaly, anemia.

• **Diagnosis**
Barium meal, CT scan of abdomen, panendoscopy, fecal occult blood.

• **Disease Severity**
Weight loss, tumor characteristics or depth of invasion, cell type, cardiac tumor, cachexia, ascites, abdominal pain, peritonitis secondary to perforation, degree of local extension, associated adenopathy, and previous gastric surgery.

• **Concept and Application**
Malignant changes of the gastric epithelium. Premalignant conditions are atrophic gastritis, intestinal metaplasia, dysplastic gastric polyp, and pernicious anemia.

• **Management**
Radical gastric resection, irradiation, chemotherapy.

F. Gastric Volvulus

• **H&P Keys**
Retching, inability to vomit; epigastric distention; inability to pass nasogastric tube; chronic crampy abdominal pain.

• **Diagnosis**
Barium upper gastrointestinal series, endoscopy.

• **Disease Severity**
Duration of symptoms, perforation or gangrene of stomach or shock.

• **Concept and Application**
Presence of paraesophageal hiatus hernia or shock. Eventration of left hemidia-phragm, rotation around the longitudinal axis (organoaxial volvulus), or mesenteric axial volvulus.

• **Management**

Acute. IV fluids, antibiotics, derotation, anterior gastropexy and gastrostomy.

Chronic. Anterior gastropexy and antireflux procedure, division of gastrocolic ligament.

G. Appendicitis

• **H&P Keys**
Periumbilical pain shifting to right lower quadrant, anorexia, nausea and vomiting, low-grade fever, tender right lower quadrant, tender on rectal examination.

• **Diagnosis**
History and physical, leukocytosis, ultrasound (especially in children).

• **Disease Severity**
White blood cell count, high fever, peritonitis, elderly, pregnancy, morbidity resulting from delayed diagnosis.

- **Concept and Application**
  Obstruction of appendix lumen and bacterial invasion.

- **Management**
  Fluid resuscitation, antibiotics, appendectomy.

H. Ulcerative Colitis

- **H&P Keys**
  Abdominal cramps, bloody diarrhea, weight loss, rectal urgency, abdominal tenderness, fever. Rule out anemia.

- **Diagnosis**
  Colonoscopy, barium enema, rectum always involved.

- **Disease Severity**
  Dehydration, malnutrition, cecal perforation, massive lower gastrointestinal bleeding, frequent relapses, systemic manifestations (total colonic involvement, failure of medical treatment). A definite increased risk of colon carcinoma exists.

- **Concept and Application**
  Immunologic injury to colon mucosa. Defect of suppressor T-cells in gut wall, possible infectious etiology, true cause remains uncertain.

- **Management**

  Acute. Bed rest, sulfasalizine, steroids, nothing by mouth. Total parenteral nutrition, subtotal colectomy and ileostomy.

  Chronic. Sulfasalazine, steroids, immunosuppressive agents, panproctocolectomy with J-pouch.

I. Crohn's Disease

- **H&P Keys**
  Crampy abdominal pain, diarrhea, perianal fistula and abscess, extraintestinal manifestation, abdominal mass, rectal bleeding less common than with ulcerative colitis.

- **Diagnosis**
  Proctosigmoidoscopy, colonoscopy, barium enema and isotope scanning.

- **Disease Severity**
  Severe anal disease, extraintestinal manifestation, malnutrition, abdominal mass, intraabdominal abscesses, failure of medical treatment, amount of small bowel and colon involved.

- **Concept and Application**
  Immunologic mechanism that leads to inflammatory reaction and damage; cytopathic effect of transmissible agent.

- **Management**

  Medical. Bed rest; low-residue, high-protein diet; sulfasalazine, metronidazol, aminosalicylates delivered orally or rectually. 6 mercaptopurine and cyclosporin may be employed in refractory cases.

  Surgical. Small-bowel resection, segmental colectomy, stricturoplasty. Surgical is indicated only for the complications of Crohn's. Unlike ulcerative colitis surgery is not definitive treatment.

J. Acute Mesenteric Ischemia

- **H&P Keys**
  Abdominal pain, diarrhea, rectal bleeding, atrial fibrillation, minimal abdominal findings, pain often out of proportion to physical exam findings. Abdominal pain in the setting of low cardiac output.

- **Diagnosis**
  White blood cell count, ABG, lactic acid, angiography.

- **Disease Severity**
  Fever, abdominal tenderness, guarding, hypotension, leukocytosis, base deficit, elevated lactic acid, disseminated intravascular coagulation, pulmonary dysfunction, diffuse peritonitis, associated cardiac comorbidity.

- **Concept and Application**
  Embolic and thrombotic occlusion of mesentery vessels, thrombosis of mesenteric veins, severe splanchnic vasoconstriction.

- **Management**
  Intravenous fluids, antibiotics, thromboembolectomy, bowel resection, anticoagula-

tion, intra-arterial papaverine. Treatment of cardiac etiology with arrhythmia control, long-term anticoagulation.

K. Small Bowel Obstruction

• **H&P Keys**
Colicky abdominal pain, vomiting, failure to pass flatus or feces; abdominal distention, visible peristalsis, high-pitched bowel sound, dehydration. Rule out previous surgery.

• **Diagnosis**
Plain abdominal roentgenograms (air-fluid levels), barium upper GI series with small bowel follow through.

• **Disease Severity**
Poor urine output, leukocytosis, unremitting pain, high fever, localized peritonitis.

• **Concept and Application**
Narrowing or occlusion of bowel lumen, proximal bowel distention with gas and fluid. This distension leads to increased intestinal wall pressure with resulting lymphatic then venous destruction eventually causing arterial insufficiency and gangrene of the bowel. Adhesions, hernia, tumor are the most common etiologies.

• **Management**
Fluid and electrolyte resuscitation, nasogastric decompression, Foley catheterization, laparotomy, and correction of cause with or without bowel resection.

L. Large-Bowel Obstruction

• **H&P Keys**
Crampy abdominal pain; nausea and vomiting; obstipation; abdominal distention; visible peristalsis; high-pitched, frequent bowel sounds; abdominal tenderness; abdominal mass, cachexia.

• **Diagnosis**
Plain roentgenogram of abdomen, gastrografin enema, colonoscopy.

• **Disease Severity**
Poor urine output, leukocytosis, intermittent pain, presence of carcinoma.

• **Concept and Application**
Narrowing or occlusion of bowel lumen, proximal bowel distention with gas and fluid, gangrenous bowel resulting from vascular compromise.

• **Management**

Medical. Fluid and electrolyte resuscitation, nasogastric decompression, monitoring urine output.

Surgical. Decompression, colostomy or cecostomy, colectomy with colostomy or primary resection with anastomosis performed much less commonly.

M. Diverticulitis

• **H&P Keys**
Localized abdominal pain, especially left lower quadrant tenderness, constipation, increase frequency of defecation, nausea and vomiting, low-grade fever, mild abdominal distention, mucus per rectum, blood noted in stools. Patient usually has abnormal bowel function.

• **Diagnosis**
Plain abdominal films, CT scan of the abdomen and pelvis, colonoscopy is rarely employed in the acute setting.

• **Disease Severity**
WBC, perforation, hemorrhage, abscess formation, fecal peritonitis, septic shock.

• **Concept and Application**
Raised intracolonic pressure and abdominal colonic contraction leading to pulsion diverticulum; entrapped fecalith causes obstruction of the diverticulum and resulting inflamation with potential perforation.

• **Management**

Medical. Nothing by mouth, systemic antibiotics, fluid-electrolyte resuscitation.

Surgical. Drainage of abscess, colectomy (Hartman's procedure), colectomy with primary anastomosis done less frequently.

N. Rectal Tumor

- **H&P Keys**
  Rectal bleeding, mucous discharge, change of bowel habits, tenesmus, rectal mass, hepatomegaly, ascites.

- **Diagnosis**
  Colonoscopy, barium enema, flexible sigmoidoscopy, endorectal ultrasound scan, MRI, CT scan of pelvis and abdomen.

- **Disease Severity**
  Anemia, abnormal liver function tests, location of tumor, tumor differentiation, fixity of tumor.

- **Concept and Application**
  Malignant change in adenoma, genetic predisposition to malignant change, mutational activation of genes by carcinogenic agents.

- **Management**
  Low anterior section, abdominoperineal resection, radiation, chemotherapy, local excision for superficial lesions.

O. Hemorrhoids

- **H&P Keys**
  Rectal bleeding and pain, mucous discharge, prolapse spontaneously or with defecation, perianal itching, anal verge normal or hypertrophic, visible prolapsed hemorrhoids.

- **Diagnosis**
  Rectal examination, proctosigmoidoscopy, barium enema.

- **Disease Severity**
  Degree of hemorrhoidal prolapse, coexisting Crohn's disease, failure of conservative measures.

- **Concept and Application**
  Prolapse of normal mucosal cushion, increased anal canal pressure.

- **Management**
  High-fiber diet, warm sitz baths, sclerotherapy, rubber band ligation, cryosurgery, hemorrhoidectomy. Be sure to rule out coexistent rectal or sigmoid pathology.

P. Anal-Rectal Abscesses

- **H&P Keys**
  Deep buttock pain or rectal pain, fever, perianal mass.

- **Diagnosis**
  Rectal-perianal examination, CT scan sometimes indicated.

- **Disease Severity**
  Coexisting Crohn's disease, diffuse spread of abscess, extension into adjacent anatomic space, presence of complex fistula.

- **Concept and Application**
  Invasion of perirectal spaces by pathogenic organisms; infection of anal crypts, hair follicles, or sebaceous cysts. Supratenator, perianal, intersphinctenic, and ischicanal abscesses.

- **Management**
  Examination under anesthesia, antibiotics, warm sitz baths, local wound care, incision and drainage are paramount.

Q. Anorectal Fistula

- **H&P Keys**
  Chronic purulent discharge from perianal opening, history of perianal abscess.

- **Diagnosis**
  Rectal examination, anoscopy, proctoscopy, rectal ultrasound fistulography.

- **Disease Severity**
  Co-existing Crohn's, complex or high fistulas, TB, incontinence, HIV status.

- **Concept and Application**
  Injury or infected anal crypts.

- **Management**
  Examination under anesthesia. Lay open the fistula and use seton; if associated with diverticulitis, perform colon resection, Goodsall's rule.

R. Pilonidal Cyst

- **H&P Keys**
  Purulent drainage from sacrococcygeal sinus; pain, tender mass, induration, hair emerging from opening.

- **Diagnosis**
  Physical examination.

- **Disease Severity**
  Hirsutism, multiple tracts, multiple recurrence, poor postoperative follow-up.

- **Concept and Application**
  Macerated skin, suction effect of buttock when walking, loose hair embedded in skin.

- **Management**
  Incision and drainage of abscess; wide local excision of sinus tract; healing by primary closure, secondary intention, local flaps.

S. Benign Neoplasm of Small Bowel

- **H&P Keys**
  Asymptomatic, occult GI bleeding, bowel obstruction (crampy abdominal pain, bloating, vomiting), dysphagia, early satiety, constipation.

- **Diagnosis**
  Upper GI series and small bowel follow-through, esophagogastroduodenoscopy, CT scan of the abdomen and pelvis.

- **Disease Severity**
  Massive GI bleeding, nonviable bowel secondary to intussusception.

- **Concept and Application**
  Benign smooth-muscle tumor.

- **Management**
  Enucleation, wedge excision depending on size and symptomatology.

T. Colon Polyps

- **H&P Keys**
  Rectal bleeding, altered bowel habits, mucus discharge from rectum, rectal mass, heme-positive stools, family history, anemia.

- **Diagnosis**
  Colonoscopy, barium enema, complete blood count (CBC).

- **Disease Severity**
  Family history, size of polyp, histological variant, degree of dysplasia, multiple adenomas.

- **Concept and Application**
  Neoplasia of intestinal epithelium (tubular villous), abnormal mixture of normal tissue (hamartomas).

- **Management**
  Polypectomy, bowel resection, panproctocolectomy and J-pouch (for familial polyposis).

U. Duodenal Atresia

- **H&P Keys**
  Bile-stained vomiting, post-feeding vomiting, distended upper abdomen, passage of meconium, antepartum polyhydramnios, stigmata of Down's syndrome (30%).

- **Diagnosis**
  Plain roentgenogram ("double-bubble" sign), upper GI series and follow-through, barium enema, evaluate cardiac system with echocardiography.

- **Disease Severity**
  Prematurity, associated anomalies (eg, congenital heart disease), low birth weight, trisomy 21.

- **Concept and Application**
  Hypoplasia or atresia of duodenum at level of ampulla, annular pancreas.

- **Management**
  Elevate head of bed, nasogastric decompression; correct fluid and electrolyte imbalance; duodenoduodenostomy, decompression gastrostomy; correct associated malrotation; chromosomal studies.

V. Malrotation

- **H&P Keys**
  Biliary vomiting, hematemesis, heme-positive nasogastric aspirate, failure to thrive, mild abdominal distention, passage of meconium.

- **Diagnosis**
  Plain roentgenogram of abdomen ("double-bubble" sign), upper GI series, barium enema.

- **Disease Severity**
  Hematemesis, bloody stools, abdominal guarding or rigidity, heart rate, blood pressure, leukocytosis, ABG, mentation.

- **Concept and Application**
Abnormality of usual embryonic rotation and fixation. Types: (1) nonrotation (midgut suspended by superior mesenteric vessels), (2) incomplete rotation (narrow small-bowel mesentery, adhesive Ladd's bands), (3) reversed rotation (retroarterial cecal rotation), and (4) anomalous fixation of mesentery.

- **Management**
Fluid and electrolyte correction, nasogastric decompression, antibiotics, surgical derotation of bowel, division of Ladd's bands, widen base of mesentery, fixation of cecum, appendectomy.

W. Hirschsprung's Disease

- **H&P Keys**
Failure to pass meconium, chronic constipation, bile-stained vomiting, reluctance to feed, diarrhea, irritability, abdominal distention, palpable stool in lower abdomen, stool expulsion after rectal examination, male infant.

- **Diagnosis**
Plain abdominal roentgenogram, barium enema, rectal biopsy and rectal manometry.

- **Disease Severity**
Diarrhea, abdominal guarding, abdominal distention, malnutrition; length of bowel involved.

- **Concept and Application**
Absence of cephalocaudal growth of parasympathetic myenteric nerve cells, functional obstruction, rectum always involved.

- **Management**
Rectal tube and colonic washing, colostomy, endorectal pull-through.

X. Imperforate Anus

- **H&P Keys**
Anal dimple but no orifice; ectopic anal opening or fistula; meconium in vagina, urethra, or urine.

- **Diagnosis**
Physical examination, test urine for meconium, Rice-Wangensteen radiographic technique, ultrasound study kidneys and heart, sacrum roentgenogram. Associated in 70% with other abnormalities.

- **Disease Severity**
Associated anomalies, acidosis, neurologic deficit, agenesis of sacral vertebrae, incontinence.

- **Concept and Application**
Abnormal growth and fusion of embryonic anal hillocks, faulty division of the cloaca by urorectal septum.

- **Management**
Posterior sagittal anoplasty, sigmoid colostomy, division of fistula, repeated anal dilation.

VIII. DISEASES OF THE GALLBLADDER AND LIVER

A. Biliary Atresia

- **H&P Keys**
Jaundice, dark urine, pale-colored stools, hepatomegaly, splenomegaly, usually in 2- to 4-week-old infants.

- **Diagnosis**
Rose bengal nuclear medicine scan, hepato-iminodiacetic acid (HIDA) scan, serum lipoprotein X, abdominal ultrasound; needle biopsy of liver, exploratory laparotomy, cholangiography. Must rule out α-antitrypsin disease.

- **Disease Severity**
Jaundice, fever, cirrhosis, sepsis, esophageal varices, liver failure, delayed diagnosis, age (less than 12 weeks).

- **Concept and Application**
Acquired absence of patent bile ducts, periportal fibrosis, cirrhosis.

- **Management**
IV fluids, vitamin K, Roux-en-Y-hepatico-jejunostomy, liver transplantation.

B. Acute Cholecystitis

- **H&P Keys**
Right upper-quadrant pain, radiation into interscapular area, nausea and vomiting, anorexia, fever, history of fatty food intolerance. Mild icterus, right upper-quadrant tenderness, and guarding, palpable gallbladder.

- **Diagnosis**
Plain roentgenogram of abdomen, ultrasound HIDA scan, liver function tests.

- **Disease Severity**
Unremitting fever; leukocytosis; elevated amylase, jaundice; free perforation; palpable gallbladder, suggesting empyema or pericholecystic abscess; chills; common duct stones; diabetes mellitus; response to therapy.

- **Concept and Application**
Obstruction of cystic duct with stone, secondary bacterial invasion, lysolecithin-induced inflammation.

- **Management**

Acute. IV fluids, nasogastric tube, antibiotics, cholecystostomy, and cholecystectomy.

Chronic. Cholecystectomy.

C. Choledochal Cyst

- **H&P Keys**
Abdominal pain, episodic jaundice, mass in right upper-quadrant, fever, dark urine, pale stools.

- **Diagnosis**
Ultrasound of abdomen, CT scan of abdomen, endoscopic retrograde cholangiopancreatography (ERCP), percutaneous transhepatic cholangiography.

- **Disease Severity**
Cirrhosis, fever, jaundice, recurrent pancreatitis, portal hypertension.

- **Concept and Application**
Persistence of embryonic hepaticopancreatic duct, regurgitation of pancreatic juice in bile duct, cystic changes in bile duct, fibrosis, inflammation. If untreated, risk of carcinoma is increased.

- **Management**
Excision of choledochal cyst, cholecystectomy and biliary reconstruction with a Rouxen Y limb.

D. Choledocholithiasis

- **H&P Keys**
Biliary colic, pruritus, chills, fever, jaundice, dark urine, pale stools, and right upper-quadrant tenderness, nausea and vomitting.

- **Diagnosis**
Liver function tests (LFTs), ultrasound, ERCP, percutaneous transhepatic cholangiography (PTC), amylase, lipase.

- **Disease Severity**
Heart rate, hypertension, hemobilia, leukocytosis, amylase, presence of hepatic abscess, biliary cirrhosis, liver failure, portal hypertension, coexistent diabetes mellitus.

- **Concept and Application**
Stones originating in gallbladder; primary stones arising in intrahepatic duct or common bile duct.

- **Management**

Acute. IV fluids, IV antibiotics, nasociliary drainage, ERCP and sphincterotomy, extracorporeal shockwave lithotripsy (ESWL), cholecystectomy and common bile duct exploration, transduodenal sphincteroplasty, choledochoduodenostomy.

Chronic. Antibiotics, drainage procedures as described above, hepatic lobectomy.

E. Carcinoma of the Gallbladder

- **H&P Keys**
Right upper-quadrant pain, jaundice, weight loss, right upper-quadrant mass, fever.

- **Diagnosis**
LFTs, ultrasound scan, CT scan of abdomen and pelvis.

- **Disease Severity**
Weight loss, malnutrition, age, depth of tumor invasion, incidental finding, nonresectibility.

- **Concept and Application**
Eighty percent of cases associated with gallstones. Porcelain gallbladder may be present.

- **Management**
Cholecystectomy, radical region lymphadenectomy and wedge excision of gallbladder bed. Surgery most often is palliative.

F. Hepatic Adenoma

- **H&P Keys**
Right upper-quadrant pain, asymptomatic, palpable hepatic mass, hemoperitoneum, hypotension, use of oral contraceptives, female sex.

- **Diagnosis**
Ultrasound scan, CT scan of the abdomen, tecnecium colloid sulfur colloid scan, angiography, aspiration biopsy.

- **Disease Severity**
Blood pressure, heart rate, abdominal distention, abdominal guarding, large adenoma (greater than 6 cm).

- **Concept and Application**
Encapsulated homogeneous mass of hepatocyte, no bile ducts or central vein present.

- **Management**

Adenoma Less than 6 cm. Observation, discontinue oral contraceptive.

Adenoma Greater than 6 cm. Surgical resection.

G. Focal Nodular Hyperplasia

- **H&P Keys**
Most often asymptomatic, much less tendency to hemorrhage than adenomas. Can present similarly if symptomatic.

- **Diagnosis**
Ultrasound scan, CT. Tecnecium colloid sulfur colloid aspiration biopsy.

- **Disease Severity**
Depends on the reason for presentation, hemodynamic factors.

- **Concept and Application**
Histologically normal appearing hepatocytes, bile ducts, four Kupfer cells.

- **Management**
Conservative observation.

IX. DISEASE OF THE PANCREAS

A. Acute Pancreatitis

- **H&P Keys**
Epigastric pain with back pain, nausea and vomiting, retching, hypotension, fever, left pleural effusion, abdominal tenderness, abdominal mass, jaundice, abdominal distention, Cullen's sign, Grey Turner's sign. Rule out alcohol abuse.

- **Diagnosis**
Amylase, lipase, ultrasound scan of the abdomen, CT scan of the abdomen, plain roentgenogram, ERCP.

- **Disease Severity**
Age, blood glucose, WBC, lactic dehydrogenase, aspartate transaminase, calcium level, urea, hematocrit, excess base, arterial P_{O_2}. Estimated fluid sequestered greater than 6 L. Fibrinogen, methemalbumin, respiratory rate, urine output, persistent fever, abdominal mass, jaundice, hematemesis, and hemoperitoneum.

- **Concept and Application**
Enzymatic digestion of gland, duct obstruction (gallstones and protein), chemical injury to the gland.

- **Management**
Fluid replacement, GI rest, calcium and magnesium replacement. ERCP, analgesia, cholecystectomy, biliary drainage, debridement of necrotic pancreatic tissue. Oxygen supplement with mechanical ventilation and parenteral nutrition.

B. Pancreatic Carcinoma

- **H&P Keys**
Vague abdominal pain, back pain, weight loss, pruritus, jaundice, abdominal mass,

hepatomegaly, migratory thrombophlebitis, sudden onset of diabetes mellitus.

- **Diagnosis**
Ultrasound of the abdomen, CT scan of the abdomen, ERCP, pandescopy, aspiration biopsy of pancreatic mass, angiography, lymph node capsular invasion, distant metastasis, vascular invasion.

- **Concept and Application**
Malignant change in the pancreatic duct, increased risk with severe smoking and consumption of fat and fried foods.

- **Management**

Curative. Pancreaticoduodenectomy, total pancreatectomy, distal pancreatectomy, intra-operative irradiation, external-beam radiation, multidrug chemotherapy.

Palliative. Biliary enteric bypass and enterostomy, biliary stent, analgesia, splanchnic plexus nerve block.

C. Gastrinoma

- **H&P Keys**
Severe peptic ulcer symptoms, diarrhea, previous ulcer operation.

- **Diagnosis**
Basal acid output/maximal acid-output ratio, serum gastrin level, secretin provocative test, UGI endoscopy, CT scan, transhepatic portal vein sampling, intraoperative endoscopic ultrasound, gastrinoma triangle (cystic duct, junction of second and third portions of the duodenum and the junction of the head and neck of the pancrease).

- **Disease Severity**
Refractory peptic ulcer disease, hemorrhage, perforated ulcer, extremely high gastrin levels (greater than 5000 pg/ml, multiple tumors, associated multiple endocrine neoplasia Type I. Malignant potential reported in 50% to 70%.

- **Concept and Application**
Hypersecretion of gastric acid caused by excessive production of gastrin by tumor.

- **Management**
Omeprazole, H_2-receptor antagonist, Streptozotocin and 5-fluorouracil (for malig-

nancy), gastrectomy. Resection of the tumor with pancreatico-duodenectomy common.

X. HERNIA

A. Inguinal Hernia

- **H&P Keys**
Aching in groin; bulge or lump in groin, with or without one in the scrotum, mass in the groin.

- **Diagnosis**
Physical examination: Herniography.

- **Disease Severity**
Uncorrected chronic cough, prostatism or constipation, large indirect hernia, nonreducible hernia, abdominal distention, recurrent hernia, leukocytosis, fever, tenderness, history of chronic obstructive pulmonary disease (COPD), presence of incarceration or strangulation.

- **Concept and Application**
Persistent peritoneal diverticulum, increased intra-abdominal pressure, weakness of transversalis fascia, patent process vaginalis.

- **Management**
Standard or laproscopic herniography.

B. Femoral Hernia

- **H&P Keys**
Groin discomfort, lump in the groin, mass below inguinal ligament, medial to the vessels.

- **Diagnosis**
Physical examination.

- **Disease Severity**
Intestinal obstruction, tender and irreducible hernia.

- **Concept and Application**
Protrusion of intra-abdominal contents through femoral canal.

- **Management**
Excision of sac, closure of femoral canal. For intestinal obstruction, exploratorylap-

arotomy and possible bowel resection, often requires mesh.

C. Umbilical Hernia

- **H&P Keys**
  Bulge in umbilicus; fascial defect felt.

- **Diagnosis**
  Physical examination.

- **Disease Severity**
  Associated diseases such as cirrhosis and intra-abdominal tumor.

- **Concept and Application**
  Gradual yielding of the umbilical scar tissue.

- **Management**
  Younger than 6 years, observation. Older than 6 years, repair fascial defect.

D. Incisional (Ventral) Hernia

- **H&P Keys**
  Pain; swelling adjacent to scar.

- **Diagnosis**
  History and physical examination.

- **Disease Severity**
  Large multiple defects, intercurrent disease, bowel obstruction, age, sepsis, general debility, steroids, nutrition; history of COPD.

- **Concept and Application**
  Disruption of fascial closure resulting from poor surgical technique, wound infection, age, general debility, type of incision or suture material, nutrition.

- **Management**
  Weight reduction to correct intercurrent disease, improved nutrition, therapeutic pneumoperitoneum, direct fascial repair, mesh placement.

E. Hernia with Obstruction

- **H&P Keys**
  Pain at site of hernia, abdominal pain, vomiting, obstipation, fever, tachycardia, pros-

tration, abdominal distention, hypoactive bowel sounds, oliguria.

- **Diagnosis**
  Physical examination, plain roentgenogram, high-resolution ultrasound scan.

- **Disease Severity**
  Fever, urine output, heart rate, blood pressure, abdominal guarding, mentation, age.

- **Concept and Application**
  Intra-abdominal contents present within rigid confines of hernia, fascial neck compromises blood supply. Edematous intestinal segment.

- **Management**
  IV fluids, nasogastric tube decompression, monitoring of urine output, antibiotics, correction of electrolyte imbalance. Surgery to release hernia content, resect bowel, repair hernia.

F. Diaphragmatic Hernia

- **H&P Keys**
  Gasping respiration, cyanosis, heart sound displaced to right, absent breath sound on left, bowel sounds on affected hemithorax, scaphoid abdomen.

- **Diagnosis**
  Chest x-ray, antenatal ultrasound scan, upper GI series.

- **Disease Severity**
  Associated anomalies, ABG, cyanosis, respiratory rate, prolonged mechanical ventilation, response to therapy.

- **Concept and Application**
  Incomplete diaphragm, persistence of pleuroperitoneal hiatus, impaired pulmonary development.

- **Management**
  Nasogastric tube decompression, mechanical ventilation, arterial line, Priscoline® (pulmonary vasodilator), extracorporeal membrane oxygenation. Surgery to reduce herniated bowel and repair diaphragmatic defect.

19

Ill-Defined Symptom Complex

Mary Ann Kuzma, MD, and Debra Feldman, MD

I. SYMPTOMS REFERABLE TO THE CIRCULATORY SYSTEM

A. Palpitations

- **H&P Keys**
  Onset, duration, timing, and frequency of palpitations; precipitating and alleviating factors; associated symptoms of chest pain, dyspnea, light-headedness; history of heart disease or murmur, diabetes, or thyroid disease; risk factors for coronary artery disease; medication use; tachycardia, hypotension, fever; evidence of congestive heart failure; evidence of thyroid disease; murmur or rub.

- **Diagnosis**
  Studies: Electrocardiogram (ECG); serum electrolytes, complete blood count (CBC), drug levels, thyroid studies if indicated; Holter monitor and echocardiography if cardiac cause is suspected. Cardiac causes include arrhythmias; valvular heart disease; cardiomyopathy, pericarditis, congestive heart failure. Other causes include anxiety, fever, thyrotoxicosis, pregnancy, hypoglycemia, drugs (alcohol, nicotine, cocaine, caffeine, decongestants, theophylline, epinephrine), and pheochromocytoma.

- **Disease Severity**
  Cardiac arrhythmia associated with hypotension.

- **Concept and Application**
  Palpitations are often a normal physiologic response to emotional or physical activity. Those from cardiac disease are often associated with tachycardia or arrhythmias.

- **Management**
  Remove precipitating factors if possible, reassure patient if process is benign, treat underlying disease.

B. Murmurs

- **H&P Keys**
  Associated symptoms of chest pain, palpitations, dyspnea, dizziness; history of hypertension, rheumatic or cardiac disease, anemia or thyroid disease; fever, wide pulse pressure; nature of carotid upstroke; other heart sounds; timing, location, quality, intensity, and radiation of murmur; evidence of congestive heart failure.

- **Diagnosis**
  Studies: ECG, chest roentgenogram, echocardiography if cardiac workup is appropriate. Cause can be innocent or physiologic etiologies, valvular heart disease, or septal defects.

- **Disease Severity**
  Severity depends on nature and extent of underlying cardiac etiology.

- **Concept and Application**
  Results from vibrations in heart and great vessels caused by turbulent blood flow.

- **Management**
  Reassure patient if etiology is innocent or benign. Treat underlying cardiac disease if appropriate.

II. SYMPTOMS REFERABLE TO THE RESPIRATORY SYSTEM

A. Dyspnea

- **H&P Keys**
  Associated symptoms of chest pain, palpitations, cough, fever, weight loss; duration, timing, and frequency of dyspnea; relation of dyspnea to exertion; smoking history; occupational or environmental exposures; past or present history of pulmonary or cardiac disease; patient's general appearance with regard to respiratory difficulty; abnormal vital signs; lung percussion and auscultation; abnormal cardiac rhythm or auscultation; signs of congestive heart failure; abdominal mass or distention; mental status assessment.

- **Diagnosis**
  History and physical exam findings key to making diagnosis. Chest roentgenogram, ECG, arterial blood gases, pulmonary function tests, exercise stress testing, echocar-

diography, ventilation-perfusion scan only if indicated. Pulmonary causes include asthma or emphysema; bronchitis, pneumonia, or lung abscess; pneumothorax; pulmonary embolism; malignancy (primary lung cancer or lung metastases); interstitial lung disease; pulmonary hypertension; large pulmonary effusion. Cardiac causes are ischemic heart disease, left-sided heart failure, arrhythmias, pericardial tamponade. Other causes include neurological or muscular disorders affecting the respiratory muscles, abdominal distention from ascites or marked obesity, anxiety, deconditioning, and upper-airway infection or obstruction.

- **Disease Severity**
  Decreased mentation, tachycardia, hypotension; signs of congestive heart failure; hypoxemia, hypercarbia, ECG or chest roentgenogram abnormalities.

- **Concept and Application**
  Sensation of dyspnea produced by differing mechanisms depending on the specific underlying disease.

- **Management**
  Treat underlying disease process, and provide supplemental oxygen or mechanical ventilation if appropriate.

B. Stridor

- **H&P Keys**
  Associated symptoms of fever, cough, dyspnea, dysphagia, odynophagia, hoarseness, weight loss; neck and oropharynx exam, gag reflex, indirect mirror exam, if possible.

- **Diagnosis**
  Arterial blood gases or pulse oximetry, lateral roentgenogram of neck if infection is suspected. In adults, flexible fiber-optic endoscopy of airway. Infectious causes of intralaryngeal lesions are acute bacterial epiglottitis and laryngotracheobronchitis (croup). Other types of intralaryngeal lesions are caused by malignancy, foreign body, trauma, benign tumors, and smoke inhalation.

- **Disease Severity**
  Patient's inability to handle oral secretions, coupled with dyspnea or hypoxemia, indicates near-complete airway obstruction and requires emergency intubation or tracheotomy.

- **Concept and Application**
  Stridor indicates *marked* upper airway obstruction, inspiratory stridor indicates airway obstruction above the vocal cords, and mixed or expiratory stridor usually indicates an obstruction below the vocal cords.

- **Management**
  Remove obstructing lesion if possible. Control airway. Hospitalize and provide supplemental oxygen. Administer intravenous (IV) antibiotics (third-generation cephalosporin) or steroids (of questionable benefit if infectious cause).

C. Cough

- **H&P Keys**
  Frequency, duration, and timing of cough; color and nature of sputum; other upper-respiratory tract symptoms; fever, dyspnea, orthopnea, anorexia, weight loss, vomiting; associated heartburn or postnasal drip; smoking history; environmental or occupational precipitants; past or present history of pulmonary, cardiac, sinus, or allergic disease; exposure to tuberculosis (TB); medications; tachypnea; evidence of otitis pharyngeal erythema or exudates, sinus tenderness; lymphadenopathy; percussion and auscultation of lungs; signs of congestive heart failure.

- **Diagnosis**
  Studies: Emphasis on history and physical exam. Chest roentgenogram if pneumonia, malignancy, pulmonary edema, TB, bronchiectasis, or sarcoidosis is suspected. If sputum is purulent, gram stain and culture. If chest roentgenogram is negative, consider pulmonary function tests. If malignancy still suspected, CT scan of chest, bronchoscopy, or both. Pulmonary causes include pneumonia or tracheobronchitis, asthma, irritants (pollutants, cigarette smoke), chronic obstructive pulmonary dis-

ease, lung cancer, tuberculosis, pulmonary edema, bronchiectasis, or sarcoidosis. Other causes are reflux; postnasal drip or rhinitis; pharyngitis, otitis, sinusitis, impacted cerumen; and angiotensin-converting enzyme (ACE) inhibitors.

- **Disease Severity**
Presence of dyspnea, fever, tachypnea, weight loss; evidence of congestive heart failure; worsening bronchospasm; or hypoxia.

- **Concept and Application**
Afferent cough receptors located in the nose, larynx, lungs, stomach, sinuses, pharynx, or auditory canals respond to mechanical, inflammatory, chemical, and thermal stimulants. Therapy is directed at removing these stimulants.

- **Management**
Treat underlying etiology if known. Initiate trial of H_2 blockers if reflux is suspected. Administer antihistamines or topical steroids if allergic rhinitis is suspected. Administer antitussives if patient is unable to sleep.

D. Hemoptysis

- **H&P Keys**
Duration of symptoms and appearance of expectorated blood and sputum; associated symptoms of chest pain, fever, weight loss, hematuria; exposure to tuberculosis; smoking history or asbestos exposure; history of rheumatic fever or heart murmur; history of bleeding disorder, anticoagulant use, or blunt trauma; lymphadenopathy; chest wall exam and lung auscultation; heart murmur; signs of congestive heart failure.

- **Diagnosis**
Studies: Chest roentgenogram, coagulation studies, culture and stain for acid-fast bacilli if sputum is available, CT scan of chest if hemoptysis is significant, and bronchoscopy if tumor is suspected or if patient requires surgery to stop the bleeding. Infectious causes include bronchitis, TB (with cavitary disease), aspergilloma, lung abscess, and necrotizing pneumonia. Pulmonary causes

include pulmonary embolism (with infarction), malignancy, bronchiectasis, arterial or venous malformations, bronchial adenoma, pulmonary contusion, pulmonary edema (usually just blood-streaked sputum, not gross hemoptysis), and pulmonary vasculitis (Goodpasture's, Wegener's). Other cause is bleeding diathesis, including excessive anticoagulant therapy.

- **Disease Severity**
Massive hemoptysis is defined as cough producing more than 250 cc of blood in 24 hours. Minor amounts of hemoptysis can accompany cough associated with a respiratory infection.

- **Concept and Application**
Inflammation, ulceration, or injury to any part of the tracheobronchial mucosa can result in hemoptysis. Pulmonary vascular injury also causes hemoptysis. Bleeding disorders associated with hemoptysis are usually accompanied by an underlying bronchopulmonary lesion.

- **Management**
Once the diagnosis is established, treat underlying cause.

III. SYMPTOMS REFERABLE TO THE GENITOURINARY SYSTEM

A. Renal Colic

- **H&P Keys**
Onset, location, duration, and radiation of pain; associated symptoms of nausea or vomiting, hematuria, dysuria, inability to void, or fever; past history of nephrolithiasis, systemic illness, or urinary infections; dietary and medication history; family history of nephrolithiasis; lymphadenopathy or organomegaly.

- **Diagnosis**
Studies: Urinalysis; serum blood urea nitrogen (BUN), creatinine, calcium, and uric acid; kidney, ureter, and bladder roentgenogram; and IV pyelogram. Causes include nephrolithiasis, pyelonephritis, renal

embolic infarction, and abdominal or pelvic mass or infection.

- **Disease Severity**
Severity of pain, nausea, and vomiting. Presence of fever.

- **Concept and Application**
Nonradiating pain usually indicates upper-tract disease, and pain radiating to the groin usually indicates ureteral disease. Ureteral obstruction causes hyperperistalsis (mechanism of pain).

- **Management**
Hydrate, control pain. Treat underlying disease process.

B. Dysuria

- **H&P Keys**
Duration and timing of dysuria; associated symptoms of urinary frequency, hematuria, nocturia, fever, flank or abdominal pain, vaginal or urethral discharge, nausea and vomiting, or dyspareunia; risk factors for sexually transmitted disease (STD); history of diabetes, sickle cell disease; recurrent urinary tract infections, or renal calculi; abnormal vital signs; costovertebral angle tenderness; suprapubic tenderness; pelvic or prostatic examination.

- **Diagnosis**
Studies: Urinalysis; urine culture if pyuria is present. Cervical cultures in women if urine analysis negative; urethral cultures in men. Urologic evaluation with cystoscopy, IV pyelogram, or ultrasound if no evidence of infection. Causes include acute bacterial cystitis or pyelonephritis; urethritis; vulvovaginitis; renal calculi; urethral irritant, stricture, tumor, or foreign body; and trauma.

- **Disease Severity**
Fever and severe costovertebral angle tenderness. Need to rule out obstruction associated with infection.

- **Concept and Application**
Irritation or inflammation of bladder or urethral mucosa leads to intense burning sensation.

- **Management**
Antibiotics as indicated by exam and cultures, STD counseling, and treatment of underlying disease.

C. Oliguria and Anuria

- **H&P Keys**
Associated qualitative changes in the urine; associated symptoms of fever, rash, vomiting, diarrhea, blood loss, weight loss, travel; past or present history of renal, cardiac, hepatic, pelvic, vascular, or neurologic disease; family history of renal disease; history of trauma or surgical procedures; recent radiologic procedures; medication use; volume depletion or overload; elevated blood pressure or hypotension; retinopathy; signs of congestive heart failure; abdominal or pelvic mass; prostatic enlargement; abnormal mental status.

- **Diagnosis**
Urinalysis (macro- and microscopic evaluation); urinary indexes (sodium, osmolality); serum electrolytes, glucose, BUN, creatinine, CBC; ultrasound, IV pyelogram, cystoscopy, and voiding cystourethrogram if needed to evaluate site of obstruction. Prerenal causes include hemorrhage, gastrointestinal (GI) losses, renal losses; vasodilatation secondary to drugs, sepsis, or anaphylaxis; and "third-spacing" of fluids (congestive heart failure, burns, hypoalbuminemia, pancreatitis). Renal causes include acute tubular necrosis, vascular disease, glomerulonephritis or interstitial nephritis, end-stage renal disease, bilateral cortical necrosis, hemolytic-uremic syndrome, and paraprotein or crystal-mediated disease. And postrenal causes include bilateral ureteral obstruction, bladder outlet obstruction, urethral obstruction, and congenital malformation of the kidney.

- **Disease Severity**
Malignant hypertension or congestive heart failure.

- **Concept and Application**
Anuria should not be attributed to primary renal disease without evaluating the pa-

tency of the bladder, ureters, urethra, and renal veins and arteries.

- **Management**
Catheterize bladder. Alleviate obstruction and discontinue nephrotoxic drugs. Fluid challenge and optimize arterial blood volume and cardiac status. Manage electrolyte and acid-base abnormalities. Treat hypertension aggressively. Measure intake-output carefully. Hemodialyze if volume overload or electrolyte or acid-base disturbances are life-threatening. Treat underlying disease.

D. Proteinuria

- **H&P Keys**
Associated urinary symptoms; associated systemic symptoms: recent sore throat, rash, joint pain, fever, fatigue, anorexia; past or present history of renal disease or urinary tract infections; history of HIV infection, hypertension, or diabetes; medication use (particularly analgesics); family history of renal disease; elevated blood pressure; rash, lymphadenopathy, or joint effusions; edema; retinopathy; heart murmur; organomegaly or mass.

- **Diagnosis**
Studies: Urinalysis (dipstick evaluation), followed by microscopic examination. Twenty-four-hour urine protein measurement. Serum electrolytes, glucose, BUN, creatinine, albumin, cholesterol, CBC. Serum complement levels, antinuclear antibody (ANA), and antistreptococcal antibodies and serum and urine protein electrophoresis. Renal ultrasound, intravenous pyelogram (IVP), or biopsy if indicated. Renal causes include exercise (induced or orthostatic proteinuria); urinary tract infection; glomerular, interstitial, or tubular disease; and polycystic kidney disease. Proteinuria also is associated with the following systemic illnesses: diabetes mellitus, malignancy, systemic lupus erythematosis, preeclampsia, amyloidosis, sarcoidosis, cryoglobulinemia, HIV infection, infectious endocarditis and hepatitis, syphilis, and drug-induced illness (ACE inhibitors, cephalosporins, heroin, penicillamine).

- **Disease Severity**
Massive proteinuria (>3.5 g per day).

- **Concept and Application**
Glomerular proteinuria secondary to injury of basement membrane leads to increased protein permeability. Tubular proteinuria secondary to decreased tubular protein reabsorption.

- **Management**
Benign, transient, or exercise-induced proteinuria requires no further workup. Discontinue drug associated with proteinuria. Treat underlying renal or systemic illness responsible for the condition.

IV. ILL-DEFINED PRESENTATIONS

A. Lymphadenitis

- **H&P Keys**
Pain at site of recent trauma or wound; associated symptoms of fever, malaise, anorexia; contact with cats; immunocompromised patient; tachycardia; enlarged tender regional lymph nodes; nearby erythema, rash, or abscess.

- **Diagnosis**
Studies: CBC with differential; blood and wound cultures. Causes include superficial thrombophlebitis, cellulitis, and cat-scratch fever.

- **Disease Severity**
Systemic manifestations (fever, malaise).

- **Concept and Application**
Lymph node inflammation.

- **Management**
Heat, elevation, and analgesics. Antibiotic therapy (penicillin, nafcillin, or cephalosporin). Incision and drainage of abscess if present.

B. Dizziness and Giddiness

- **H&P Keys**
Onset, duration, frequency, and intensity of episodes; associated symptoms of nausea, ear pain, tinnitus, hearing loss, dysphagia,

diplopia, dysarthria, hemiparesis; precipitating and relieving factors; history of anemia or cardiac, cerebrovascular, thyroid, or psychiatric disease; recent viral illness; medication use; orthostatic hypotension or tachycardia; nystagmus; evidence of cerumen impaction, middle-ear disease, or hearing loss; carotid bruit; aortic stenosis murmur; abnormal neurologic exam; evidence of congestive heart failure or arrhythmia.

- **Diagnosis**
  Studies: Provocative testing; CBC and electrolytes if metabolic abnormality is suspected; audiological evaluation and electronystagmography if vestibular disorder is suspected; and magnetic resonance imaging (MRI), if further testing indicated. Vestibular disorders include benign postural vertigo, otitis, Ménière's disease, tumors, and vestibular neuronitis and ototoxic drugs. Systemic causes include arrhythmia and aortic stenosis; cerebellar ischemia or stroke and basilar insufficiency; anxiety, depression, and psychoses; multiple sclerosis; anemia; hypoglycemia; hypoxia; and drug side effects. Other causes are carotid sinus hypersensitivity and hyperventilation.

- **Disease Severity**
  Depends on specific etiology, degree of associated symptoms, and whether patient is incapacitated by dizziness.

- **Concept and Application**
  Vestibular disorders result from interruption of vestibular nerve, frequently at its endpoint in the inner ear.

- **Management**
  Treat underlying disease; avoid precipitating factors; and treat symptoms with meclizine and antiemetics if needed. Reassure and educate patient if etiology is benign.

C. Malaise and Fatigue

- **H&P Keys**
  Duration, associated symptoms of fever, arthralgias, dyspnea, weight loss; recent illness; changes in lifestyle, occupation, or sleep; history of anemia, malignancy, cardiac, pulmonary, renal, or endocrine disease; psychiatric history of depression or anxiety disorder; history of medication; pharyngeal erythema or exudates; lymphadenopathy; rash, pallor, or jaundice; thyroid enlargement; evidence of arrhythmia or congestive heart failure; abdominal tenderness or mass; focal findings on neurologic exam; and slow deep tendon reflexes.

- **Diagnosis**
  Studies: CBC, electrolytes, BUN, creatinine, glucose; thyroid function tests only if history or physical exam points to thyroid disease. Causes include overexertion or inadequate sleep; anxiety or depression; side effect of medication; mononucleosis, tuberculosis, hepatitis, HIV infection, or endocarditis; anemia; hypothyroidism; chronic cardiopulmonary, connective tissue, or renal disease; malignancy; and chronic fatigue syndrome.

- **Disease Severity**
  Accompanying symptoms if depression is suspected, and severity and extent of underlying organic etiology.

- **Concept and Application**
  Malaise and fatigue accompany most illnesses, both organic and emotional.

- **Management**
  Treat underlying etiology and educate patient.

D. Septic Shock

- **H&P Keys**
  Recent wound or symptoms of skin, respiratory, gastrointestinal, urinary tract infections; immunocompromised condition; medication use; decreased urine output; fever, tachypnea, tachycardia, hypothermia, or hypotension; change in mental status; cool extremities; and decreased or absent peripheral pulses.

- **Diagnosis**
  Blood, urine, sputum cultures; electrolytes, BUN, creatinine, CBC, coagulation studies;

arterial blood gases; chest roentgenogram, ECG; lactate level, liver function tests.

- **Disease Severity**
Hypotension longer than 1 hour, inadequate response to volume, requirement of pressors, high lactate level, and prolonged oliguria.

- **Concept and Application**
Results from interactions between microbes, leukocytes, humoral mediators, and vascular endothelium. Endotoxins cause activation of complement system, coagulation cascade, and numerous other mediators that lead to marked vasodilatation and myocardial depression.

- **Management**
Place patient in Trendelenburg position. Replace volume and insert urinary catheter to monitor urine output. Monitor cardiac rhythm and central venous pressure. Administer broad-spectrum antibiotics and vasopressor drugs, dopamine, or both. Provide supplemental oxygen. Manage electrolyte and acid-base abnormalities.

E. Enlarged Lymph Nodes

- **H&P Keys**
Associated symptoms are fever, anorexia, sore throat, weight loss, cough, dyspnea, edema, red eye, and rash; history of malignancy, connective tissue disease, or immunocompromised condition; exposure to cats or TB; risk factors for HIV infection; smoking history; location and physical characteristics of peripheral nodes; joint effusion or inflammation; rash; and hepatomegaly or splenomegaly.

- **Diagnosis**
Studies: CBC with differential. Throat culture; monospot if pharyngitis or cervical or submandibular adenopathy is present. Rapid plasma reagin, HIV, ANA, rheumatoid factor. Chest roentgenogram. Lymph node biopsy if there is still no diagnosis and if suspicion of malignancy or serious infectious process is still high. Causes of generalized disorder are mononucleosis, HIV, and syphilis; malignancy; connective tissue

disease; lipodoses; and drug reaction to dilantin, hydralazine, or allopurinol. Causes of regionalized disorder include local infection; reactive hyperplasia; pharyngitis, syphilis, herpes, chancroid, cat-scratch fever, rubella; malignancy; and granulomatous disease.

- **Disease Severity**
Extent and etiology of underlying disease govern severity. Nodes in excess of 3 cm often indicate malignancy. Lymphadenopathy in patients older than 50 years.

- **Concept and Application**
Mechanisms responsible for lymph node enlargement include antigenic response of lymphocytes and macrophages, infectious infiltration of inflammatory cells, proliferation of malignant lymphocytes or macrophages within the lymph node, and invasion of lymph node by malignant cells.

- **Management**
Treat underlying infection or malignancy.

F. Chest Pain

- **H&P Keys**
Quality, location, radiation, and duration of pain; associated symptoms such as dyspnea, diaphoresis, fever, cough, rash; aggravating and relieving factors; history of recent trauma or surgical procedure; relation to meals; past or present history of cardiac, pulmonary, esophageal, or rheumatologic disease; risk factors for ischemic heart disease; current medication or alcohol use; signs of anxiety or depression; evidence of tachycardia, arrhythmia, tachypnea, hypotension, hypertension, fever, or weight loss; chest auscultation; localized tenderness and pain with movement; and unilateral leg edema.

- **Diagnosis**
Studies: History and physical examination are keys. Also, chest roentgenogram, rib films, ECG, barium swallow, if appropriate. Cardiac causes include myocardial ischemia or infarction and pericarditis. Pulmonary causes include pulmonary embolism, pneumonia or tracheobronchitis, pneumothorax,

and pleurisy. Vascular cause is aortic aneurysm or dissection. And gastrointestinal (GI) causes include esophagitis or gastroesophageal reflux; aspirin or nonsteroidal anti-inflammatory drugs (NSAIDs) related; peptic ulcer disease, gallbladder, or pancreatic disease; costochondritis or muscle, bone, or ligament strain; panic attacks, anxiety, or somatization disorder; breast disease; and herpes zoster.

- **Disease Severity**
  Dependent on specific disease etiology and associated symptoms.

- **Concept and Application**
  Scientific concepts are listed under specific disease etiology.

- **Management**
  Treat underlying disease, fix reversible factors, and manage pain.

G. Gastrointestinal Hemorrhage

- **H&P Keys**
  Presence of hematemesis, vomiting of "coffee ground" material; melanotic stools, hematochezia; onset and duration of symptoms; accompanying symptoms of dizziness, rapid heartbeat, weakness, weight loss, nausea, anorexia; predisposing conditions; medications (especially aspirin, NSAIDs, glucocorticoids); alcohol abuse; liver disease; history of previous GI bleeding or malignancy, diverticulitis, vomiting, or inflammatory bowel disease. Pallor and cool skin may be present if patient is in shock.

  Pulse will reveal tachycardia; blood pressure may be elevated, normal, or low, depending on degree of blood loss. Oral cavity may contain blood or be pale in color, abdomen may be tender or rigid if perforation is present, rectal exam may reveal melanotic stool hematochezia or hemoccult positive stool.

- **Diagnosis**
  For upper GI hemorrhage: CBC, prothrombin time/partial prothrombin time (PT/PTT). Nasogastric tube localizes bleeding to upper GI tract. If bleeding is rapid,

may need emergency upper endoscopy; otherwise upper endoscopy when stable. Angiography if bleeding is rapid and site is still unknown. Causes include esophagitis, esophageal cancer, esophageal tear (Mallory-Weiss), esophageal varices, gastric ulcer, gastritis, gastric cancer, gastric varices, and duodenal ulcer. For lower GI hemorrhage: CBC, PT/PTT, anoscopy, sigmoidoscopy. If bleeding is rapid, angiography and radio-labeled red blood cell scan. If patient stabilizes, colonoscopy to detect underlying lesion. Causes include hemorrhoids, anal fissures, anal fistulas, infectious proctitis, trauma to rectal vault, colonic cancer, ruptured colonic diverticulum, Meckel's diverticulum, colonic angiodysplasias, infectious diarrhea, ischemic colitis, and inflammatory bowel disease.

- **Disease Severity**
  Degree of volume loss, assessed by orthostasis, hypotension, signs of shock, is most important indicator of severe disease. Hemoglobin and hematocrit, evidence of inadequate oxygenation of tissue (ie, lactic acidosis or symptoms of angina).

- **Management**
  For acute GI bleeding, establish IV access for rapid delivery of fluid if necessary; central venous access may be required in presence of hemodynamic compromise. IV fluid replacement with normal saline or blood as tolerated. Regular monitoring of hemoglobin and hematocrit to detect ongoing or recurrent bleeding. For rapid upper GI hemorrhage, upper endoscopy with sclerosis of varices; coagulation of bleeding ulcers with laser, thermocoagulation, or electrocautery may be necessary. If bleeding persists and is severe, use of arterial vasoconstrictors can be attempted. Angiography with local vasoconstrictors or embolization of bleeding site also can be attempted. Depending on the rate of bleeding and the site, surgery may be indicated. For rapid lower GI bleeding, arteriography, followed by infusion of vasoconstrictors at the bleeding site, may be necessary. Emergency surgery also may be necessary. For less severe acute bleeding, watchful

waiting is indicated because most GI hemorrhages are self-limited. Replacement of blood may be indicated if patient's underlying medical condition will not permit the wait to allow the bone marrow to replenish the blood supply. Iron should be replaced. Patients should not be fed orally until their condition is stable. For chronic bleeding, if no hemodynamic compromise is evident and history, physical, and available studies suggest a slow chronic blood loss, management is aimed at uncovering the condition causing the blood loss. Patients should receive iron replacement.

H. Diarrhea

- **H&P Keys**

General medical history; onset, duration, and pattern of symptoms (establish whether acute or chronic); relationship of diarrhea to food intake and its characteristics (color, quantity, formed, excessive odor, presence of blood or mucus); other GI symptoms accompanying diarrhea (nausea, vomiting, abdominal pain, flatulence, bloating); weight loss; medication history (especially recent use of antibiotic); dietary history (especially lactose, sorbitol use, unusual foods before onset of acute diarrhea); history of substance abuse; psychological and psychiatric history (stressors, eating disorder); previous abdominal surgery; travel history; and risk factors for HIV disease. Complete physical exam, including vital signs (fever, blood pressure, orthostatic changes), weight, oral mucosa (moist or dry), axillary sweat, abdominal exam (tenderness, distention, mass), rectal exam (blood, mucus, fecal impaction).

- **Diagnosis**

Causes of acute diarrhea (less than 2 weeks) include viral, bacterial, or parasite infection; medications; diverticulitis; ischemic colitis; and inflammatory bowel disease. If no fever or only low-grade fever and no bloody diarrhea or dehydration are present on physical exam, no further testing is needed. However, if patient looks ill, has high fever, bloody diarrhea, or dehydra-

tion, studies include CBC, serum electrolytes, stool exam for white blood cells, ova, and parasites; stool culture; *Clostridium difficile* toxin; and liver function tests (if elevated, check viral serology). In the elderly, radiologic studies may be indicated for acute diverticulitis and ischemic colitis. For chronic diarrhea, most patients should have CBC, serum electrolytes, total protein, albumin, pancreatic enzymes, liver function tests, stool exam for ova and parasites. Further testing may include colonoscopy, upper endoscopy with biopsy, fecal fat quantification if malabsorption is suspected, specific tests for type of malabsorption, and blood levels of secreted substances that could cause diarrhea. Causes include inflammatory bowel disease; malabsorption from pancreatic insufficiency, lactose intolerance, bacterial overgrowth, amyloidosis, celiac sprue, intestinal bypass surgery, Whipple's disease; secretory substances from carcinoid tumor, Zollinger-Ellison syndrome, villous adenoma, medullary carcinoma of thyroid, vasoactive intestinal peptide secreting adenoma; changes in bowel motility (diabetes mellitus, irritable bowel syndrome, neurologic disease); obstruction (fecal impaction, malignant tumor); and medications.

- **Concept and Application**

Many mechanisms are possible for this symptom. For example, damage to intestinal mucosa from infection, toxins, inflammatory diseases, irradiation, or vascular disease. Medications also cause diarrhea by a variety of mechanisms. Malabsorption causes undigested solute to be delivered to the intestine, stimulating secretory function of the bowel. Neurologic or idiopathic conditions may cause changes in intestinal motility.

- **Management**

Identify underlying cause of diarrhea. Treat symptoms with psyllium, opiate antidiarrheals (avoid in cases of acute infection or inflammatory bowel disease), and clonidine for diabetic diarrhea.

I. Reyes Syndrome 2-16yr

- **H&P Keys**

  Age of patient (most likey in children ages 2 to 16 years); recent <u>viral illness</u> (upper respiratory, GI, varicella); nausea and vomiting; depressed mental status; seizures. Examine patient for increased respiratory rate, hepatomegaly, and altered mental status (from lethargy to agitation to decorticate posturing to decerebrate posturing to flaccid).

- **Diagnosis**

  Serum electrolytes (<u>metabolic acidosis with respiratory alkalosis</u>), liver function tests (extremely high aspartate transaminase, alanine transaminase, and lactic dehydrogenase [LDH]; moderate increases in bilirubin), elevated arterial ammonia levels, prolonged PT/PTT, low serum glucose. CT or MRI scan of head to rule out other causes of change in mental status, and liver biopsy if diagnosis is uncertain.

- **Disease Severity**

  Arterial ammonia greater than 300. Prognosis is worse with increasing degree of depressed mental status on admission.

- **Concept and Application**

  Pathology is unknown. Epidemiologically associated with use of aspirin with a viral infection. Involves mitochondria of brain or liver causing cerebral edema.

- **Management**

  Reduce cerebral edema by increasing serum osmolarity with hyperosmolar solution. Elevate patient's head 30%. If patient is posturing, will need intracranial monitoring, possible intubation and hyperventilation to decrease serum pH, and osmotic agents and barbiturates. Monitor serum electrolytes, serum glucose, PT/PTT, ammonia levels. Administer an EEG to monitor improvement. Treat seizures with anticonvulsant. Avoid lumbar puncture if possible.

J. Dyspepsia

- **H&P Keys**

  Onset, severity, pattern, duration of symptoms; abdominal pain and pressure; gas-siness or bloating; excessive belching; burning sensation in chest; weight loss; psychological stressors; dietary history (symptoms often follow ingestion of food or specific foods); early satiety; medication history. Physical exam is usually nonspecific.

- **Diagnosis**

  In patients younger than 40 years, diagnostic testing reserved for those who do not respond to symptomatic and dietary therapy.

  In older patients, especially those with abdominal pain, imaging studies of the upper and lower GI tracts, pancreas, and biliary tract by endoscopy or radiologic studies should be done as directed by history and physical exam. If no etiology for the symptoms can be uncovered after directed set of exams, dyspepsia becomes a likely diagnosis.

  GI disease or systemic disease may generate similar symptoms, but dyspepsia is diagnosis of exclusion.

- **Disease Severity**

  Determined by the patient's complaints. No study is available to quantitate severity.

- **Concept and Application**

  Unknown and likely multifactorial. Hypotheses include a functional illness secondary to a psychological disorder or a subtle motility disorder.

- **Management**

  Attempt to restrict the patient's diet on the basis of dietary history. Also can attempt a trial of H_2-blockers or antacids as well as a trial of medications to improve gastric motility. Counsel the patient regarding the nature of symptoms; psychological counseling also may be appropriate.

K. Abdominal Pain

- **H&P Keys**

  Onset, character, location, pattern, duration, intensity of pain; maneuvers that elicit or relieve pain; nausea, vomiting, constipation, diarrhea; weight loss, anorexia; concurrent or recent infections; history of trauma, peptic ulcer disease, alcohol use, pancreatitis, biliary disease, previous abdominal surgeries, malignancy, or kidney stones; medications; dietary history; gynecologic history; general medical illness (especially diabetes, vascular disease, sickle cell anemia). Physical exam includes general appearance of patient and vital signs. Inspection of abdomen for signs of distention and retroperitoneal hemorrhage (eg, flank ecchymoses); gentle palpation to localize tenderness, detect rebound tenderness, and identify masses and organomegaly; auscultation to detect presence and character of bowel sounds and percussion to detect shifting dullness of ascites; cough test for peritoneal inflammation. Rectal exam to check for pain suggesting pelvic peritonitis and for obvious or occult blood. Gynecologic exam to check for pain suggesting pelvic peritonitis, purulent cervical discharge, and cervicitis.

• **Diagnosis**
Studies: Depend on patient's clinical status and which diagnoses seem most likely after the history and physical exam. Initially, CBC, electrolytes, BUN and creatinine, pancreatic enzymes, liver function tests, and urinalysis. Further blood testing would depend on outcome of previous tests and clinical picture. Other studies may include obstruction series, abdominal ultrasound, water-soluble contrast or barium enema, angiography, CT scan of abdomen and pelvis, endoscopy of GI tract, radionuclide studies, laparoscopy, aspiration of peritoneal fluid.

• **Concept and Application**
Abdominal pain has multiple causes, including the following: traumatic rupture of abdominal organs, inflammatory bowel disease, abdominal abscess, irritable bowel disease, trauma to abdominal musculature, peptic ulcer disease (with or without perforation), pancreatitis, appendicitis, hepatitis, ruptured viscus or diverticuli, acute cholecystitis, ascending cholangitis, intestinal obstruction, ureteral obstruction (extrinsic or intrinsic), aortic aneurysm rupture, intestinal ischemia, bowel infarction, ectopic

pregnancy, pelvic inflammatory disease, ruptured ovarian cyst, torsion of ovary or testicle, diabetic ketoacidosis, sickle-cell crisis, porphyria, C1 esterase deficiency, familial Mediterranean fever, embolic disease (from platelets, infection, cholesterol), vasculitis, and toxins.

• **Disease Severity**
Acute onset, autonomic stimulation (tachycardia, tachypnea), hemodynamic instability, signs of peritoneal inflammation, signs of perforation, severity of pain, metabolic acidosis, signs of obstruction.

• **Management**
Acute abdominal pain is more likely to represent a serious condition needing rapid diagnosis and treatment: Massive hemorrhage requires immediate surgery; hemodynamic instability requires central venous access and careful monitoring as diagnostic and treatment plans are developed and intravenous fluids should be administered to maintain intravascular volume.

Avoid pain medications that might mask clinical course of underlying condition; use antibiotics, depending on suspected cause of pain and likelihood of surgical intervention. Other management strategies would be based on the underlying condition causing abdominal pain. Chronic abdominal pain can usually be approached with less urgency. Outpatient evaluation on the basis of symptoms and exam can be done if no acceleration of abdominal symptoms has occurred.

L. Nausea and Vomiting

• **H&P Keys**
Onset and duration of symptoms (acute versus chronic), character of vomitus (color, contents, blood, or "coffee grounds"), relationship to eating, history or symptoms of eating disorders, accompanying GI symptoms (diarrhea, abdominal pain, constipation), weight loss, signs of infection (fever, myalgias, cough, dysuria, frequency), medication history, substance abuse history,

pregnancy, vertigo, tinnitus, history or symptoms of central nervous system disease, chest pain, history of cardiac disease, psychological stressors, previous surgical history (especially GI surgery: eg, vagotomy, gastric stapling). Physical exam includes general appearance, vital signs, signs of dehydration (orthostasis, dry mucous membranes, absence of axillary sweat), abdominal exam, complete exam for systemic disease that may cause nausea and vomiting.

- **Diagnosis**
  Studies: Serum electrolytes, BUN and serum creatinine, CBC, liver function tests, pancreatic enzymes, urine or serum pregnancy test. Further tests depend on results of history and physical; may include endoscopy and radiologic studies of GI tract, ultrasound of abdomen, obstruction series, stool examination for pathogens, CT of abdomen, gastric emptying study, ECG, additional blood studies. GI causes include gastric outlet obstruction, gastroparesis, peptic ulcer disease, upper GI tract bleeding, appendicitis, intestinal obstruction, cholecystitis, pancreatitis, peritonitis, perforation, and infection (viral or bacterial or parasitosis). Other causes include renal failure, infection of any organ system, cardiac disease (myocardial infarction, congestive heart failure), CNS disease (tumor, encephalitis, meningitis, hydrocephalus), migraine headaches, labrynthitis, Ménière's disease, endocrine disease (diabetic ketoacidosis, adrenal insufficiency, hyperthyroidism), pregnancy, medications, toxins, psychiatric disease and psychological stress.

- **Concept and Application**
  Vomiting center, in lateral reticular formation, controls acts of vomiting. Inputs to this center arise from chemoreceptor trigger zone in floor of fourth ventricle, GI tract, cerebral cortex, higher midbrain, labrynthine apparatus, and other parts of body. Output from vomiting center goes to phrenic nerve, spinal nerves, and vagus nerve to larynx, pharynx, esophagus, and stomach.

- **Management**
  Recognize the underlying condition. Treat symptoms with dopamine antagonists metoclopramide and cisapride (are not useful for motion sickness and inner-ear dysfunction), antihistamines and anticholinergics (are useful for motion sickness and labrynthitis), corticosteroids, lorazepam and tetrahydrocannabinoids (used to treat chemotherapy-induced nausea and vomiting), odansetron, phenothiazine derivatives (useful for mild-to-moderate nausea).

M. Dysphagia

- **H&P Keys**
  Difficulty swallowing (solids, liquids, or both) or moving foods from mouth to esophagus; pain on swallowing (odynophagia); symptoms of gastroesophageal reflux; coughing or choking on swallowing; sensation of food or medications getting stuck in middle of chest or at xyphoid process; course of dysphagia (onset, duration: did difficulty swallowing solids precede difficulty swallowing liquids? Are symptoms progressive or intermittent?), weight loss; history of aspiration of a foreign body, aspiration pneumonia, ingested contents aspirating through the nose, neurologic disease, ingestion of caustic substances (eg, lye), cigarette smoking, iron deficiency anemia, or irradiation of head, neck, or esophagus; hoarseness of voice; or substance abuse. Physical symptoms include inflammatory or exudative lesions of mouth and/or tongue, cervical adenopathy, thyromegaly, neck mass, fine or coarse extrabreath sounds. Neurologic exam to detect cerebrovascular accident or neuromuscular disease.

- **Diagnosis**
  Diagnostic tests should include ear, nose, and throat exam, with laryngoscopy, cineradiographic barium swallow, upper endoscopy, esophageal motility studies, chest roentgenogram, CT of chest as indicated by history and physical exam. Causes include oropharyngeal dysphagia (difficulty

moving food from mouth to pharynx to esophagus as result of neurologic disease such as cerebrovascular accident or upper and lower motor neuron disease), myopathy, cricopharyngeal achalasia, Zencker's diverticulum, or tumors; esophageal dysphagia (difficulty swallowing within the esophagus) caused by obstructing lesions such as strictures, benign tumors, malignant tumor, neuromuscular disease, achalasia of lower esophageal sphincter, motility disorders, or lesion of upper stomach.

- **Disease Severity**
  Dysphagia for solids progressing to dysphagia for liquids suggests an expanding obstructive lesion. Weight loss suggests significant impairment.

- **Concept and Application**
  Swallowing is complex process involving cerebral cortex; input from GI tract, brainstem swallowing center, and cranial nerves V, VII, IX, X, XII, and smooth and striated muscles. Neuromuscular lesions, inflammatory conditions, tumors, esophageal diverticulum, and infiltrative disease can cause difficulty swallowing.

- **Management**
  Dependent on underlying cause of the symptom. Achalasias and strictures may be treated with bougienage; achalasia may require myotomy. Esophageal cancers may be treated by resection, radiation therapy, or chemotherapy, depending on the stage; palliation is by laser therapy or bougienage. Neurologic conditions may respond to rehabilitation or may require nasogastric, gastric, or jejunal feedings.

N. Jaundice

- **H&P Keys**
  Onset and duration of symptoms; presence of yellow coloring of skin or sclera and darkening of urine; abdominal pain; fever; pruritus; acholic stools; weight loss; changes in bowel movements; anorexia; arthralgias; medications; substance abuse (especially alcohol); or history of congestive heart failure, malignancy, cholelithiasis, liver disease, or travel to areas where hepatitis is endemic. Physical exam should include color of skin (yellow to green), skin excoriations, and skin stigmata of hepatic cirrhosis (spider angiomata, palmar erythema), vital signs (fever), lymphadenopathy, signs of congestive heart failure (jugular venous distention, pulmonary congestion, enlarged heart, pedal edema), and abdominal exam (liver size may be small, normal, or enlarged; edge of liver may be smooth or nodular; liver may be tender or nontender; pancreatic mass or gallbladder may be palpable; splenomegaly may be present with cirrhosis.

- **Diagnosis**
  Studies: Bilirubin levels (direct = conjugated, indirect = unconjugated); liver function tests (increased alkaline phosphatase and gamma glutamyl transferase suggest obstruction; increased aminotransferases suggest hepatocellular disease). CBC and PT/PTT; viral serology and drug screen if indicated by history and physical exam. Ultrasound of liver, CT scan of abdomen, liver biopsy, percutaneous cholangiography, endoscopic retrograde cholangiopancreatography may be indicated. Serum bilirubin usually equal to or greater than 2.0 mg/dL for detectable jaundice. Unconjugated bilirubinemia (80% to 90% of total bilirubin) is associated with hemolysis, absorption of hematoma, ineffective erythropoiesis, Gilbert syndrome, neonatal jaundice, Crigler-Najjar syndrome, and medications. Conjugated bilirubinemia (50% of total bilirubin) is associated with hepatitis, cirrhosis, biliary cirrhosis, medications, alcoholic liver disease, sepsis, Dubin-Johnson syndrome, Rotor's syndrome, cholestatic jaundice of pregnancy, cholelithiasis, sclerosing cholangitis, pancreatitis, malignancy, biliary atresia, biliary stricture, postoperative, and benign recurrent cholestasis.

- **Disease Severity**
  May be reflected by degree of liver enzyme elevation but is not always directly correlated. Decreased synthetic activity usually reflects significant liver damage.

- **Concept and Application**
  Increased unconjugated bilirubin is secondary to increased production (diminished uptake into liver, diminished conjugation). Increased conjugated bilirubinemia is the result of hepatocellular damage or intrahepatic or extrahepatic obstruction.

- **Management**
  Aim is relieving underlying cause of jaundice or symptoms of underlying condition.

O. Ascites   *Transudative vs exudative*

- **H&P Keys**
  Onset and duration of abdominal swelling or distention, abdominal pain, weight loss, anorexia, shortness of breath, orthopnea, pedal edema, symptoms of reflux and burning, skin rashes, malaise and weakness, cloudy urine, alcohol intake, or history of malignancy, heart, liver, or renal disease. Physical exam includes vital signs, orthostasis. Skin exam for spider angiomata and palmar erythema. Neck exam for jugular venous distention and supraclavicular adenopathy. Lung exam for rales or dullness to auscultation, percussion, or both, suggesting pulmonary edema or pleural effusion. Heart exam for enlargement, S3, and irregular rhythm. Abdominal exam to inspect for distention, abdominal mass, auscultation for bowel sounds, and palpation for fluid wave, shifting dullness, abdominal mass, tenderness, liver size, and splenic enlargement. Gynecologic exam for pelvic masses and tenderness.

- **Diagnosis**
  Studies: Tests to establish ascites if uncertain from physical exam; ultrasound or CT scan of abdomen. Once ascites is confirmed, paracentesis of abdominal fluid to check for protein, lactic dehydrogenase (LDH), cell count, gram stain and culture, and triglycerides if indicated to differentiate transudate from exudative effusion. Peritoneal biopsy may be indicated for tuberculosis (TB). CBC, liver function tests, serum electrolytes, BUN, and creatinine; PT/PTT; chest roentgenogram. Additional studies such as liver biopsy, Doppler ultra-

sound, laparoscopy, and angiography may be indicated to establish etiology. Causes include cirrhotic liver disease, congestive heart failure, nephrotic syndrome, malignancy (either primary or secondary), spontaneous bacterial peritonitis, trauma, TB, parasites, hepatic vein thrombosis, benign ovarian tumors, and pancreatic pseudocyst.

- **Concept and Application**
  Ascites fluid can be secondary to increased hydrostatic forces such as hepatic congestion from congestive heart failure or decreased oncotic pressure that generally presents with transudative fluid. Exudative ascites fluid is usually secondary to disease affecting peritoneum directly, such as tumor or infection.

- **Management**
  Treatment of ascites depends on underlying cause. Treat with bed rest and salt and fluid restriction if ascites is symptomatic. Administer potassium-sparing diuretics or, if unresponsive, loop diuretics or thiazide. Monitor for electrolyte abnormalities and dehydration. Therapeutic paracentesis can be performed if patient does not have intravascular volume depletion; large-volume paracentesis can be performed while replacing albumin intravascularly with careful hemodynamic monitoring. Shunting may be indicated in recurrent cirrhotic ascites that is unresponsive to medical management.

P. Weight Loss

- **H&P Keys**
  Documentation or confirmation of weight loss (intentional or involuntary); food history; associated symptoms of anorexia, nausea or vomiting, dysphagia, diarrhea, abdominal pain, fever, night sweats, polyuria; life stressors; history of malignancy, thyroid problem, diabetes, depression, or cardiac, pulmonary, or GI disease; recent travel; medication and alcohol use; poor dentition; lymphadenopathy; thyroid mass or enlargement; jaundice or rash; abnormal abdominal exam; peripheral neuropathy.

- **Diagnosis**
Studies: Electrolytes, glucose, BUN, creatinine. Hemoccult, chest roentgenogram, liver function tests if malignancy is suspected. Stool samples if GI loss is suspected, and thyroid function tests if thyroid disease is suspected. Causes include decreased intake resulting from malignancy, depression or anxiety, anorexia nervosa, inadequate access to food, drug or alcohol intake, HIV infection, liver disease, hypercalcemia, or severe infection, dementia, cardiopulmonary, or renal disease. Normal or increased intake resulting from malignancy, diabetes, hyperthyroidism, fever, GI disease (malabsorption), or anxiety.

- **Disease Severity**
Depends on underlying etiology. In the elderly, involuntary weight loss exceeding 5% within 1 year.

- **Concept and Application**
Principal mechanisms are inadequate intake, excessive metabolic needs, or nutrient losses.

- **Management**
Treat underlying disease. Fix reversible factors. Administer mineral and vitamin supplements or supplement diet with enteral or parenteral nutrition, if indicated.

BIBLIOGRAPHY

Goroll AH. *Primary Care Medicine.* 2nd ed. Philadelphia: JB Lippincott Co; 1987.

Isselbacher KJ. *Harrison's Principles of Internal Medicine.* 13th ed. New York: McGraw-Hill, Inc; 1994.

Mengal MB. *Ambulatory Medicine.* Norwalk, CT: Appleton & Lange; 1993.

Tierney LM. *Current Medical Diagnosis and Treatment.* Norwalk, CT: Appleton & Lange; 1993.

20

Otolaryngology and Respiratory System Diseases

Jeffrey M. Finkelstein, MD, DMD, FACS

I. DISEASES OF THE EAR

A. Infectious Otitis Externa

- **H&P Keys**
  Pain in the external canal that can be enhanced by tragal pressure or by tugging on the auricle. Erythema of the ear canal and evidence of debris and swelling within the canal on otoscopy, occasional erythema of the pinna, and swelling in the post auricular space. History of ear trauma, exposure to high humidity, or swimming. Sensations of fullness, tinnitus, and hearing loss; occasional sensations of disequilibrium, itching of external canal.

- **Diagnosis**
  Direct examination, identification of offending organism by gram-stain and/or culture.

- **Disease Severity**
  Pain, fever, degree of swelling, closure of ear canal, regional soft-tissue swelling and erythema, and lymphadenopathy.

- **Concept and Application**
  Contamination of the external canal by contaminated water or trauma of the ear canal by manipulation permits invasion of offending organism; organisms are usually mixed, bacterial, or fungal. Implies failure of the piloapocrine system and the protective effect of cerumen.

- **Management**
  Acute: Cleansing of ear canal, inspect eardrum to rule out middle-ear disease, place a wick to carry otic drops to the canal and maintain in place; otic drops usually containing 2% acetic acid to change pH of canal, hydrocortisone to reduce inflammation and swelling, and a specific topical antibiotic usually to cover gram-positive as well as gram-negative organisms; pain management is important, and antibiotics should be administered if the infection has extended beyond the confines of the canal to produce lymphadenopathy, soft-tissue involvement, and fever. Subsequent prophylaxis requires keeping the ear dry and using prophylactic (acetic acid or alcohol) drops to decontaminate the ear after bathing or swimming in the future.

B. Malignant Otitis Externa   Loss X, XI, XII

- **H&P Keys**
  Auricular pain, discharge, hearing loss, feeling of fullness, granular tissue within the external auditory canal. Usually a history of immunocompromise such as diabetes mellitus, old age, or HIV infection. Presence of lymphadenopathy and evidence of infiltration into surrounding soft tissues; loss of cranial function, including facial nerve (VII) and cranial nerves X, XI, XII.

- **Diagnosis**
  Should include culturing the external auditory canal for offending organism, computed tomography (CT) scan to determine extent of bony destruction and infiltration into surrounding soft tissues. Possibly, subsequent magnetic resonance imaging (MRI) to evaluate presence of intracranial disease, and gallium scan to detect presence of bony involvement of surrounding structures.

- **Disease Severity**
  Expanding soft-tissue involvement with intracranial spread and decreased function of cranial nerve.

- **Concept and Application**
  Severe infection of periauricular soft tissue and bone in immunocompromised host, with rapidly expanding and infiltrating infection with potential for cranial nerve destruction, central nervous system (CNS) involvement. Most common organism is *Pseudomonas aeruginosa*.

- **Management**
  Intravenous antibiotics, with judicious debridement as necessary. Despite aggressive treatment, still significant percentage of mortality.

C. Acute Otitis Media

- **H&P Keys**
  This infection usually occurs in all age groups but is more prevalent in children

ages 3 months to 7 years of age. Occurs more frequently during winter months and is associated with upper respiratory tract and viral infections. Symptoms and signs normally include hyperemia of the tympanic membrane with erythema, exudate within the middle-ear space, and, at times, purulent discharge from the external canal as well as pain and dizziness with decreased appetite in young children. Other signs and symptoms are hearing loss, tinnitus, and, on occasion, imbalance; fever also is a key point.

- **Diagnosis**
Direct inspection via otoscopy, culture of any purulent debris from the external canal, and tympanocentesis in infants under 3 months of age.

- **Disease Severity**
Degree of fever, pain, hearing loss, and duration of otorrhea when present. Postauricular swelling indicates spread of disease process to mastoid air cell system; the presence of adenopathy within the parotid and upper neck indicates extension into soft tissues in surrounding regions. Necrotizing otitis media, beta-hemolytic streptococci seen in patients with concomitant disease process or immunocompromise.

- **Concept and Application**
The basic etiology is eustachian tube dysfunction with bacterial spread through the eustachian tube from the nasopharynx into the middle-ear space. Most common organisms include strep pneumonia and *Haemophilus influenzae;* also *Branhamella catarrhalis,* streptococcus and staphylococcus, but less commonly; in infants gram-negative organisms such as *Esherichia coli* must be identified during tympanocentesis (most common in infants younger than 6 weeks).

- **Management**
Systemic antibiotics, usually amoxicillin (30–40 mg/kg per day for uncomplicated infections and for children under age 12; other antibiotics used are erythromycin, sulfa for children allergic to penicillin, and trimethoprim sulfamethoxazole and

cephalosporins as necessary. Myringotomy may be indicated to determine bacteriology as well as tympanocentesis (as mentioned). When purulent discharge and tympanic membrane perforation exist, topical antibiotic drops in addition to systemic antibiotics are useful. Acute otitis media may benefit from prophylactic antibiotics as well as possible myringotomy and tube placement.

D. Chronic Otitis Media

- **H&P Keys**
Chronic otitis media is a rare complication of acute otitis media. It is manifested by the presence of a tympanic membrane perforation or development of a cholesteatoma in the middle-ear space, particularly in the area of the pars flacida. The physical findings are drum perforations with persistent otorrhea, hearing loss, tinnitus, presence of retraction pockets with epithelial debris, and occasional sensations of disequilibrium and vertigo.

- **Diagnosis**
Diagnostic studies include direct otoscopy, with careful cleansing of tympanic membrane area to identify presence or absence of perforation, its position and size. The character of the middle-ear mucus membrane is seen through the perforation and the presence or absence of epithelial debris either within the middle ear or in the pars flacida area. Tuning-fork studies will suggest the reversal of the Rinne, with lateralization to the side of greatest conduction loss; and audiogram, tympanogram, CT scans of temporal bone, both axial and coronal views without contrast, help delineate the degree and severity of disease and location of bone destruction and cholesteatoma if present. Cultures are helpful in determining antibiotic therapy; chronic otitis media is produced most commonly by *P. aeruginosa* and staphylococcal organisms; not uncommonly *Proteus mirabilis* and *E. coli* may be present. Culture sensitivity is needed to determine the offending organism.

CHRONIC OTITIS MEDIA

- **Disease Severity**

  Degree of perforation and otorrhea, vertigo, degree of hearing loss, presence of facial nerve paralysis, or headache indicate the possibility of intracranial extension of middle-ear and mastoid disease.

- **Concept and Application**

  Recurrent acute otitis media or single episode of acute necrotizing otitis media produce obstruction of tympanic membrane and chronic changes in the mucus membrane of the middle ear and mastoid concomitant with eustachian tube obstruction. Organisms involved are *P. aeruginosa* (most commonly) and *Staphylococcus aureus*; occasionally, proteus species as well as *E. coli* may be isolates. In immunocompromised patients, acid-fast and fungal disease must be considered.

- **Management**

  Antibiotics directed at gram-negative organisms; treatment with antibiotics for 3 to 6 weeks; concomitant use of otic drops with broad-spectrum antibiotics, acidifying agents (2% acetic acid), and often steroids to reduce inflammation. In patients with perforation, the ear must be kept dry during washing and bathing; swimming is not allowed. If cholesteatoma is present, this is a surgical disease requiring extirpation of the cholesteatoma and sealing of the ear drum by means of tympanoplasty, with or without reconstruction of the ossicular chain if it is involved.

E. Otitis Media with Effusion (Serous Otitis Media)

- **H&P Keys**

  History is associated with multiple bouts of acute otitis media with slow resolution. Condition also should be suspected in children with language delay and decreased response to auditory cues. Signs and symptoms include decreased hearing, retracted ear drum, dullness to the tympanic membrane, and straw-colored fluid with bubbles within the middle ear space.

- **Diagnosis**

  Direct visualization via otoscopy and insufflation during pneumatic otoscopy; also tympanometry and audiometry.

- **Disease Severity**

  Degree of hearing loss, as noted on audiometry, and disability in response to auditory cues.

- **Concept and Application**

  Eustachian tube blockage, with subsequent negative pressure within the middle-ear space changing the surface tension and producing metaplasia of epithelium of middle ear to a secertory epithelium migrating from the eustachian tube orifice of the middle ear.

- **Management**

  Initial management should be observation for approximately 3 months, during which 90% resolve. Generally, antibiotics are offered initially; some suggest that antihistamine decongestants are not uniquely helpful. In adults with serous otitis media, if unilateral, one must pay careful attention to the nasopharynx to rule out nasopharyngeal lesions—again, particularly in immunocompromised hosts. If the serous otitis media does not resolve and hearing loss persists after a period of careful observation and treatment, myringotomy with aspiration of the middle ear content and subsequent placement of ventilation tubes is the treatment of choice. In adults, attempts at autoinflation with Valsalva's maneuver is often effective in resolving serous otitis media; in children with recurrent nonresolving serous otitis media, adenoidectomy with or without tonsillectomy is often recommended.

F. Cerumen (Earwax) Impaction

- **H&P Keys**

  The patient will often complain of a history of feeling of fullness in the ear; decreased hearing, often after washing; pressure in the ear; and occasional pain in the external ear.

- **Diagnosis**

  Direct visualization via otoscopy.

Menieres

- **Disease Severity**
  Quality of hearing loss and degree of cerumen impaction. Rule out foreign body within the external canal, particularly in children and retarded patients.

- **Concept and Application**
  Often occurs with physical manipulation of the ear canal, particularly with the use of cotton applicators and digging in the ears. Narrow canal with increased cerumen production and possible foreign body.

- **Management**
  Removal of cerumen by mechanical irrigation when an intact tympanic membrane is known, or use of instruments, suction, or both as appropriate to degree of impaction and quality of cerumen.

G. Vertigo

- **H&P Keys**
  Vertigo is a complex complaint; it must be determined whether the vertigo is otologic, central, or medical in origin. Determining whether the disease is peripheral is made easier by the symptom of definite sensation of movement, most often rotary. When the vertigo is paroxysmal and severe, it is more likely to be peripheral; attacks may last minutes to hours (seldom longer) and may be associated with vegetative signs such as sweating, nausea, and vomiting. Patient never loses consciousness. Conversely, central vertigo is more often mild and described as a sensation of light-headedness or unsteadiness. It is vague, without specific onset or termination, and may be constant; attacks may last weeks or months, often without an obvious nystagmus. Associated symptoms of vertigo may be nystagmus (with peripheral pathology, the nystagmus can often be seen); with irritative lesions, nystagmus is often to the side of involved ear; nystagmus with changing of direction is more often central than peripheral. Causes of vertigo of otologic origin are acute otitis media, serous otitis media, head trauma with involvement of labyrinthine apparatus, and trauma to middle ear by penetrating wound, with

dislocation of ossicles and production of vertigo and hearing loss, Cogan's syndrome, vestibular neuronitis, temporal bone fractures, acute barotrauma with perilymph fistulas and endolymphatic hydrops (Ménière's disease). Ménière's disease is a disease process involving abnormal absorption or production of endolymph, which produces a quadrad or triad of symptoms of tinnitus, vertigo, fluctuant hearing loss, and sensations of fullness or blockage in the ear; the disease process may begin suddenly with tinnitus or any of the other symptoms; vertigo is severe and unrelenting for minutes to hours; nausea and vomiting are often present.

- **Diagnosis**
  History of fluctuant hearing loss, tinnitus, vertigo, neurosensory hearing loss on audiometric evaluation, evidence of canal paresis with vestibular studies involving the affected ear, negative examinations with intracranial MRI with gadolinium for VIII nerve and neurovascular bundles. Electronystagmography documenting canal paresis or hypoactivity of affected ear.

- **Disease Severity**
  Severity of vertigo, length of episodes, frequency of attacks, degree of hearing loss.

- **Concept and Application**
  Temporal bone studies indicate presence of hydrops of the endolymphatic space with destruction of neuroepithelium thought to be secondary to abnormality of stria vascularis, endolymphatic sac mechanism, or both.

- **Management**
  For acute cases, benzodiazepam-like drugs are effective if nausea and vomiting are not a problem. For long-term management of Ménière's disease, diuretics and low-sodium diet are often effective. In patients with continuing sensations of disequilibrium who fail to respond to medical therapy, endolymphatic sac decompression; VIII nerve section; or, in patients who have nonfunctioning ears from auditory stand-

point and unilateral disease for more than 5 years, labyrinthectomy is procedure of choice; diazepams and antihistamine group such as meclizine hydrochloride, diphenhydramine hydrochloride (Benadryl), or dimenhydrinate (Dramamine).

H. Otalgia

- **H&P Keys**
Otalgia may represent pain of otologic origin or of distant disease referred to the ears, such as dental infection, pharyngitis, or tonsillitis. Symptoms include ear pain (sharp, constant, dull, or burning). Determination of duration of pain and exacerbating and remitting factors are essential. Physical examination includes inspection of the external ear, otoscopy with examination of external canal and tympanic membrane with middle ear; examination of the temporomandibular joints with direct pressure both externally and on the pterygoid muscles within the orocavity; and complete examination of the upper aerodigestive tract, nasopharynx, oropharynx, tongue, larynx, and hypopharynx.

- **Diagnosis**
If cause is not obvious, diagnostic studies such as CT scan and MRI of upper aerodigestive tract and neck are useful. Studies also include direct laryngoscopy, nasopharyngoscopy, audiologic testing, and tympanometry, as well as palpation of tonsillar fossae, tongue base, and neck. Direct laryngoscopy and cervical esophagoscopy also may be indicated.

- **Disease Severity**
Presence of tumors or lesions in the upper aerodigestive tract referring pain to the ear are of potentially great concern and may be life-threatening.

- **Concept and Application**
Direct stimulation of nerves supplying sensation to the ear via inflammatory process or direct pressure, transmission via the same nerves through the temporomandibular joint and mechanism of referred pain via myositis and muscle spasm from associated joint musculature. Referred pain

from tongue base, larynx, or pyriform sinus occurs via the vagus or glossopharyngeal nerve.

- **Management**
Management will vary, depending on underlying disease process. It may be as simple as cerumen removal or as complex as cancer extirpation and adjunctive treatments.

I. Hearing Loss

- **H&P Keys**
Obvious loss of hearing acuity is noted either by patient or by friends and family; may be associated with other otologic signs such as tinnitus or vertigo or with associated exposure to loud noise or head trauma. Hearing loss may be mild, moderate, or severe; patient may have congenital hearing loss as a result of either congenital or acquired disease, a history of head injury or recurrent ear infection, exposure to ototoxic drugs, exposure to loud noise, or infectious processes such as meningitis. Physical examination begins with an interview to determine degree of hearing loss; then otoscopy to rule out disease process in external canal or middle ear and tuning-fork studies with Rinne and Weber studies as primary modalities.

- **Diagnosis**
Audiometry, including air, bone, and speech discrimination studies; brain stem evoked potential studies when indicated; tympanometry. In children with congenital losses or rapidly progressive neural losses, CT scan of temporal bone and serologic studies for autoimmune disease as well as congenital or acquired syphilis.

- **Disease Severity**
Careful evaluation of the individual's ability to communicate. Degree of hearing loss is evinced on audiometry.

- **Concept and Application**
Conduction hearing losses are manifested primarily by evidence of congenital findings of abnormal pinna and microtia, atresia, and periauricular tags and stenosis. Concomitant

congenital abnormalities such as cleft palate, cardiac disease, and kidney abnormalities should trigger search for otic abnormality. Conduction hearing loss in children is most often of congenital or of traumatic origin in infancy. In acquired disease, acute otitis media and serous otitis media affect more than 30% of children at some point. Most common disease in young adults is otosclerosis, with gradual fixation of stapedius foot plate; it is a genetically determined disease process (Mendelian dominant with variable penetrance). Other conduction hearing losses can occur as result of longitudinal factors of the temporal bone and barotrauma with middle-ear bleeding; effusion also produces conduction hearing losses. Congenital sensorineural hearing losses may be of genetic origin (eg, Waardenburg's syndrome) or caused by congenital syphilis. Acquired neural losses may be secondary to head or ear trauma, meningitis, an autoimmune disease process, acoustic tumors, or syphilis. In the aging population, presbycusis or a gradual high-frequency sensorineural hearing loss is most often seen after age 60.

- **Management**
  For sensorineural hearing losses of acquired type and of mild to moderate or even severe degree, amplification by means of hearing aid is available. For profound losses not amenable to amplification, cochlear implant surgery is available. For conduction hearing losses secondary to middle-ear disease, aspiration of fluid and myringotomy (as noted), ossicular reconstruction by means of stapes surgery or ossiculoplasty, and tympanoplasty for correction of tympanic membrane perforations.

J. Sudden Hearing Loss

- **H&P Keys**
  History of abrupt hearing loss for minutes to hours. Presence of tinnitus and vertigo and their severity should be determined by clinical otoscopy. History should include infection, trauma, vascular problem, otologic problem, neurologic problem, history of neurotoxic drugs, possible diabetes mellitus, autoimmune disorders.

- **Diagnosis**
  Audiometric testing, including air and bone conduction, electronystagmography (ENG) and calorics, testing of auditory brain responses, CT scan and MRI of the temporal bone, blood sugar, fluorescent treponemal antibody absorption (ABS-FTA) testing and sedimentation rate, and direct examination.

- **Disease Severity**
  Degree of hearing loss as determined by audiogram; presence or absence of vertigo or tinnitus and patient's disability.

- **Concept and Application**
  Multiple etiologies with multiple mechanisms of disease: infection, including mumps; herpes zoster; syphilis; meningitis; otitis media encephalitis; vascular lesions, including embolic phenomenon, coagulopathy, cerebrovascular accident; trauma, including temporal bone fracture, barotrauma, or noise-induced trauma; otologic, including Ménière's disease, perilymph fistula, chronic otitis media, and acoustic neuroma; neurologic disease, including mul-tiple sclerosis, Cogan's syndrome; and metabolic disorders, including diabetes mellitus, drug toxicity, and autoimmune disorders.

- **Management**
  After treatment of the underlying etiology when the hearing loss is idiopathic, high-dose steroids (60 mg Prednisone per day) tapered over 2 to 3 weeks may be beneficial.

K. Barotrauma

- **H&P Keys**
  History of recent scuba diving or air flight with inability to equalize pressure between external environment and middle ear; pain, tinnitus, hearing loss, and vertigo. Physical examination may reveal hemotympanum, eardrum perforation, nystagmus, nausea, vomiting, and hearing loss.

- **Diagnosis**
  Direct inspection of ear via otoscopy and pneumatic otoscopy; audiologic and tympanometric testing; vestibular testing, including ENG.

- **Disease Severity**
  Degree of vertigo and patient's functioning, including hearing loss and duration of symptoms.

- **Concept and Application**
  Acute changes in barometric pressure and failure of the eustachian tube to function properly. A large pressure gradient across the middle ear may result in trauma and the destruction of middle ear, inner ear, or both. Eustachian tube dysfunction may be a result of infectious, anatomic, or neoplastic abnormalities. The difference in barometric pressure may result in rupture of round or oval window seals, causing acute inner-ear abnormalities that lead to hearing loss or vertigo. Disruption of the tympanic membrane or vessels within middle ear may result in tympanic membrane perforation or hemotympanum.

- **Management**
  For uncomplicated barotrauma, appropriate nasal decongestants, systemic decongestants, and watchful waiting for resolution of hemotympanum or tympanic membrane perforation. For inner-ear dysfunction, bed rest for 24 hours may result in resolution if no significant hearing loss or vertigo is present; should these symptoms persist, middle-ear exploration with patching of oval and round windows is treatment of choice. Prevention of barotrauma can be helped with appropriate use of nasal decongestants and systemic decongestants before scuba diving or flying.

L. Tinnitus

- **H&P Keys**
  History of noise in the ear, which is generated endogenously, not from the environment. Complaints are about continuous humming, hissing, or whistling. Pulsatile tinnitus that is synchronous with heartbeat may accompany hearing loss or vertigo.

- **Diagnosis**
  Tinnitus that is bilateral, symmetrical, and of reasonably long standing is most often benign and requires audiometry. Unilateral tinnitus or pulsatile tinnitus requires workup with MRI, auscultation of the chest and neck to determine presence of transmitted or carotid bruits, auscultation within the ear to determine presence or absence of lesions, and CT scan to rule out vascular lesions of the ear.

- **Disease Severity**
  Tinnitus may be extremely loud and produce inability to concentrate, sleep, or function. Tinnitus matching audiogram, CT scan, MRI, auscultation of neck, ultrasound, noninvasive studies of great vessels of neck, and transcranial Dopplers. Examination of the ear for vascular lesions involving middle ear.

- **Concept and Application**
  Tinnitus may result from cochlear disease secondary to acoustic trauma, ototoxic drugs, viral or vascular disease of the cochlea, otosclerosis, conduction hearing loss such as ossicular discontinuity secondary to trauma, and serous otitis media. Tinnitus also may be of central origin, with brain stem lesions or 8th nerve lesions secondary to acoustic tumors. Patient should have temporomandibular joint examination as well.

- **Management**
  As per etiology.

II. DISEASES OF THE MOUTH AND THROAT

A. Herpes Simplex of the Orocavity

- **H&P Keys**
  History of prodromal fever, headache, irritability, malaise, nausea, vomiting, halitosis, and tender adenopathy. Usually includes children ages 2 to 5 years.

- **Diagnosis**
  Clinical examination with Giemsa's stain evaluation of vesicular fluid revealing syncytial giant cells with intranuclear inclusions.

- **Disease Severity**
Degree of symptoms listed above.

- **Concept and Application**
Initial herpes virus Type I. Infection usually occurs in children ages 2 to 5 years.

- **Management**
Symptomatic therapy includes salt water gargles and irrigations, soft diet, antipyretics and topical anesthetics as needed. Intravenous (IV) hydration for severe debilitation.

B. Oral Thrush (Candidiasis, Monoliasis)

- **H&P Keys**
Tends to occur in patients who are immunocompromised, debilitated, diabetic, or HIV positive; have used antibiotics for prolonged periods; or are receiving radiotherapy. Also seen in normal infants. Signs and symptoms include oral pain, odynophagia, and dysphagia. Physical examination reveals erythematous and edematous mucosa with soft, white exudate, which is easily scraped, revealing red, slightly ulcerated surface. Fever and adenopathy are unusual.

- **Diagnosis**
Physical examination, gram stain revealing yeast forms, culture on Saboraud's agar.

- **Disease Severity**
Depends on underlying etiology.

- **Concept and Application**
Candida albicans occurs on 25% of normal mucosa; a normal saprophytic organism becomes pathogenic in circumstances mentioned.

- **Management**
Includes nystatin oral suspension (200 000 units per cc, 2–3 cc swish and swallow) every 4 hours until inflammation is controlled. Mycelex troches or other antifungal agents also can be used.

C. Masses in the Nasopharynx

- **H&P Keys**
History of nasal obstruction, bleeding, hearing loss, pain, and neck masses.

- **Diagnosis**
Direct examination of nasopharynx by anterior rhinoscopy, flexible intranasal endoscopy, rigid endoscopy, mirror laryngoscopy, lateral x-rays of the nasopharynx, CT scan, and MRI with gadolinium for more careful delineation. Biopsy of lesion when found with tissue diagnosis. Determination of presence or absence of immunocompromising disease process, AIDS, diabetes, post chemotherapy for malignancy.

- **Disease Severity**
Hearing loss, nasal obstruction, epistaxis, cranial nerve neuropathies and involvement, cervical lymphadenopathy, distant metastases.

- **Concept and Application**
Numerous lesions may involve nasopharynx, including lymphoepithelioma (poorly differentiated squamous cell carcinoma), chordoma, angiofibroma, lymphoma and other age-related tumors, serous otitis media secondary to eustachian tube blockage and infiltration by tumor. Tumor may invade skull base with third nerve palsy as well as other cranial nerve involvements; metastases to regional lymph nodes produces lymphadenopathies.

- **Management**
Depends on type of lesion noted. Benign processes respond most often to conservative management or surgical extirpation. Malignancies may require extirpation and irradiation, chemotherapy, or both. Lesions of the ear secondary to masses in the nasopharynx may require myringotomy and tube placement to correct serous otitis media.

D. Malignant Neoplasms of the Oropharynx and Hypopharynx

- **H&P Keys**
Usual history of tobacco and ethanol use. More common in men than women; usually occurs between ages of 50 and 80 years. Symptoms may include globus sensation, odynophagia, dysphagia, irritation with foods, referred otalgia, lump in neck, alteration of voice, weight loss. More advanced

lesions may include respiratory distress with stridor. Physical examination includes complete examination of upper aerodigestive tract, including indirect mirror examination and flexible fiberoptic nasopharyngolaryngoscopy as well as bimanual palpation of the orocavity and neck.

- **Diagnosis**
  Careful clinical examination of upper aerodigestive tract, including direct laryngoscopy, cervical esophagoscopy, nasopharyngoscopy, and bronchoscopy, with appropriate histologic examination of biopsy material. Additional studies include CT scan and MRI of head and neck region.

- **Disease Severity**
  TNM staging and extent of tumor with its location. Yielding extreme variation in disease severity.

- **Concept and Application**
  Vast majority are squamous cell carcinoma of the involved mucosa and muscle, with varying degrees of tissue involvement based on stage and invasion. Initial spread of primary tumor tends to be in cervical lymph nodes, followed by distant metastasis should disease process continue.

- **Management**
  Combined treatment using surgery, irradiation, and chemotherapy as dictated by size and extent of tumor.

E. Hoarseness

- **H&P Keys**
  Presence of infectious disorder, local use/abuse, history of smoking and ethanol use, history of arthritis, history of trauma and intubation, possible endocrinopathy, benign and malignant neoplasms, functional disorders, reflux symptomatology; physical examination would include indirect mirror examination and direct laryngoscopy as well as complete physical examination of the upper aerodigestive tract; symptoms include hoarseness, possible referred otalgia, possible throat/laryngeal pain, dysphagia, dyspnea, cough, etc.

- **Diagnosis**
  Thorough examination of the larynx using indirect and direct methods, complete examination of the upper aerodigestive tract; adjunctive radiologic studies would include CT scan, MRI scan, barium swallow, thyroid function tests, biopsy as appropriate.

- **Disease Severity**
  Due to vast etiologic sources a large variety of disease severity occurs.

- **Concept and Application**
  Disruption of normal mucosal wave of the vocal cords with creation of turbulent air flow resulting in hoarseness, edema, vocal masses and irregularities, as well as limited function or hyperfunctioning of the vocal cords may result in hoarseness.

- **Management**
  Directed toward etiology.

F. Strep Throat (Acute Tonsillitis/Pharyngitis)

- **H&P Keys**
  Sore throat, fever, malaise, anorexia, and odynophagia occurs more commonly in children. Physical findings include erythema of the pharynx and tonsils, purulent debris in tonsillar crypts and pharynx, malodorous purulence causing halitosis and bad taste, peritonsillar swelling and limited motion of the uvula and soft palate, dysphagia (with severe infections), and palpable and tender adenopathy with severe infections.

- **Diagnosis**
  Direct physical examination with visualization of the tonsils and pharyngeal walls, culture of offending organisms.

- **Disease Severity**
  Fever, tonsillar hypertrophy, dehydration, referred otalgia, odynophagia, dysphagia, dehydration, peritonsillar abscess, retropharyngeal abscess, and airway compromise. Response to therapy.

- **Concept and Application**
Bacterial infection involving the tonsils, pharynx, or both. Most common are β-hemolytic strep, *Streptococcus pyogenes*, *Haemophilus influenzae*, *Haemophilus parainfluenzae*, *Corynebacterium diphtheriae*, and *Streptococcus pneumoniae*. Other possibilities include viral diseases such as adenovirus and mononucleosis.

- **Management**
Appropriate antibiotics, oral or IV hydration, incision and drainage of peritonsillar or retropharyngeal abscesses, if present. IV hydration and antibiotics for recalcitrant infections. Recurrent tonsillitis (six episodes per calendar year) is best treated with tonsillectomy. Pain management, oral rinses, and antipyretics for fever are important.

G. Cancer of the Larynx

- **H&P Keys**
History of heavy tobacco and ethanol use or possible asbestos exposure. Occurs in males between the ages of 50 and 70 years. Symptoms include hoarseness, throat and neck pain, dysphagia, dyspnea, hemoptysis, weight loss, referred otalgia, neck mass. Physical examination may include visualization of tumor on indirect and flexible direct laryngoscopy, palpation of neck for masses, and detectable stridor, wheezing, and hoarseness.

- **Diagnosis**
Complete examination of the upper aerodigestive tract, including indirect and direct laryngoscopy, bimanual palpation, CT scan of neck and larynx, MRI.

- **Disease Severity**
Depends on TNM staging and extent of disease process.

- **Concept and Application**
Squamous cell carcinoma is most frequent malignant neoplasm of the larynx (95%). Tumor initially remains confined to the larynx, then spreads to cervical lymph nodes and ultimately metastasizes to distant areas.

- **Management**
Management includes surgery, radiation therapy, and chemotherapy, depending on extent and stage of disease.

III. DISEASES OF THE RESPIRATORY SYSTEM

A. Acute Sinusitis

- **H&P Keys**
History of recent upper respiratory tract infection associated with purulent rhinorrhea, headache, pain, and pressure over the affected sinus (cheek-maxillary, forehead-frontal, periorbital-ethmoid, and occipital headache-sphenoid). Other signs and symptoms include purulent postnasal drip, pressure and headache, nasal obstruction, referred otalgia, and orbital pain.

- **Diagnosis**
Nasal endoscopy, both standard and endoscopic; culturing of purulent discharge; sinus roentgenograms or CT scan of sinuses; sinus tap to determine presence of pus for culture and treatment.

- **Disease Severity**
Fever, chills, sinus pressure and pain; possible periorbital cellulitis, edema, proptosis, blindness, headache or intracranial complication such as meningitis, brain abscess, or cavernous sinus thrombosis.

- **Concept and Application**
Obstruction of ostea of sinuses in middle meatus (osteomeatal complex) leading to negative pressure, transudate followed by exudate, and acute infection. Presence of anatomic abnormalities such as septal deviation, concha bullosa, turbinate hypertrophy, nasal polyposis, and allergic rhinitis. Bacteriology is similar to that of acute otitis media, including *H. influenzae*, *S. aureus*, Group A beta streptococcus, pneumococcus, and more unusual organisms in immunocompromised hosts.

- **Management**
  Antibiotics such as amoxicillin or ampicillin or amoxicillin with clavulonic acid to cover suspected organisms; both systemic and topical decongestants to nasal mucosa. Surgical drainage of affected sinuses as indicated by severity of disease and degree of patient's illness. Steroids, antihistamines, or both for patients with a significant allergic component to their sinusitis.

B. Chronic Sinusitis

- **H&P Keys**
  Symptoms are persistent rhinorrhea, postnasal discharge, pressure, headache, foul smell or taste. Physical examination reveals presence of changes in nasal mucosa; history of allergy is predisposing factor; erythema and swelling of nasal mucosa and purulence are present.

- **Diagnosis**
  Intranasal examination after careful vasoconstriction both by direct examination and by fiberoptic endonasal examination, with particular reference to middle meatus, osteomeatal complex to rule out presence of polypoid changes and presence or absence of occlusion of maxillary sinus and sphenoid ethmoid sinus complex. Plain roentgenograms are not as valuable as axial and coronal CT scans without contrast of sinuses to determine degree of sinus involvement, which sinuses are in fact involved, and presence of anatomic abnormalities. Cultures for offending organism.

- **Disease Severity**
  Persistence of purulent rhinorrhea, pain, pressure, fatigue, halitosis; presence of complications of chronic sinusitis with orbital or intracranial complications.

- **Concept and Application**
  Patients who have had poorly treated acute sinusitis and patients with allergic nasal disease with edema and polypoid changes of mucus membrane that block ostea outflow tracts are predisposed to sinusitis. Anatomic abnormalities such as septal deviations and pneumatization of turbinates with blockage of osteomeatal complex.

- **Management**
  Long-term antibiotics (3 to 6 weeks) with concomitant use of intranasal steroid sprays, nasal decongestants, and correction of intranasal anatomic abnormalities. In patients who fail conservative medical management, as described above; functional endoscopic sinus surgery to remove the offending tissue blocking osteomeatal complex with ethmoidectomy, maxillary sinus antrostomy, sphenoidotomy, and frontal sinus duct reconstruction.

C. Fungal Sinusitis

- **H&P Keys**
  Immunocompromised patients, patients with chronic sinusitis, or both; presence of unremitting sinusitis following vigorous local therapy; pain and swelling about the ethmoid and eyelid areas.

- **Diagnosis**
  Diagnostic studies include biopsy, gram stain and culture of suspicious material for septate versus nonseptate hyphae, CT scan for evidence of calcifications within the sinuses, and skin testing for *Aspergillus.*

- **Disease Severity**
  Evidence of bone destructive, foul-smelling rhinorrhea, with swelling of soft tissues of cheek, eyelid, lateral face; involvement of infraorbital nerve; systemic manifestations of fatigue and debility.

- **Concept and Application**
  Patients with immunocompromised states following chemotherapy for malignant disease or with diabetes or HIV infection have decreased ability to mount immunologic response to these secondary fungal infections; decreased ability also may be secondary to prolonged use of antibiotics with overgrowth of fungi as consequence.

- **Management**
  Surgical debridement, use of appropriate antifungal agents such as amphotericin, correction of underlying immunocompromising mechanism if possible.

D. Chronic Rhinitis

- **H&P Keys**

  Long-tern nasal obstruction, postnasal discharge, sneezing, rhinorrhea, and possible purulence. Patients may complain of seasonal symptoms or have symptoms referable to emotional or temperature change. Physical examination reveals erythema of mucus membrane, often with crusting and bleeding and occasional purulence.

- **Diagnosis**

  Gram stain of nasal smears for eosinophils or polymorphonuclear cells; sinus roentgenograms, CT scan, or both to rule out occult sinusitis. Allergy studies to rule out allergic disease as primary causative factor.

- **Disease Severity**

  Persistence of nasal obstruction, postnasal discharge, pressure and pain, inability to sleep because of nasal obstruction, fatigue, loss of concentration, and loss of time from work.

- **Concept and Application**

  Symptoms may be of allergic, infectious, or vasomotor origin. Determination of presence or absence of purulence by culture sensitivities. Presence of allergy by allergy studies and by history. Nasal obstruction secondary to temperature change mechanism, positioning of head, or emotional factors (fear, anger, passion, sadness); mechanism is endogenous release of vasoactive histaminelike substances that trigger vasodilatation and activation of goblet cells within the nasal and sinus mucus membranes.

- **Management**

  Determination of etiology and direction of therapy to allergic, infectious, or vasomotor disease process; also included in that therapy would be antihistamine decongestants, steroid nasal sprays, cromolyn sodium as a nasal spray, systemic steroids, and intranasal medicaments such as lubricating drops when indicated.

E. Allergic Rhinitis

- **H&P Keys**

  Nasal obstruction and congestion, nasal puritis, rhinorrhea, sneezing, and symptoms related to seasons. History of presence or absence of animals, specific plants, flowers, molds, and conditions (eg, feather pillows) that would support the growth of molds or allergies. Physical examination may reveal swollen, pale blue nasal mucosa and turbinates with nasal obstruction and generally clear rhinorrhea, and swollen (cobblestonelike) lymphoid tissue in the posterior pharyngeal wall.

- **Diagnosis**

  Nasal smears to detect the presence of eosinophils, immunoglobulin E levels, and total eosinophil count. Allergic skin testing, RAST (radioallergosorbant test) testing, food diary with confirmation of symptoms related to specific food allergens.

- **Disease Severity**

  Degree of function during allergic periods (ie, potential loss of school or work time).

- **Concept and Application**

  The antigen/antibody reaction causing degranulation of mass cells and basophils releasing histamines, prostaglandins, and other vasoactive elements leading to symptoms of rhinorrhea, nasal congestion, puritis, and so on.

- **Management**

  If possible, avoiding specific allergen is most useful for mild-to-moderate symptoms; treatment with antihistamines, nasal steroids, systemic steroids, sympathomimetic medications as well as sodium cromolyn nasal spray are indicated. Also, immunotherapy with allergy shots for desensitization as well as diet control are useful adjuncts.

F. Epistaxis (Nosebleed)

- **H&P Keys**

  Episode can be intermittent or acute; bleeding may be from anterior nares or may produce postnasal bleeding. Patient may give history of digital trauma to nose or history of nasal obstruction, particularly in boys younger than 15 years. Bleeding may respond to anterior nares pressure or may require intranasal packing, posterior nasal packing, or both.

- **Diagnosis**
  Direct examination of nose after careful intranasal vasoconstriction and local anesthesia permits examination of anterior nares, particularly in area of Kiesselbach's (Little's) area. Postnasal space can be examined by fiberscope under local anesthesia; sinus roentgenograms or CT scans should be done to rule out intrasinus occult malignancies.

- **Disease Severity**
  Minor intermittent bleeding stops spontaneously with gentle pressure. Severe postnasal bleeding is life-threatening and requires postnasal packing, hospitalization, and intensive care observation; necessity for blood transfusion and surgical intervention with ligation of sphenopalatine or maxillary artery.

- **Concept and Application**
  Most common cause is simple drying and crusting of nasal mucosa with neovascularization of Kiesselbach's area. Sphenopalatine artery bleeding is often associated with hypertension; patients may have Rendu-Osler-Weber disease or hereditary telangiectasia. Bleeding in young male children is produced by juvenile angiofibromas and other bleeding diatheses involving platelet or other coagulation deficit secondary to either primary platelet involvements or other blood dyscrasias.

- **Management**
  Bleeding from anterior Kiesselbach's area responds well to gentle pressure or, in recurrent involvements, to cauterization using trichloroacetic acid or other oxidizing agents such as silver nitrate in dilute solutions; significant bleeding requires anterior nasal packs. Posterior bleeding requires posterior packing or intranasal balloons; unresponsive bleeding requires transfusion, ligation of offending vessels, hospitalization, and intensive care management. For

Rendu-Osler-Weber disease, bleeding from affected telangiectatic areas is controlled with cauterization or argon laser. Juvenile angiofibromas and neoplastic lesions of the sinuses require extirpation.

G. Disorders of Olfaction and Taste

- **H&P Keys**
  Anosmia (loss of sense of smell) and lack of taste and secondary to upper respiratory infection, nasal obstruction, trauma, viral infections, tumors, exposure to irritative fumes such as ammonia or other industrial pollutants.

- **Diagnosis**
  Intranasal examination after careful intranasal vasoconstriction to rule out obstructive lesions of nasal cavity and nasal vault. CT scan of sinuses to rule out sinus and intranasal involvements and MRI with gadolinium to rule out involvements of the olfactory bulb and olfactory projections into the hypocampus and temporal lobe. Taste and smell testing and examination of the tongue to rule out atrophy or abnormality of taste buds.

- **Disease Severity**
  Inability to function in environment because of inability to detect crucial odors, loss of appetite, malnutrition secondary to loss of appetite, psychic trauma because of loss of sense of taste and smell.

- **Concept and Application**
  Olfactory fibers projected into the nose from the olfactory bulb through the area of the cribiform plate; lesions of nose that obstruct air flow to these critical fibers produce a relative anosmia. Head injury with a *commotio* injury in the brain case may result in forces that shear the olfactory fibers from the olfactory nerve. Viral infections most often produce reversible neuritic change in olfactory fibers, preventing their ability to respond to olfactory stimuli. Irritation secondary to industrial solvents and pollutants also may injure the neural epithelium in the same fashion. Loss of taste most often is olfactory in origin; majority of patients do not lose chordatym-

pani function, which monitors salt, sour, sweet, and bitter. Chordatympani function can be lost following middle-ear or mastoid surgery or trauma to the temporal bone or head.

- **Management**

  Use of topical steroids for inflammatory process, removal of obstructive lesions of nose and nasal vault. Removal from environment containing noxious and polluting substances. Treatment of infectious processes when appropriate. Return of olfactory function may take from 3 weeks to 18 months.

H. Acute Upper Respiratory Infection (Most Common in Winter Months)

- **H&P Keys**

  Manifested by choryza, rhinorrhea, nasal obstruction, pharyngitis, cough, conjunctivitis, headache. Physical examination reveals conjunctivitis, nasal obstruction with boggy, pale turbinates and, initially, clear rhinorrhea. Later, purulence may occur; pharynx is diffusely red without exudate; low-grade fever and, occasionally, small, mild to moderate cervical lymphadenopathy are present.

- **Diagnosis**

  Physical examination, determination of febrile state.

- **Disease Severity**

  Degree of nasal obstruction, ear discomfort, throat pain, dysphagia, musculoskeletal symptoms.

- **Concept and Application**

  Acute upper respiratory infections are viral in origin in both adults and children, most commonly in winter months. More than 120 adenoviruses produce choryzalike symptoms; none confer any specific long-term immunity and none respond to antibiotic therapy.

- **Management**

  In acute phase, nasal and oral decongestants, steam or cool-mist vaporization, antihistamines, antipyretics, and anti-inflammatory agents such as Tylenol in young children, and aspirin or nonsteroidal anti-inflammatory agents in adults. Chicken soup and other fluids; bed rest when indicated. Purulent phase lasts 3 to 5 days and should not require antibiotics. If it lasts longer, one must consider the possibility of sinusitis as a consequence of the acute upper respiratory infection; acute otitis medias may occur in conjunction as well.

I. Wegener's Granulomatosis

- **H&P Keys**

  Lesion of upper respiratory tract may involve ear, nose, sinus, soft palate, hard palate, tongue, and larynx—most often close to midline. Patients have generally systemic symptoms, including cough and often renal-like symptoms.

- **Diagnosis**

  CT scans of sinuses and ear to determine presence of lesion, biopsy of specific lesions showing Wegener's granulomas and vasculitis chest roentgenogram. Biopsies of pulmonary lesions and renal biopsies also are indicated.

- **Disease Severity**

  Wegener's granulomatosis may progress rapidly and may involve the ear, with both facial and auditory nerve involvement; may involve the sinuses and eyes, with changes in vision; and may involve the upper airway, with airway compromise.

- **Concept and Application**

  Wegener's granulomatosis is a disease of unknown etiology manifested by the involvement of upper respiratory, pulmonary, and renal systems. Biopsies show classic granulomas and vasculitis.

- **Management**

  Use of cyclophosphamide and steroids in combination for long-term and supportive systemic therapy.

J. Cystic Fibrosis

- **H&P Keys**

  Chronic recurrent upper and lower respiratory dysfunction with nasal obstruction, nasal purulence, loss of pulmonary function, dyspnea, chronic cough, production of purulent secretions with cough. Examination reveals debilitated child or adolescent; watery nasal polypoid tissue can be seen intranasally, often extending into the nasopharynx.

- **Diagnosis**
  Direct examination shows multiple polypoid changes in young children; CT scans show polypoid and polycystic changes in all sinuses. Sweat coloid study and chest roentgenogram.

- **Disease Severity**
  The degree of nasal obstruction and purulence and their impact on patient's pulmonary status with increased dyspnea, cough, cyanosis and recurrent infection.

- **Concept and Application**
  Mucus membrane abnormalities with loss of salivary function, mucus membrane reactivity with polypoid changes within the nose and sinuses, production of abnormal mucoid elements and increased tenacity and viscosity block sinus outflow tracts and involve pulmonary system.

- **Management**
  Systemic antibiotics, intranasal removal of polyps with recurrence and sinusitis, and functional endoscopic sinus surgery for recurrent sinusitis with polyp formation. Supportive systemic therapy.

BIBLIOGRAPHY

Bailey BJ. *Head and Neck Surgery: Otolaryngology.* Philadelphia: JB Lippincott Co; 1993.

Ballenger JJ. *Disease of Nose, Throat, Ear, Head and Neck.* 14th ed. Philadelphia: Lea & Febiger; 1991.

Cummings C, Fredrickson JM, Harker LA, Krause CA, Schuller DE. *Otolaryngology: Head and Neck Surgery.* 2nd ed. St. Louis: CV Mosby Co; 1993.

DeWeese DD, Saunders WH. *Textbook of Otolaryngology.* 7th ed. St. Louis: CV Mosby Company; 1988.

Lee KJ, ed. *Essential Otolaryngology: Head and Neck Surgery.* 6th ed. Medical Examination Publishing; 1995.

Index

Lesler-Trelat sym
 sudden appearance (3-6 mo)
 Rapid ↑ in size; # of seborrheic keratoses
 assoc colon/breast cancer

CARCINOID - Episodes Flushing   GARDNER-Adeno Ca of colon
                (FACE, neck) CHEST)
             Dyspnea
             ASTHMA
             DIARRHEA
             murmur pulm stenosis

     serotonin secreting tumor
     appendix, sm intestine
     bronchus

Diaphragmatic hernia
    Foramen Bochdaleck - (L)
           post lat
           failure pleuro peritoneal canal to
                Close

    Forman of margagni = Rare
            RIGHT ANT

    Bili uncong - physiologic or path (indirect)
       conjug - pathologic. (DIRECT)

    Subaponeurtic or subgaleal hmg - crosses suture line
                    may result in Any

    Cephlahematoma does not cross suture line

   M AFP - 15-17 wk gestation
       ↑AFP = neural tube   ↓AFP trisomy

   Amnio 12-14 wk
   PUS - chromesone analysis

(A) Autosomal Dominant

MUTATION GENE CODING FOR STRUCTURAL PROTEIN

50% chance passing on

MARFAN
myotonic dystrophy

tuberosis sclerosis

(B) AUTOSOMAL RECESSIVE:

MUTATIONS IN GENES CODING FOR ENZYMES.
NEEDS BOTH TO DISPLAY problem

CF (CFTR)

inborn errors of metabolism

PKU; Defect phenylalanine hydroxylase
Prevents conversion phen→tyn.

hypopigment - tyr need for
melelin.

mucopoly saccharidose

deficit of liposomal enzymes responsible for
intracellular catabolism of mucopolysaccharides
AR except HUNTERS (MPS II) - X link recessive

Glycogen storage - lack enzymes in glycogen breakdown

McArdles - skeletal phosphorylase
late childhood, adol adult
Fatigue, cramp, myoglobinuria

(C) X link: always maternal in origin

Hemophilic
Duchenne musc dys
Fragile X
color blindness

Turner XO

Klinfelter XXY
small testicles

Cri du Chat - 5p

Retinoblastoma - deletion chm 13 (13q14)

Prader Willi - del 15 (q11-q13)
Dm - hypoventilation - obesity
appetite d/o - central obesity

Herpangine
    Enterovirus
        Coxsackie A, B
        Echovirus
        Summer/fall

    fever, ST, pain ⊤ swallow
    1-2 mm vesicles

Cervical adenitis
    1) CAT scratch - B hensalae
      atypical mycobact
      EBV
      measles
      Rubella
      Mycoplasm TB
      Franuselic
      Yersenvi
      Candida
        Histo
        Toxo

Rocky mtn - Tcycline
        Chloramphenic

  Lyme: early doxycycline
        Amoxi
    Late Rocephin
      PCN G

Erythema Infectiosum
    5th - Parvo

Parvo preg → Death
      feb.

LDL= Total choc − (LDL + TG/5)

LDL= Total choc − (LDL + TG/5)

Erythema nodosum

Painful red nodules (septal panniculitis)
associated c̄
- cocci diomyocosis
- Histoplasmosis
- VIRAL
- TB
- Strept. infection
- SARcoidosis
- estrogen/BCP
- inflammatory bowel dz

Erythema multiforme ≡ Steven Johnson

- ↑TARGETOID lesion
- affects cutaneous, mucosal surfaces
- Follow HSV; myioplasma infection
  or Drugs (like sulfa)

Hypercalcemia

All pt c̄ ↑Ca++ must be worked up

Malignancy or 1° Hyperparathyroidism ~90%

Sensitivity   POST.   TP/All people c̄ d3
Specificity   TN/All people s̄ d3

PPV   TP/People who test for d3

$$PPV = a / a+b$$

Neg P V: $d / c+d$

Odds RATO:
Relative Risk

Expose

$$OR = ad/bc$$

RR   Disease risk in exposed / disease risk in
              unexpose

$$RR \left[a/a+b / c / (c+d) \right]$$

APPLETON & LANGE REVIEW SERIES

Health Related

Appleton & Lange's Review of Cardiovascular-Interventional Technology
Vitanza
1995, ISBN 0-8385-0248-2

Appleton & Lange's Review for the Chiropractic National Boards, Part I
Shanks
1992, ISBN 0-8385-0224-5

Appleton & Lange's Review for the Dental Assistant, 3/e
Andujo
1992, ISBN 0-8385-0135-4

Appleton & Lange's Review for the Dental Hygiene National Board Review, 4/e
Barnes and Waring
1995, ISBN 0-8385-0230-X

Appleton & Lange's Review for the Medical Assistant, 4/e
Palko and Palko
1994, ISBN 0-8385-0197-4

Medical Technology Examination Review, 2/e
Hossaini
1984, ISBN 0-8385-6283-3

Appleton & Lange's Review of Pharmacy, 5/e
Hall and Reiss
1993, ISBN 0-8385-0162-1
Appleton & Lange's Review for the

Appleton & Lange's Review for the Radiography Examination, 2/e
Saia
1993, ISBN 0-8385-0058-7

Radiography: Program Review & Exam Preparation (PREP)
Saia
1996, ISBN 0-8385-8244-3

Appleton & Lange's Review for the Surgical Technology Examination, 4/e
Allmers and Verderame
1996, ISBN 0-8385-0270-9

Appleton & Lange's Review for the Ultrasonography Examination, 2/e
Odwin
1993, ISBN 0-8385-9073-X

First Aid

1996 First Aid for the USMLE Step 1
A Student-to-Student Guide
Bhushan, Le, and Amin
1996, ISBN 0-8385-2597-0

First Aid for the USMLE Step 2
A Student-to-Student Guide
Go, Curet-Salim, and Fullerton
1996, ISBN 0-8385-2591-1

First Aid for the Wards
A Student-to-Student Guide
Le, Bhushan, and Amin
1996, ISBN 0-8385-2596-2

First Aid for the Match
A Student-to-Student Guide
Le, Bhushan, and Amin
1996, ISBN 0-8385-2596-2

Instant Exam

The Instant Exam Review for the USMLE Step 2, 2/e
Goldberg
1996, ISBN 0-8385-4328-6

The Instant Exam Review for the USMLE Step 3
Goldberg
1994, ISBN 0-8385-4334-0

Comprehensive A&L Reviews

Appleton & Lange's Review for the USMLE Step 1, 2/e
Barton
1996, ISBN 0-8385-0265-2

Appleton & Lange's Review for the USMLE Step 2, 2/e
Catlin
1996, ISBN 0-8385-0266-0

Appleton & Lange's Review for the USMLE Step 3, 2/e
Jacobs
1997, ISBN 0-8385-0305-5

Basic Science

Appleton & Lange's Review of Anatomy for the USMLE Step 1, 5/e
Montgomery
1995, ISBN 0-8385-0246-6

Appleton & Lange's Review of Epidemiology & Biostatistics for the USMLE
Hanrahan and Madupu
1994, ISBN 0-8385-0244-X

Appleton & Lange's Review of Microbiology and Immunology for the USMLE Step 1, 3/e
Yotis
1996, ISBN 0-8385-0273-3

Appleton & Lange's Review of General Pathology, 3/e
Lewis and Barton
1993, ISBN 0-8385-0161-3

Clinical Science

Appleton & Lange's Review of Internal Medicine
Goldlist
1996, ISBN 0-8385-0251-2

Appleton & Lange's Review of Obstetrics and Gynecology, 5/e
Julian, et al.
1995, ISBN 0-8385-0231-8

Appleton & Lange's Review of Pediatrics, 5/e
Lorin
1993, ISBN 0-8385-0057-9

Appleton & Lange's Review of Psychiatry, 5/e
Easson
1994, ISBN 0-8385-0247-4

Public Health and Preventive Medicine Review, 2/e
Penalver
1984, ISBN 0-8385-5936-2

Specialty Board Reviews

The MGH Board Review of Anesthesiology, 4/e
Dershwitz
1994, ISBN 0-8385-8611-4

(More on Reverse)

APPLETON & LANGE QUICK REVIEW SERIES

Health Related

MEPC: Medical Assistant
Examination Review, 4/e
Dreizen and Audet
1989, ISBN 0-8385-5772-4

MEPC: Medical Record,
Examination Review, 6/e
Bailey
1994, ISBN 0-8385-6192-6

MEPC: Occupational Therapy
Examination Review, 5/e
Dundon
1988, ISBN 0-8385-7204-9

MEPC: Optometry
Examination Review, 4/e
Casser et al.
1994, ISBN 0-8385-7449-1

MEPC: Physician Assistant
Examination Review, 3/e
Rahr and Niebuhr
1996, ISBN 0-8385-8094-7

Comprehensive A & L Reviews

MEPC: USMLE Step 1 Review
Fayemi
1995, ISBN 0-8385-6269-8

MEPC: USMLE Step 2 Review
Jacobs
1996, ISBN 0-8385-6270-1, A6270-1

MEPC: USMLE Step 3 Review
Chan
1996, ISBN 0-8385-6339-2, A6339-4

Basic Science

MEPC: Anatomy, 10/e
A USMLE STEP 1 Review
Wilson
1995, ISBN 0-8385-6218-3

MEPC: Biochemistry, 11/e
A USMLE STEP 1 Review
Glick
1995, ISBN 0-8385-5779-1

MEPC: Microbiology, 11/e
A USMLE Step 1 Review
Kim
1995, ISBN 0-8385-6308-2

MEPC: Pathology, 10/e
A USMLE STEP 1 Review
Fayemi
1994, ISBN 0-8385-8441-1

MEPC: Pharmacology, 8/e
A USMLE STEP 1 Review
Krzanowski et al.
1995, ISBN 0-8385-6227-2

MEPC: Physiology, 9/e
A USMLE STEP 1 Review
Penney
1995, ISBN 0-8385-6222-1

Clinical Science

MEPC: Neurology, 10/e
A USMLE Step 2 Review
Slosberg
1993, ISBN 0-8385-5778-3

MEPC: Pediatrics, 9/e
A USMLE Step 2 Review
Hansbarger
1995, ISBN 0-8385-6223-X

**MEPC: Preventive Medicine and
Public Health, 10/e**
A USMLE Step 2 Review
Hart
1996, ISBN 0-8385-6319-8

MEPC: Psychiatry, 10/e
A USMLE Step 2 Review
Chan and Prosen
1995, ISBN 0-8385-5780-5

MEPC: Surgery, 11/e
A USMLE Step 2 Review
Metzler
1995, ISBN 0-8385-6195-0

Specialty Board Reviews

MEPC: Anesthesiology, 9/e
Specialty Board Review
Dekornfeld and Sanford
1995, ISBN 0-8385-0256-3

MEPC: Otolaryngology
Specialty Board Review
Head & Neck Surgery
Willett and Lee
1995, ISBN 0-8385-7580-3

MEPC: Neurology, 4/e
Specialty Board Review
Giesser and Kanof
1995, ISBN 0-8385-8650-3

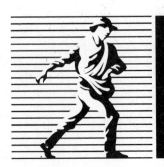

To order or for more information,
visit your local health science bookstore
or call Appleton & Lange toll free at
1-800-423-1359.